THE COMPLETE GUIDE TO
SPORTS NUTRITION
7TH EDITION

Anita Bean

BLOOMSBURY

LONDON · NEW DELHI · NEW YORK · SYDNEY

Published by Bloomsbury Publishing Plc
50 Bedford Square, London WC1B 3DP
www.bloomsbury.com

Seventh edition 2013
Sixth edition 2009; reprinted 2010 and 2012
Fifth edition 2006
Fourth edition 2003
Third edition 2000; reprinted 2001
Second edition 1996; reprinted 1997 (twice), 1998, 1999, 2000
First edition 1993; reprinted 1994, 1995

ISBN (print): 978 1 4081 7457 9
ISBN (Epub): 978 1 4081 8252 9
ISBN (EPDF): 978 1 4081 8251 2

A CIP catalogue record for this book is available from the British Library.

Acknowledgements
Commissioning Editor: Charlotte Croft
Editor: Sarah Cole
Designer: James Watson
Illustration on page 9 by Tina Howe
All other illustrations by Clive Goodyer

Cover photograph courtesy of Shutterstock
Photographs © Shutterstock
Author photograph © Grant Pritchard

Lucozade, Rice Krispies, Cornflakes, Gatorade, Shredded Wheat, Bran Flakes, Cheerios, Weetabix, Crunchy Nut Cornflakes, Golden Grahams, Isostar, Fanta, Mars Bar, Just Right Cereal, Power Bar, Alpen and All Bran are all registered trademarks.

Typeset in Adobe Caslon by seagulls.net
Printed and bound in India by Replika Press Pvt. Ltd.

10 9 8 7 6 5 4 3 2 1

CONTENTS

ACKNOWLEDGEMENTS

Many people have contributed directly and indirectly to this book. These include the many sportspeople, coaches and scientists whom I have had the privilege to meet and work with over the years. They have provided me with inspiration, knowledge and precious insights into sport. I value their suggestions, comments and honesty.

I would also like to thank Simon, my husband, for his patience; and Chloe and Lucy, my two wonderful (and sporty) daughters for making me believe that anything is possible.

Finally, this book would not have been written without the vision and enthusiasm of the editorial team at Bloomsbury. I am grateful for their diligence and support over the last 20 years.

FOREWORD

I know from first-hand experience just how important good nutrition is for sports performance. It's always been a crucial part of my training strategy and has, undoubtedly, helped me achieve the success I've enjoyed. I've learned over the years that I have to fuel my body properly otherwise I wouldn't have the energy or the strength to push my body through gruelling workouts and races.

My biggest nutritional challenge has always been eating enough food. In training, I burn 5000–6000 calories a day, which is a vast amount of food! And definitely not easy to fit in around training and everything else. I've worked out – often through trial and error – how much I have to eat, the right times to eat and which are the best foods for fast recovery.

There are so many things to think about before a big race but, for me, nutrition is right up there near the top. I have to plan what I'm going to eat and drink beforehand and make sure I have the right amounts of carbs, protein and fats. It's not always easy, especially when I'm travelling or competing in other countries – I have to check beforehand that I'll be able to get all the food and drink I need.

That's why this book is such a useful resource to me. It explains clearly and concisely the science of nutrition for sport. It's helped me with my training and competitions. And it's answered loads of questions I've had about my diet. Anita has managed to make a complex subject accessible and exciting.

Her advice is accurate and, importantly, it's also realistic and achievable. So it's hardly surprising that, since it was first published in 1993, *The Complete Guide to Sports Nutrition* has become the top-selling book on sports nutrition in the UK. I would thoroughly recommend it to anyone who wants to get more out of their sport. I've learned a lot from this book and I'm confident it will help you, whether you're just training for fitness or getting ready for the next Olympics.

**James Cracknell OBE, MSc,
British international rowing double
Olympic champion and world record holder.**

PREFACE TO THE SEVENTH EDITION

This book was first published in 1993, when the science of sports nutrition was in its infancy and there was little reliable nutrition information available to athletes. Since then our knowledge of sport and exercise nutrition has increased, new guidelines have evolved and research continues to be published. The idea of this book has always been to translate the science of nutrition into practical information that athletes can understand and use. I've attempted to provide science-based facts and recommendations in an easy-to-digest format, and avoid simply listing opinions or anecdotes. All the information is backed with carefully selected scientific references, which are listed at the back of the book. Over the years I am happy to say that this book has remained a trusted reference and practical handbook for many athletes, coaches and sports professionals.

So what's new? This seventh edition brings together the latest research and information on sport and exercise nutrition. It includes the consensus recommendations of leading sports organisations, such as the International Olympic Committee, the American College of Sports Medicine and the American Dietetic Association, as well as findings of eminent sports nutrition researchers.

There is now overwhelming evidence that diet significantly influences athletic performance. As a former athlete and having worked closely with many athletes, I know first-hand how important diet is in supporting any training programme and helping athletes reach their goals. Any improvement in performance, whether it's speed, strength, endurance or power, requires consistent and hard training as well as good nutrition.

Since the publication of the 6th edition, research in sports nutrition has focused on recovery nutrition and nutrient timing. There have been new recommendations on the optimal amount of protein to be consumed after exercise as well as the timing and type of protein. Milk has come under the nutritional spotlight in recent years with a growing amount of evidence supporting its role as a recovery food. This is particularly exciting given the enormous array of expensive engineered recovery supplements out there! If a natural and inexpensive food can be proven to improve recovery and performance, then this has to be great news for every athlete.

Scientists have also made progress in the quest for giving elite athletes the edge in long-duration competitions, with the development of sports drinks containing 'multiple transportable carbohydrates' that allow the body to absorb 90 g instead of 60 g carbohydrate per hour. Other changes include the abolition of advice to drink ahead of thirst and a warning against over-hydration during long events. There are no longer hard and fast guidelines on fluid intake and, in practice, athletes have to find a compromise between preventing dehydration and ensuring they don't over-hydrate.

I've watched with equal fascination and scepticism as more and more sports supplements appear on the market. Science continues to disprove the claims of most, which I am happy to report in this book. However, there is some sound evidence on the benefits of vitamin D, beetroot juice and buffers (bicarbonate and β-alanine). Finally, it's worth mentioning the new research on low carbohydrate diets during training followed by a high carbohydrate prior to competition ('train low, compete high'), and keeping an eye on emerging trends towards higher fat diets instead of the low fat diets once believed beneficial for athletes.

I hope that you will find the information in this book useful and it will help you achieve whatever you are aiming for in sport.

Anita Bean

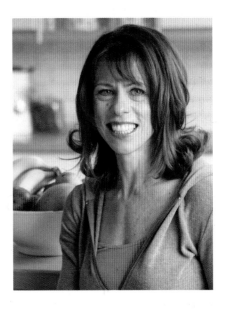

AN OVERVIEW OF SPORTS NUTRITION

1

There is universal scientific consensus that diet affects performance. A well-planned eating strategy will help support any training programme, whether you are training for fitness or for competition; promote efficient recovery between workouts; reduce the risk of illness or overtraining, and help you to achieve your best performance.

Of course, everyone has different nutritional needs and there is no single diet that suits all. Some athletes require more calories, protein or vitamins than others; and each sport has its unique nutritional demands. But it is possible to find broad scientific agreement as to what constitutes a healthy diet for sport generally. The following guidelines are based on the conclusions of the International Olympic Committee Consensus Conference on Sports Nutrition in 2003 and 2010 (IOC, 2011; IOC 2003); the Joint Position Statement of the American College of Sports Medicine, American Dietetic Association, and Dietitians of Canada (ACSM/ADA/DC, 2009) and the 2007 consensus statement of the International Association of Athletic Federations (IAAF, 2007).

The 2010 IOC Statement is significant because it highlights the importance of nutrition strategies in optimising elite performance. It recognises the advances in sports nutrition research since 2003, including the new concept of energy availability (energy intake minus the energy cost of exercise); the importance of protein timing and intakes of 15–25g protein after training to aid long-term maintenance or gain of muscle; greater intakes of carbohydrate (90 g/hr) for exercise over 3 hours; the importance of vitamin D for performance; and the need for a personalised hydration plan to prevent dehydration as well as hyponatraemia. The process leading to publication was extremely thorough and drew on the combined expertise of many of the world's leading sports nutrition experts.

1. ENERGY

It is crucial that athletes meet their energy (calorie) needs during hard periods of training in order to achieve improvements in performance and maintain good health. Failure to consume sufficient energy can result in muscle loss, reduced performance, slow recovery, disruption of hormonal function (in females) and increased risk of fatigue, injury and illness. Researchers have recently identified the concept of energy availability, defined as dietary intake minus exercise energy expenditure, or the amount of energy available to the body to perform all other functions after exercise training expenditure is subtracted. It has been suggested that 30 kcal/kg fat-free mass (FFM)/ day should be the lower threshold of energy availability in females (fat free mass includes muscles, organs, fluid and bones.)

Your daily calorie needs will depend on your genetic make-up, age, weight, body composition, your daily activity and your training programme. It is possible to estimate the number of calories you need daily from your body weight (BW) and your level of daily physical activity.

Step 1: Estimate your basal metabolic rate (BMR)

As a rule of thumb, BMR uses 22 calories for every kg of a woman's body weight and 24 calories per kg of a man's body weight.

Women: BMR = weight in kg x 22
Men: BMR = weight in kg x 24

For a more accurate method for calculating BMR, see p. 146.

Step 2: Work out your physical activity level (PAL)

This is the ratio of your overall daily energy expenditure to your BMR – a rough measure of your lifestyle activity.

- Mostly inactive or sedentary (mainly sitting): 1.2
- Fairly active (include walking and exercise 1–2 x week): 1.3
- Moderately active (exercise 2–3 x weekly): 1.4

Your BMR is the number of calories you burn at rest (to keep your heart beating, your lungs breathing, to maintain your body temperature, etc). It accounts for 60–75% of the calories you burn daily. Generally, men have a higher BMR than women.

Physical activity includes all activities from doing the housework to walking and working out in the gym. The number of calories you burn in any activity depends on your weight, the type of activity and the duration of that activity.

- Active (exercise hard more than 3 x weekly): 1.5
- Very active (exercise hard daily): 1.7

Step 3: Multiply your BMR by your PAL to work out your daily calorie needs

Daily calorie needs = BMR x PAL
This figure gives you a rough idea of your daily calorie requirement to maintain your weight. If you eat fewer calories, you will lose weight; if you eat more then you will gain weight.

2. CARBOHYDRATE

Carbohydrate is an important fuel for exercise. It is stored as glycogen in your liver and muscles, and must be re-stocked each day. Approximately 100 g glycogen (equivalent to 400 kilocalories) may be stored in the liver, and up to 400 g glycogen (equivalent to 1600 kilocalories) in muscle cells. The purpose of liver glycogen is to maintain steady blood sugar levels. When blood glucose dips, glycogen in the liver breaks down to release glucose into the bloodstream. The purpose of muscle glycogen is to fuel physical activity.

The more active you are and the greater your muscle mass, the higher your carbohydrate needs. While high-carbohydrate diets (more than 60% of energy intake) have been recommended in the past, experts now prefer to express carbohydrate requirements in terms of grams per kg body weight. Guidelines for daily intakes range from 3 to 7 g per kg of body weight per day for low and moderate intensity daily training lasting up to one hour. Depending on the fuel cost of the training schedule, a serious athlete may need to consume between 7–12 g of carbohydrate per kg body weight each day (350–840 g per day for a 70 kg athlete) to ensure adequate glycogen stores.

To promote rapid post-exercise recovery, experts recommend consuming 1.0–1.5 g carbohydrate per kg BW per hour within 30 minutes after exercise and then at 2-hour intervals up to 6 hours. If you plan to train again within 8 hours, it is important to begin refueling as soon as possible after exercise. Moderate and high glycaemic index (GI) carbohydrates (*see* p. 32) will promote faster recovery during this period. However, for recovery periods of 24 hours or longer, the type and timing of carbohydrate intake is less critical, although you should choose nutrient-dense sources wherever possible.

It is recommended that the pre-exercise meal provides 1–4 g carbohydrate per kg body weight, depending on exercise intensity and duration, and that this should be consumed between 1 and 4 hours before exercise.

During exercise lasting less than 45 minutes, there is no performance advantage to be gained by consuming additional carbohydrates. For intense exercise lasting between 45 and 75 minutes, very small amounts of carbohydrates are likely to be beneficial. This may be as little as a single sweet or simply swilling (not swallowing) a carbohydrate drink in your mouth. Interestingly, studies have found that a carbohydrate mouth rinse can improve performance in events lasting approximately one hour even when that carbohydrate is not consumed. But for exercise lasting longer than about one hour, consuming between 30 and 60 g carbohydrate helps maintain your blood glucose level, spare muscle glycogen stores, delay fatigue and increase your endurance. The amount

Table 1.1	Guidelines for daily carbohydrate intake
Activity level	**Recommended carbohydrate intake**
Very light training (low intensity or skill based exercise)	3–5 g/ kg BW daily
Moderate intensity training (approx 1 h daily)	5–7 g/ kg BW daily
Moderate–high intensity training (1–3 h daily)	7–12 g / kg BW daily
Very high intensity training (> 4 h daily)	10–12 g / kg BW daily

Source: Burke, 2007

depends on the intensity and duration of exercise, and is unrelated to body size.

The longer and the more intense your workout or event, the greater your carbohydrate needs. Previously, it was thought that the body could absorb only a maximum of 60 g carbohydrate per hour. However, recent research suggests that it may be higher – as much as 90 g, a level that would be appropriate during intense exercise lasting more than 3 hours. The 2010 IOC Consensus Statement highlights the use of mixtures of several carbohydrates (e.g. glucose, fructose and sucrose) to increase the rate of carbohydrate uptake and oxidation during exercise. A 2:1 mixture of glucose + fructose is generally associated with minimal GI distress. Choose high GI carbohydrates (e.g. sports drinks, energy gels and energy bars, bananas, fruit bars, cereal or breakfast bars), according to your personal preference and tolerance.

3. PROTEIN

Amino acids from proteins form the building blocks for new tissues and the repair of body cells. They are also used for making enzymes, hormones and antibodies. Protein also provides a (small) fuel source for exercising muscles.

Athletes have higher protein requirements than non-active people. Extra protein is needed to compensate for the increased muscle breakdown that occurs during and after intense exercise, as well as to build new muscle cells. The IOC, IAAF and the ACSM/ADA/DC consensus statements all recommend between 1.2 and 1.7 g protein/kg BW/day for athletes, which equates to 84–119 g daily for a 70 kg person. This is considerably more than a sedentary person, who requires 0.75 g protein/kg BW daily. However, the timing as

well as the amount of protein is crucial when it comes to promoting muscle repair and growth. It is best to distribute protein intake throughout the day rather than consuming it in just one or two meals. Experts recommend consuming 20–25 g protein with each main meal as well as immediately after exercise.

Several studies have found that eating carbohydrate and protein together immediately after exercise enhances recovery and promotes muscle building. The types of protein eaten after exercise are important – high quality proteins, particularly fast-absorbed proteins (such as whey) are considered optimal for recovery.

Some athletes eat high protein diets in the belief that extra protein leads to increased strength and muscle mass, but this isn't true – it is stimulation of muscle tissue through exercise not extra protein that leads to muscle growth. As protein is found in so many foods, most people – including athletes – eat a little more protein than they need. This isn't harmful – the excess is broken down into urea (which is excreted) and fuel, which is either used for energy or stored as fat if your calorie intake exceeds your output.

4. FAT

Some fat is essential – it makes up part of the structure of all cell membranes, your brain tissue, nerve sheaths and bone marrow and it cushions your organs. Fat in food also provides essential fatty acids and the fat-soluble vitamins A, D and E, and is an important source of energy for exercise. The IOC does not make a specific fat recommendation, but the American College of Sports Medicine (ACSM) and American Dietetic Association recommend fat provides 20–35% of calorie intake for athletes, which is consistent with the UK government recommendation of less than 35% for the general population.

The Department of Health recommends that the proportion of energy from saturated fatty acids be less than 11%, with the majority coming from unsaturated fatty acids. Omega-3s may be particularly beneficial for athletes, as they help increase the delivery of oxygen to muscles, improve endurance and may speed recovery, reduce inflammation and joint stiffness.

5. HYDRATION

You should ensure you are hydrated before starting training or competition and aim to minimise dehydration during exercise. Severe dehydration can result in reduced endurance and strength, and heat-related illness. The IOC and the ACSM/ADA/DC advise matching your fluid intake to your fluid losses as closely as possible and limiting dehydration to no more than 2% loss of body weight (e.g. a body weight loss of no more than 1.5 kg for a 75 kg person).

Additionally, experts caution against overhydrating yourself before and during exercise, particularly in events lasting longer than 4 hours. Drinking too much water may dilute your blood so that your sodium levels fall. Although this is quite rare, it is potentially fatal. The American College of Sports Medicine and USA Track & Field advise drinking when you're thirsty or drinking only to the point at which you're maintaining your weight, not gaining weight.

Sports drinks containing sodium are advantageous when sweat losses are high – for example, during intense exercise lasting more than 60–120 minutes – because their sodium content will promote water retention and prevent hyponatraemia.

After exercise, both water and sodium need to be replaced to re-establish normal hydration. This can be achieved by normal eating and drinking practices if there is no urgent need for recovery. But for rapid recovery or if you are severely dehydrated, it is recommended you drink 450–675 ml of fluid for every 500 g of body weight loss during exercise. You can replace fluid and sodium losses with rehydration drinks or water plus salty foods.

6. VITAMINS AND MINERALS

While intense exercise increases the requirement for several vitamins and minerals, there is no need for supplementation provided you are eating a balanced diet and consuming adequate energy to maintain body weight. The IOC, IAAF and ACSM/ADA/DC believe most athletes are well able to meet their needs from food rather than supplements. There's scant proof that vitamin and mineral supplements improve performance, although supplementation may be warranted in athletes eating a restricted diet or when food intake or choices are limited – for example, due to travel. However, athletes should be particularly aware of their needs for calcium, iron and vitamin D, as low intakes are relatively common among female athletes. The role of vitamin D in muscle structure and function, and the risk of deficiency, has been highlighted by the IOC and ASCM/ADA/DC. Those who have low vitamin D intakes and get little exposure to the sun may need to take vitamin D supplements.

Similarly, there is insufficient evidence to recommend antioxidant supplementation for athletes. Caution against antioxidant supplements is currently advised during training, as oxidative stress may be beneficial to the muscles' adaptation to exercise. The IOC also cautions against the indiscriminate use of supplements and warns of the risk of contamination with banned substances. Only a few have any performance benefit; these include creatine, caffeine, and sodium bicarbonate. For the majority, there is little evidence to support their use as ergogenic aids (Maughan *et al.*, 2011).

7. PRE-COMPETITION DIET

What you eat and drink during the week before a competition can make a big difference to your performance, particularly for endurance events and competitions lasting more than 90 minutes. The aim of your pre-competition eating strategy is to maximise muscle glycogen stores and ensure proper hydration.

This can be achieved by tapering your training while maintaining or increasing carbohydrate (7–10 g/kg BW/day). Small frequent meals are better than big meals. Make sure that you drink at least 2 litres per day. Avoid unfamiliar foods and drinks and stick to a well-rehearsed eating plan on the day of the event.

HOW TO PLAN YOUR TRAINING DIET

Use this fitness food pyramid as a base for developing your daily training diet. It divides food into seven categories: fruit; vegetables; carbohydrate-rich foods; calcium-rich foods; protein-rich foods; healthy fats and junk foods.

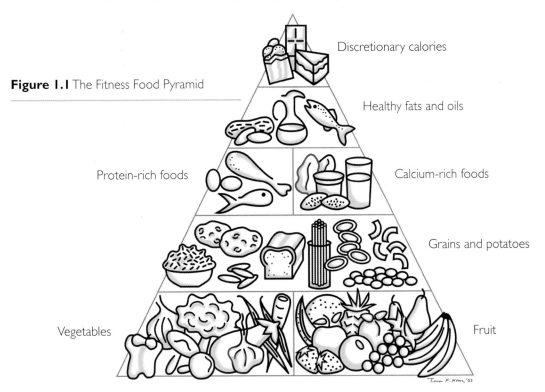

Figure 1.1 The Fitness Food Pyramid

Discretionary calories

Healthy fats and oils

Protein-rich foods

Calcium-rich foods

Grains and potatoes

Vegetables

Fruit

Table 1.2	What counts as one portion?		
Food group	**Number of portions each day**	**Food**	**Portion size**
Vegetables	3–5	1 portion = 80 g (about the amount you can hold in the palm of your hand)	
		Broccoli	2–3 spears/ florets
		Cauliflower	
		Carrots	1 carrot
		Other vegetables	2 tablespoons
		Tomatoes	5 cherry tomatoes
Fruit	2–4	1 portion = 80 g (about the size of a tennis ball)	
		Apple, pear, peach, banana	1 medium fruit
		Plum, kiwi fruit, satsuma	1–2 fruit
		Strawberries	8–10
		Grapes	12–16
		Tinned fruit	3 tablespoons
		Fruit juice	1 medium glass
Grains and potatoes	4–6	1 portion = about the size of your clenched fist	
		Bread	2 slices (60 g)
		Roll/ bagel/ wrap	1 item (60 g)
		Pasta or rice	5 tablespoons (180 g)
		Breakfast cereal	1 bowl (40–50 g)
		Potatoes, sweet potatoes, yams	1 fist-sized (150 g)
Calcium-rich foods	2–4	1 portion = 200 ml milk	
		Milk (dairy or calcium-fortified soya milk)	1 medium cup (200 ml)
		Cheese	Size of 4 dice (40 g)
		Tofu	Size of 4 dice (60 g)
		Yoghurt/ fromage frais	1 pot (150 ml)
Protein-rich foods	2–4	1 portion = size of a deck of cards (70 g)	
		Lean meat	3 slices
		Poultry	2 medium slices/ 1 breast
		Fish	1 fillet (115–140 g)
		Egg	2
		Lentils/ beans	5 tablespoons (150 g)
		Tofu/ soya burger or sausage	1–2
Healthy fats and oils	1–2	1 portion = 1 tablespoon	
		Nuts and seeds	2 tablespoons (25 g)
		Seed oils, nut oils	1 tablespoon (15 ml)
		Avocado	Half avocado
		Oily fish*	Deck of cards (140 g)

*Oily fish is very rich in essential fats so just 1 portion a week would cover your needs

The foods in the lower layers of the pyramid should form the main part of your diet while those at the top should be eaten in smaller quantities.

- Include foods from each group in the pyramid each day.
- Make sure you include a variety of foods within each group.
- Aim to include the suggested number of portions from each food group each day.

FRUIT AND VEGETABLES
5–9 portions a day
Fruit and vegetables contain vitamins, minerals, fibre, antioxidants and other phytonutrients, which are vital for health, immunity and optimum performance.

GRAINS AND POTATOES
4–6 portions a day
A diet rich in wholegrain foods – bread, breakfast cereals, rice, pasta, porridge oats – beans, lentils and potatoes maintains high glycogen (stored carbohydrate) levels, needed to fuel hard training. Aim for at least half of all grains eaten to be wholegrains. Note: portion sizes here (60 g bread) are twice those recommended by the Food Standards Agency (25 g bread), as these are more realistic for active people.

CALCIUM-RICH FOODS
2–4 portions a day
Including dairy products, nuts, pulses and tinned fish in your daily diet is the easiest way to get calcium, which is needed for strong bones.

PROTEIN-RICH FOODS
2–4 portions a day
Regular exercisers need more protein than inactive people (see pp. 56–60), so include lean meat, poultry, fish, eggs, soya or Quorn in your daily diet. Beans, lentils, dairy foods and protein supplements can also be counted towards your daily target.

HEALTHY FATS AND OILS
1–2 portions a day
The oils found in nuts, seeds, rapeseed oil, olive oil, flax seed oil, sunflower oil, and oily fish may improve endurance and recovery as well as protect against heart disease (see pp. 134–139).

DISCRETIONARY CALORIES
These are the calories that you have left after you have eaten all the fruit, vegetables, grains, protein-rich foods, calcium-rich foods and healthy fats recommended for the day. The more active you are, the more discretionary calories are allowed. For most regular exercisers this is likely to be around 200–300 calories worth of treats such as biscuits, cakes, puddings, alcoholic drinks, chocolate or crisps, but these extra calories also need to account for any added sugar in sports drinks and energy bars, or the jam you spread on your toast, or sugar you add to coffee or tea.

ENERGY FOR EXERCISE

2

When you exercise, your body must start producing energy much faster than it does when it is at rest. The muscles start to contract more strenuously, the heart beats faster to pump blood around the body more rapidly, and the lungs work harder. All these processes require extra energy. Where does it come from, and how can you make sure you have enough to last through a training session?

Before we can fully answer such questions, it is important to understand how the body produces energy, and what happens to it. This chapter looks at what takes place in the body when you exercise, where extra energy comes from, and how the fuel mixture used differs according to the type of exercise. It explains why fatigue occurs, how it can be delayed, and how you can get more out of training by changing your diet.

WHAT IS ENERGY?

Although we cannot actually see energy, we can see and feel its effects in terms of heat and physical work. But what exactly is it?

Energy is produced by the splitting of a chemical bond in a substance called adenosine triphosphate (ATP). This is often referred to as the body's 'energy currency'. It is produced in every cell of the body from the breakdown of carbohydrate, fat, protein and alcohol – four fuels that are transported and transformed by various biochemical processes into the same end product.

WHAT IS ATP?

ATP is a small molecule consisting of an adenosine 'backbone' with three phosphate groups attached.

Energy is released when one of the phosphate groups splits off. When ATP loses one of its phosphate groups it becomes adenosine diphosphate, or ADP. Some energy is used to carry out work (such as muscle contractions), but most (around three-quarters) is given off as heat. This

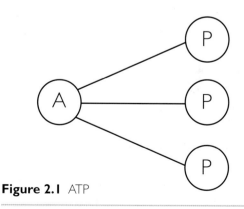

Figure 2.1 ATP

is why you feel warmer when you exercise. Once this has happened, ADP is converted back into ATP. A continual cycle takes place, in which ATP forms ADP and then becomes ATP again.

THE INTER-CONVERSION OF ATP AND ADP

The body stores only very small amounts of ATP at any one time. There is just enough to keep up basic energy requirements while you are at rest – sufficient to keep the body ticking over. When you start exercising, energy demand suddenly increases, and the supply of ATP is used up within a few seconds. As more ATP must be produced to continue exercising, more fuel must be broken down.

WHERE DOES ENERGY COME FROM?

There are four components in food and drink that are capable of producing energy:

- carbohydrate
- protein
- fat
- alcohol.

When you eat a meal or have a drink, these components are broken down in the digestive system into their various constituents or building blocks. Then they are absorbed into the bloodstream. Carbohydrates are broken down into small, single sugar units: glucose (the most common unit), fructose and galactose. Fats are broken down into fatty acids, and proteins into amino acids. Alcohol is mostly absorbed directly into the blood.

The ultimate fate of all of these components is energy production, although carbohydrates,

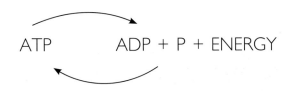

Figure 2.2 The relationship between ATP and ADP

proteins and fats also have other important functions.

Carbohydrates and alcohol are used mainly for energy in the short term, while fats are used as a long-term energy store. Proteins can be used to produce energy either in 'emergencies' (for instance, when carbohydrates are in short supply) or when they have reached the end of their useful life. Sooner or later, all food and drink components are broken down to release energy. But the body is not very efficient in converting this energy into power. For example, during cycling, only 20% of the energy produced is converted into power. The rest becomes heat.

HOW IS ENERGY MEASURED?

Energy is measured in calories or joules. In scientific terms, one calorie is defined as the amount of heat required to increase the temperature of 1 gram (or 1 ml) of water by 1 degree centigrade (°C) (from 14.5 to 15.5 °C). The SI (International Unit System) unit for energy is the joule (J). One joule is defined as the work required to exert a force of one Newton for a distance of one metre.

As the calorie and the joule represent very small amounts of energy, kilocalories (kcal or Cal) and kilojoules (kJ) are more often used. As their names suggest, a kilocalorie is 1000 calories and a kilojoule 1000 joules. You have probably seen these units on food labels. When we mention calories in the everyday sense, we are really talking about Calories with a capital C, or kilocalories. So, food containing 100 kcal has enough energy potential to raise the temperature of 100 litres of water by 1 °C.

To convert kilocalories into kilojoules, simply multiply by 4.2. For example:

- 1 kcal = 4.2 kJ
- 10 kcal = 42 kJ

To convert kilojoules into kilocalories, divide by 4.2. For example, if 100 g of food provides 400 kJ, and you wish to know how many kilocalories

that is, divide 400 by 4.2 to find the equivalent number of kilocalories:

- 400 kJ ÷ 4.2 = 95 kcal

WHY DO DIFFERENT FOODS PROVIDE DIFFERENT AMOUNTS OF ENERGY?

Foods are made of different amounts of carbohydrates, fats, proteins and alcohol. Each of these nutrients provides a certain quantity of energy when it is broken down in the body. For instance, 1 g of carbohydrate or protein releases about 4 kcal of energy, while 1 g of fat releases 9 kcal, and 1 g of alcohol releases 7 kcal.

THE ENERGY VALUE OF DIFFERENT FOOD COMPONENTS

1 g provides:

- carbohydrate 4 kcal (17 kJ)
- fat 9 kcal (38 kJ)
- protein 4 kcal (17 kJ)
- alcohol 7 kcal (29 kJ).

Fat is the most concentrated form of energy, providing the body with more than twice as much energy as carbohydrate or protein, and also more than alcohol. However, it is not necessarily the 'best' form of energy for exercise.

All foods contain a mixture of nutrients, and the energy value of a particular food depends on the amount of carbohydrate, fat and protein it contains. For example, one slice of wholemeal bread provides roughly the same amount of energy as one pat (7 g) of butter. However, their composition is very different. In bread, most energy (75%) comes from carbohydrate,

Metabolism

Metabolism is the sum of all the biochemical processes that occur in the body. There are two directions: anabolism is the formation of larger molecules; catabolism is the breakdown of larger molecules into smaller molecules. Aerobic metabolism includes oxygen in the processes; anaerobic metabolism takes place without oxygen. A metabolite is a product of metabolism. That means that anything made in the body is a metabolite.

The body's rate of energy expenditure is called the metabolic rate. Your basal metabolic rate (BMR) is the number of calories expended to maintain essential processes such as breathing and organ function during sleep. However, most methods measure the resting metabolic rate (RMR), which is the number of calories burned over 24 hours while lying down but not sleeping.

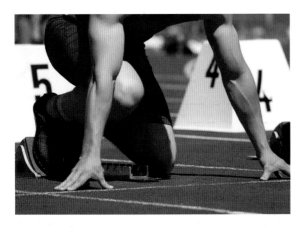

while in butter, virtually all (99.7%) comes from fat.

HOW DOES MY BODY STORE CARBOHYDRATE?

Carbohydrate is stored as *glycogen* in the muscles and liver, along with about three times its own weight of water. Altogether there is about three times more glycogen stored in the muscles than in the liver. Glycogen is a large molecule, similar to starch, made up of many glucose units joined together. However, the body can store only a relatively small amount of glycogen – there is no endless supply! Like the petrol tank in a car, the body can hold only a certain amount.

The total store of glycogen in the average body amounts to about 500 g; with approximately 400 g in the muscles and 100 g in the liver. This store is equivalent to 1600–2000 kcal – enough to last one day if you were to eat nothing. This is why a low-carbohydrate diet tends to make people lose quite a lot of weight in the first few days. The weight loss is almost entirely due to loss of glycogen and water. Endurance athletes have higher muscle glycogen concentrations compared with sedentary people. Increasing your muscle mass will also increase your storage capacity for glygocen.

The purpose of liver glycogen is to maintain blood glucose levels at rest and during prolonged exercise.

Small amounts of glucose are present in the blood (approximately 15 g, which is equivalent to 60 kcal) and in the brain (about 2 g or 8 kcal) and their concentrations are kept within a very narrow range, both at rest and during exercise. This allows normal body functions to continue.

HOW DOES MY BODY STORE FAT?

Fat is stored as *adipose* (fat) tissue in almost every region of the body. A small amount of fat, about 300–400 g, is stored in muscles – this is called intramuscular fat – but the majority is stored around the organs and beneath the skin. The amount stored in different parts of the body depends on genetic make-up and individual hormone balance. The average 70 kg person stores 10–15 kg fat. Interestingly, people who store fat mostly around their abdomen (the classic pot-belly shape) have a higher risk of heart disease than those who store fat mostly around their hips and thighs (the classic pear shape).

Unfortunately, there is little you can do to change the way that your body distributes fat. But you can definitely change the *amount* of fat that is stored, as you will see in Chapter 8.

You will probably find that your basic shape is similar to that of one or both of your parents. Males usually take after their father, and females after their mother. Female hormones tend to favour fat storage around the hips and thighs, while male hormones encourage fat storage around the middle. This is why, in general, women are 'pear shaped' and men are 'apple shaped'.

HOW DOES MY BODY STORE PROTEIN?

Protein is not stored in the same way as carbohydrate and fat. It forms muscle and organ tissue, so it is mainly used as a building material rather than an energy store. However, proteins *can* be broken down to release energy if need be, so muscles and organs represent a large source of potential energy.

WHICH FUELS ARE MOST IMPORTANT FOR EXERCISE?

Carbohydrates, fats and proteins are all capable of providing energy for exercise; they can all be transported to, and broken down in, muscle cells. Alcohol, however, cannot be used directly by muscles for energy during exercise, no matter how strenuously they may be working. Only the liver has the specific enzymes needed to break down alcohol. You cannot break down alcohol faster by exercising harder either – the liver carries out its job at a fixed speed. Do not think you can work off a few drinks by going for a jog, or by drinking a cup of black coffee!

Proteins do not make a substantial contribution to the fuel mixture. It is only during very prolonged or very intense bouts of exercise that proteins play a more important role in giving the body energy.

The production of ATP during most forms of exercise comes mainly from broken down carbohydrates and fats.

Table 2.1 illustrates the potential energy available from the different types of fuel that are stored in the body.

WHEN IS PROTEIN USED FOR ENERGY?

Protein is not usually a major source of energy, but it may play a more important role during the latter stages of very strenuous or prolonged exercise as glycogen stores become depleted. For example, during the last stages of a marathon or a long-distance cycle race, when glycogen stores are exhausted, the proteins in muscles (and organs) may make up around 10% of the body's fuel mixture.

During a period of semi-starvation, or if a person follows a low-carbohydrate diet, glycogen would be in short supply, so more proteins would be broken down to provide the body with fuel. Up to half of the weight lost by someone following a

Fuel stores	Potential energy available (kcal)		
	Glycogen	Fat	Protein
Liver	400	450	400
Adipose tissue (fat)	0	135,000	0
Muscle	1200	350	24,000

Table 2.1 Fuel reserves in a person weighing 70 kg

Source: Cahill, 1976.

low-calorie or low-carbohydrate diet comes from protein (muscle) loss. Some people think that if they deplete their glycogen stores by following a low-carbohydrate diet, they will force their body to break down more fat and lose weight. This is not the case: you risk losing muscle as well as fat, and there are many other disadvantages, too. These are discussed in Chapter 9.

HOW IS ENERGY PRODUCED?

The body has three main energy systems it can use for different types of physical activity. These are called:

1. the ATP–PC (phosphagen) system
2. the anaerobic glycolytic, or lactic acid, system
3. the aerobic system – comprising the glycolytic (carbohydrate) and lipolytic (fat) systems.

At rest, muscle cells contain only a very small amount of ATP, enough to maintain basic energy needs and allow you to exercise at maximal intensity for about 1 second. To continue exercising, ATP must be regenerated from one of the three energy systems, each of which has a very different biochemical pathway and rate at which it produces ATP.

HOW DOES THE ATP–PC SYSTEM WORK?

This system uses ATP and phosphocreatine (PC) that is stored within the muscle cells, to generate energy for maximal bursts of strength and speed that last for up to 6 seconds. The ATP–PC system would be used, for example, during a 20-metre sprint, a near-maximal lift in the gym, or a single jump. Phosphocreatine is a high-energy compound formed when the protein, creatine, is linked to a phosphate molecule (*see* box 'What is creatine?'). The PC system can be thought of as a back-up to ATP. The job of PC is to regenerate ATP rapidly (*see* Fig. 2.3). PC breaks down into creatine and phosphate, and the free phosphate

What is creatine?

Creatine is a compound that's made naturally in our bodies to supply energy. It is mainly produced in the liver from the amino acids glycine, arginine and methionine. From the liver it is transported in the blood to the muscle cells where it is combined with phosphate to make phosphocreatine (PC).

The muscle cells turnover about 2–3 g of creatine a day. Once PC is broken down into ATP (energy), it can be recycled into PC or converted into another substance called creatinine, which is then removed via the kidneys in the urine.

Creatine can be obtained in the diet from fish (tuna, salmon, cod), beef and pork (approx. 3–5 g creatine/kg uncooked fish or meat). That means vegetarians have no dietary sources. However, to have a performance-boosting effect, creatine has to be taken in large doses. This is higher than you could reasonably expect to get from food. You would need to eat at least 2 kg of raw steak a day to load your muscles with creatine.

The average-sized person stores about 120 g creatine, almost all in skeletal muscles (higher levels in fast-twitch muscle fibres, see p. 20). Of this amount, 60–70% is stored as PC, 30–40% as free creatine.

bond transfers to a molecule of ADP forming a new ATP molecule. The ATP–PC system can release energy very quickly, but, unfortunately, it is in very limited supply and can provide only 3–4 kcal. After this the amount of energy produced by the ATP–PC system falls dramatically, and ATP must be produced from other fuels, such as glycogen or fat. When this happens, other systems take over.

HOW DOES THE ANAEROBIC GLYCOLYTIC SYSTEM WORK?

This system is activated as soon as you begin high-intensity activity. It dominates in events lasting up to 90 seconds, such as a weight training set in the gym or a 400–800 m sprint. In order to meet sudden, large demands for energy, glucose bypasses the energy producing pathways that would normally use oxygen, and follows a different route that does not use oxygen. This saves a good deal of time. After 30 seconds of high-intensity exercise this system contributes up to 60% of your energy output; after 2 minutes its contribution falls to only 35%.

The anaerobic glycolytic system uses carbohydrate in the form of muscle glycogen or glucose as fuel. Glycogen is broken down to glucose, which rapidly breaks down in the absence of oxygen to form ATP and lactic acid (*see* Fig. 2.4). Each glucose molecule produces only two ATP molecules under anaerobic conditions, making it a very inefficient system. The body's glycogen stores dwindle quickly, proving that the benefits of a fast delivery service come at a price. The gradual build-up of lactic acid will eventually cause fatigue and prevent further muscle contractions. (Contrary to popular belief, it is not lactic acid, but the build up of hydrogen ions and

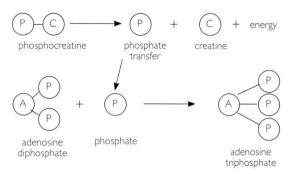

Figure 2.3 PC splits to release energy to regenerate ATP rapidly

What happens to the lactic acid?

Lactic acid produced by the muscles is not a wasted by-product. It constitutes a valuable fuel. When the exercise intensity is reduced or you stop exercising, lactic acid has two possible fates. Some may be converted into another substance called pyruvic acid, which can then be broken down in the presence of oxygen into ATP. In other words, lactic acid produces ATP and constitutes a valuable fuel for aerobic exercise. Alternatively, lactic acid may be carried away from the muscle in the bloodstream to the liver where it can be converted back into glucose, released back into the bloodstream or stored as glycogen in the liver (a process called gluconeogenesis). This mechanism for removing lactic acid from the muscles is called the lactic acid shuttle.

This explains why the muscle soreness and stiffness experienced after hard training is not due to lactic acid accumulation. In fact, the lactic acid is usually cleared within 15 minutes of exercise.

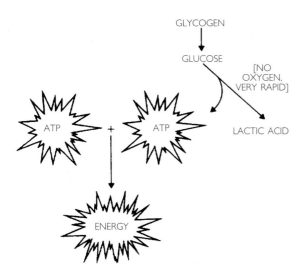

Figure 2.4 Anaerobic energy system

acidity that causes the 'burning' feeling during or immediately after maximal exercise – see p. 18.)

HOW DOES THE AEROBIC SYSTEM WORK?

The aerobic system can generate ATP from the breakdown of carbohydrates (by glycolysis) and fat (by lipolysis) in the presence of oxygen (*see* Fig. 2.5). Although the aerobic system cannot produce ATP as rapidly as can the other two anaerobic systems, it can produce larger amounts. When you start to exercise, you initially use the ATP–PC and anaerobic glycolytic systems, but after a few minutes your energy supply gradually switches to the aerobic system.

Most of the carbohydrate that fuels aerobic glycolysis comes from muscle glycogen. Additional glucose from the bloodstream becomes more important as exercise continues for longer than 1 hour and muscle glycogen concentration dwindles. Typically, after 2 hours of high-intensity exercise

(greater than 70% VO_2max), almost all of your muscle glycogen will be depleted. Glucose delivered from the bloodstream is then used to fuel your muscles, along with increasing amounts of fat (lipolytic glycolysis). Glucose from the bloodstream may be derived from the breakdown of liver glycogen or from carbohydrate consumed during exercise.

In aerobic exercise, the demand for energy is slower and smaller than in an anaerobic activity, so there is more time to transport sufficient oxygen from the lungs to the muscles and for glucose to generate ATP with the help of the oxygen. Under these circumstances, one molecule of glucose can create up to 38 molecules of ATP. Thus, aerobic energy production is about 20 times more efficient than anaerobic energy production.

Anaerobic exercise uses only glycogen, whereas aerobic exercise uses both glycogen and fat, so it can be kept up for longer. The disadvantage, though, is that it produces energy more slowly.

Fats can also be used to produce energy in the aerobic system. One fatty acid can produce

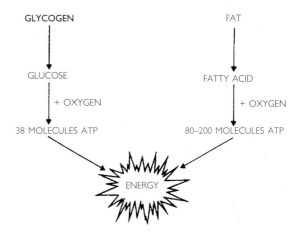

Figure 2.5 Aerobic energy system

between 80 and 200 ATP molecules, depending on its type (*see* Fig. 2.5). Fats are therefore an even more efficient energy source than carbohydrates. However, they can only be broken down into ATP under aerobic conditions when energy demands are relatively low, and so energy production is slower.

MUSCLE FIBRE TYPES AND ENERGY PRODUCTION

The body has several different muscle fibre types, which can be broadly classified into fast-twitch (FT) or type II, and slow-twitch (ST) or type I (endurance) fibres. Both muscle fibre types use all three energy systems to produce ATP, but the FT fibres use mainly the ATP–PC and anaerobic glycolytic systems, while the ST fibres use mainly the aerobic system.

Everyone is born with a specific distribution of muscle fibre types; the proportion of FT fibres to ST fibres can vary quite considerably between individuals. The proportions of each muscle fibre type you have has implications for sport. For example, top sprinters have a greater proportion of FT fibres than average and thus can generate explosive power and speed. Distance runners, on the other hand, have proportionally more ST fibres and are better able to develop aerobic power and endurance.

HOW DO MY MUSCLES DECIDE WHETHER TO USE CARBOHYDRATE OR FAT DURING AEROBIC EXERCISE?

During aerobic exercise the use of carbohydrate relative to fat varies according to a number of factors. The most important are:

1. the intensity of exercise
2. the duration of exercise
3. your fitness level
4. your pre-exercise diet.

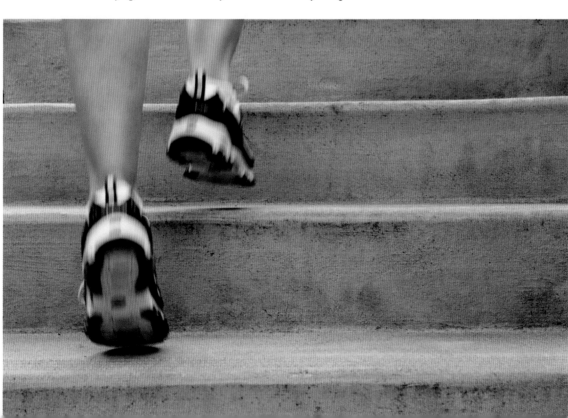

Intensity

The higher the intensity of your exercise, the greater the reliance on muscle glycogen (*see* Fig. 2.6). During anaerobic exercise, energy is produced by the ATP–PC and anaerobic glycolytic systems. So, for example, during sprints, heavy-weight training and intermittent maximal bursts during sports like football and rugby, muscle glycogen, rather than fat, is the major fuel.

During aerobic exercise you will use a mixture of muscle glycogen and fat for energy. Exercise at a low intensity (less than 50% of VO$_2$max) is fuelled mainly by fat. As you increase your exercise intensity – for example, as you increase your running speed – you will use a higher proportion of glycogen than fat. During moderate-intensity exercise (50–70% VO$_2$max), muscle glycogen supplies around half your energy needs; the rest comes from fat. When your exercise intensity exceeds 70% VO$_2$max, fat cannot be broken down and transported fast enough to meet energy demands, so muscle glycogen provides at least 75% of your energy needs.

Duration

Muscle glycogen is unable to provide energy indefinitely because it is stored in relatively small quantities. As you continue exercising, your muscle glycogen stores become progressively lower (*see* Fig. 2.7). Thus, as muscle glycogen concentration drops, the contribution that blood glucose makes to your energy needs increases. The proportion of fat used for energy also increases but it can never be burned without the presence of carbohydrate.

On average, you have enough muscle glycogen to fuel 90–180 minutes of endurance activity; the higher the intensity, the faster your muscle

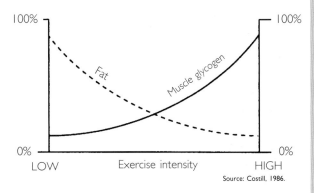

Source: Costill, 1986.

Figure 2.6 Fuel mixture/exercise intensity

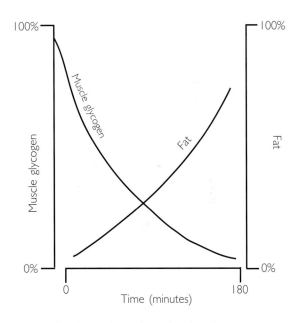

Figure 2.7 Fuel mixture/exercise duration

glycogen stores will be depleted. During interval training, i.e. a mixture of endurance and anaerobic activity, muscle glycogen stores will become depleted after 45–90 minutes. During mainly anaerobic activities, muscle glycogen will deplete within 30–45 minutes.

Once muscle glycogen stores are depleted, protein makes an increasing contribution to energy needs. Muscle proteins break down to provide amino acids for energy production and to maintain normal blood glucose levels.

Fitness level

As a result of aerobic training, your muscles make a number of adaptations to improve your performance, and your body's ability to use fat as a fuel improves. Aerobic training increases the numbers of key fat-oxidising enzymes, such as hormone-sensitive lipase, which means your body becomes more efficient in breaking down fat into fatty acids. The number of blood capillaries serving the muscle increases so you can transport the fatty acids to the muscle cells. The number of mitochondria (the sites of fatty acid oxidation) also increases, which means you have a greater capacity to burn fatty acids in each muscle cell. Thus, improved aerobic fitness enables you to break down fat at a faster rate at any given intensity, thus allowing you to spare glycogen (*see* Fig. 2.8). This is important because glycogen is in much shorter supply than fat. By using proportionally more fat, you will be able to exercise for longer before muscle glycogen is depleted and fatigue sets in.

Pre-exercise diet

A low-carbohydrate diet will result in low muscle and liver glycogen stores. Many studies have shown that initial muscle glycogen concentration is critical to your performance and that low muscle glycogen can reduce your ability to sustain exercise at 70% VO_2max for longer than 1 hour (Bergstrom *et al.*, 1967). It also affects your ability to perform during shorter periods of maximal power output.

When your muscle glycogen stores are low, your body will rely heavily on fat and protein. However, this is not a recommended strategy for fat loss, as you will lose lean tissue. (See Chapter 9 for appropriate ways of reducing body fat.)

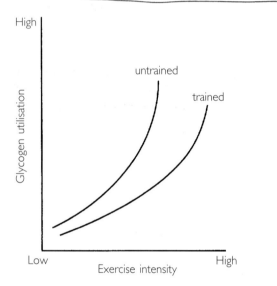

Figure 2.8 Trained people use less glycogen and more fat

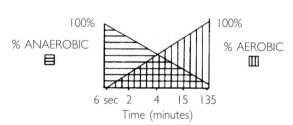

Figure 2.9 Percentage contribution of energy systems during exercise of different durations

WHICH ENERGY SYSTEMS DO I USE IN MY SPORT?

Virtually every activity uses all three energy systems to a greater or lesser extent. No single energy system is used exclusively and at any given time energy is being derived from each of the three systems (*see* Fig. 2.9). In every activity, ATP is always used and is replaced by PC. Anaerobic glycolysis and aerobic energy production depend on exercise intensity.

For example, during explosive strength and power activities lasting up to 5 seconds, such as a sprint start, the existing store of ATP is the primary energy source. For activities involving high power and speed lasting 5–30 seconds, such as 100–200 m sprints, the ATP–PC system is the primary energy source, together with some muscle glycogen broken down through anaerobic glycolysis. During power endurance activities such as 400–800 m events, muscle glycogen is the primary energy source and produces ATP via both anaerobic and aerobic glycolysis. In aerobic power activities, such as running 5–10 km, muscle glycogen is the primary energy source producing ATP via aerobic glycolysis. During aerobic events lasting 2 hours or more, such as half- and full marathons, muscle glycogen, liver glycogen, intra-muscular fat and fat from adipose tissue are the main fuels used. The energy systems and fuels used for various types of activities are summarised in Table 2.2.

Table 2.2 The main energy systems used during different types of exercise		
Type of exercise	**Main energy system**	**Major storage fuels used**
Maximal short bursts lasting less than 6 sec	ATP–PC (phosphagen)	ATP and PC
High intensity lasting up to 30 sec	ATP–PC Anaerobic glycolytic	ATP and PC Muscle glycogen
High intensity lasting up to 15 min	Anaerobic glycolytic Aerobic	Muscle glycogen
Moderate–high intensity lasting 15–60 min	Aerobic	Muscle glycogen Adipose tissue
Moderate–high intensity lasting 60–90 min	Aerobic	Muscle glycogen Liver glycogen Blood glucose Intra-muscular fat Adipose tissue
Moderate intensity lasting longer than 90 min	Aerobic	Muscle glycogen Liver glycogen Blood glucose Intra-muscular fat Adipose tissue

WHAT HAPPENS IN MY BODY WHEN I START EXERCISING?

When you begin to exercise, energy is produced without oxygen for at least the first few seconds, before your breathing rate and heart can catch up with energy demands. Therefore, a build-up of lactic acid takes place. As the heart and lungs work harder, getting more oxygen into your body, carbohydrates and fats can be broken down aerobically. If you are exercising fairly gently (i.e. your oxygen supply keeps up with your energy demands), any lactic acid that accumulated earlier can be removed easily since there is now enough oxygen around.

If you continue to exercise aerobically, more oxygen is delivered around the body and more fat starts to be broken down into fatty acids. They are taken to muscle cells via the bloodstream and then broken down with oxygen to produce energy.

In effect, the anaerobic system 'buys time' in the first few minutes of an exercise, before the body's slower aerobic system can start to function.

For the first 5–15 minutes of exercise (depending on your aerobic fitness level) the main fuel is carbohydrate (glycogen). As time goes on, however, more oxygen is delivered to the muscles, and you will use proportionally less carbohydrate and more fat.

On the other hand, if you begin exercising very strenuously (e.g. by running fast), lactic acid quickly builds up in the muscles. The delivery of oxygen cannot keep pace with the huge energy demand, so lactic acid continues to accumulate and very soon you will feel fatigue. You must then either slow down and run more slowly, or stop. Nobody can maintain a fast run for very long.

If you start a distance race or training run too fast, you will suffer from fatigue early on and be forced to reduce your pace considerably. A head start will not necessarily give any benefit at all. Warm up *before* the start of a race (by walking, slow jogging, or performing gentle mobility exercises), so that the heart and lungs can start to work a little harder, and oxygen delivery to the muscles can increase. Start the race at a moderate pace, gradually building up to an optimal speed. This will prevent a large 'oxygen debt' and avoid an early depletion of glycogen. In this way, your optimal pace can be sustained for longer.

The anaerobic system can also 'cut in' to help energy production, for instance when the demand for energy temporarily exceeds the body's oxygen supply. If you run uphill at the same pace as on the flat, your energy demand increases. The body will generate extra energy by breaking down glycogen/glucose anaerobically. However, this can be kept up for only a short period of time, because there will be a gradual build-up of lactic acid. The lactic acid can be removed aerobically afterwards, by running back down the hill, for example.

The same principle applies during fast bursts of activity in interval training, when energy is produced anaerobically. Lactic acid accumulates and is then removed during the rest interval.

WHAT IS FATIGUE?

In scientific terms, fatigue is an inability to sustain a given power output or speed. It is a mismatch between the demand for energy by the exercising muscles and the supply of energy in the form of ATP. Runners experience fatigue when they are no longer able to maintain their speed; footballers are slower to sprint for the ball and their technical ability falters; in the gym, you can no longer lift the weight; in an aerobics class, you will be unable to maintain the pace and intensity. Subjectively, you will find that exercise feels much harder to perform, your legs may feel hollow and it becomes increasingly hard to push yourself.

WHY DOES FATIGUE DEVELOP DURING ANAEROBIC EXERCISE?

During explosive activities involving maximal power output, fatigue develops due to ATP and PC depletion. In other words, the demand for ATP exceeds the readily available supply.

During activities lasting between 30 seconds and 30 minutes, fatigue is caused by a different mechanism. The rate of lactic acid removal in the bloodstream cannot keep pace with the rate of lactic acid production. This means that during high-intensity exercise lasting up to half an hour there is a gradual increase in muscle acidity, which reduces the ability of the muscles to maintain intense contractions. It is not possible to continue high-intensity exercise indefinitely because the acute acid environment in your muscles would inhibit further contractions and cause cell death. The burning feeling you experience when a high concentration of lactic acid develops is a kind of safety mechanism, preventing the muscle cells from destruction.

Reducing your exercise intensity will lower the rate of lactic acid production, reduce the build-up, and enable the muscles to switch to the aerobic energy system, thus enabling you to continue exercising.

WHY DOES FATIGUE DEVELOP DURING AEROBIC EXERCISE?

Fatigue during moderate and high-intensity aerobic exercise lasting longer than 1 hour occurs when muscle glycogen stores are depleted. It's like running out of petrol in your car. Muscle glycogen is in short supply compared with the body's fat stores. Liver glycogen can help maintain blood glucose levels and a supply of carbohydrate to the exercising muscles, but stores are also very limited and eventually fatigue will develop as a result of both muscle and liver glycogen depletion and hypoglycaemia (*see* Fig. 2.10).

During low to moderate-intensity exercise lasting more than three hours, fatigue is caused by additional factors. Once glycogen stores have been exhausted, the body switches to the aerobic lipolytic system where fat is able to supply most (not all) of the fuel for low-intensity exercise. However, despite having relatively large fat reserves, you will not be able to continue exercise indefinitely because fat cannot be converted to energy fast enough to keep up with the demand by exercising muscles. Even if you slowed your pace to enable the energy supplied by fat to meet the energy demand, other factors will cause you to fatigue. These include a rise in the concentration of the brain chemical serotonin, which results in an overall feeling of tiredness, acute muscle damage, and fatigue due to lack of sleep.

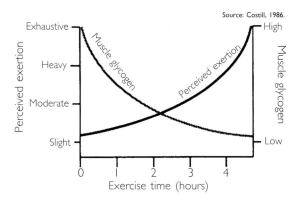

Figure 2.10 The increase in perceived exertion as glycogen stores become depleted

HOW CAN I DELAY FATIGUE?

Glycogen is used during virtually every type of activity. Therefore the amount of glycogen stored in your muscles and, in certain events, your liver, before you begin exercise will have a direct affect on your performance. The greater your pre-exercise muscle glycogen store, the longer you will be able to maintain your exercise intensity, and delay the onset of fatigue. Conversely, sub-optimal muscle glycogen stores can cause earlier fatigue, reduce your endurance, reduce your intensity level and result in smaller training gains.

You may also delay fatigue by reducing the rate at which you use up muscle glycogen. You can do this by pacing yourself, gradually building up to your optimal intensity.

SUMMARY OF KEY POINTS

- The body uses three energy systems: (1) the ATP–PC, or phosphagen, system; (2) the anaerobic glycolytic, or lactic acid, system; (3) the aerobic system, which comprises both glycolytic (carbohydrate) and lipolytic (fat) systems.
- The ATP–PC system fuels maximal bursts of activity lasting up to 6 seconds.
- Anaerobic glycolysis provides energy for short-duration high-intensity exercise lasting from 30 seconds to several minutes. Muscle glycogen is the main fuel.
- The lactic acid produced during anaerobic glycolysis is a valuable fuel for further energy production when exercise intensity is reduced.
- The aerobic system provides energy from the breakdown of carbohydrate and fat for sub-maximal intensity, prolonged exercise.
- Factors that influence the type of energy system and fuel usage are exercise intensity and duration, your fitness level and your pre-exercise diet.
- The proportion of muscle glycogen used for energy increases with exercise intensity and decreases with exercise duration.
- For most activities lasting longer than 30 seconds, all three energy systems are used to a greater or lesser extent; however, one system usually dominates.
- The main cause of fatigue during anaerobic activities lasting less than 6 seconds is ATP and PC depletion; during activities lasting between 30 seconds and 30 minutes, it is lactic acid accumulation and muscle cell acidity.
- Fatigue during moderate and high-intensity exercise lasting longer than 1 hour is usually due to muscle glycogen depletion. For events lasting longer than 2 hours, fatigue is associated with low liver glycogen and low blood sugar levels.
- For most activities, performance is limited by the amount of glycogen in the muscles. Low pre-exercise glycogen stores lead to early fatigue, reduced exercise intensity and reduced training gains.

FUELLING BEFORE, DURING AND AFTER EXERCISE

3

Carbohydrate is needed to fuel almost every type of activity and the amount of glycogen stored in your muscles and liver has a direct effect on your exercise performance. A high muscle-glycogen concentration will allow you to train at your optimal intensity and achieve a greater training effect. A low muscle-glycogen concentration, on the other hand, will lead to early fatigue, reduced training intensity and sub-optimal performance.

Clearly, then, glycogen is the most important and most valuable fuel for any type of exercise. This chapter explains what happens if you fail to eat enough carbohydrate and glycogen levels become depleted. It shows you how to calculate your precise carbohydrate requirements and considers the latest research on the timing of carbohydrate intake in relation to training.

Each different carbohydrate produces a different response in the body, so this chapter gives advice on which types of carbohydrate foods to eat. It presents comprehensive information on the glycaemic index (GI), a key part of every athlete's nutritional tool box. Finally, it considers the current thinking on carbohydrate loading before a competition.

THE RELATIONSHIP BETWEEN MUSCLE GLYCOGEN AND PERFORMANCE

The importance of carbohydrates in relation to exercise performance was first demonstrated in 1939. Christensen and Hansen found that a high-carbohydrate diet significantly increased endurance. However, it wasn't until the 1970s that scientists discovered that the capacity for endurance exercise is related to pre-exercise glycogen

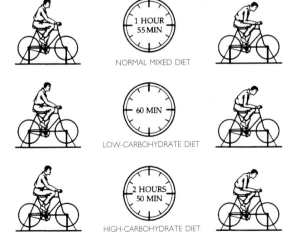

Figure 3.1 The effect of carbohydrate intake on performance

stores and that a high-carbohydrate diet increases glycogen stores.

In a pioneering study, three groups of athletes were given a low-carbohydrate diet, a high-carbohydrate diet or moderate-carbohydrate diet (Bergstrom *et al.*, 1967). Researchers measured the concentration of glycogen in their leg muscles and found that those athletes eating the high-carbohydrate diet stored twice as much glycogen as those on the moderate-carbohydrate diet and seven times as much as those eating the low-carbohydrate diet. Afterwards, the athletes were instructed to cycle to exhaustion on a stationary bicycle at 75% of VO_2max. Those on the high-carbohydrate diet managed to cycle for 170 minutes, considerably longer than those on the moderate-carbohydrate diet (115 minutes) or the low-carbohydrate diet (60 minutes) (*see* Fig 3.1).

HOW MUCH CARBOHYDRATE SHOULD I EAT PER DAY?

Sports nutritionists and exercise physiologists consistently recommend that regular exercisers consume a diet containing a relatively high percentage of energy from carbohydrate and a relatively low percentage of energy from fat (ACSM/ADA/DC, 2009; IOC, 2011). There is plentiful evidence that such a diet enhances endurance and performance for exercise lasting longer than one hour.

This recommendation is based on the fact that carbohydrate is very important for endurance exercise since carbohydrate stores – as muscle and liver glycogen – are limited. Depletion of these stores results in fatigue and reduced performance. This can easily happen if your pre-exercise glycogen stores are low. In order to get the most out

Can high fat diets increase endurance?

While most of the research on diet and endurance has focused on the role of carbohydrate, a number of studies have considered whether a high fat diet might enhance the muscles' ability to burn fat. The thinking behind this research is that since fat is a major fuel during prolonged endurance exercise, a high fat diet may be able to 'train' the muscles to burn more fat during exercise, conserving precious glycogen and giving muscles greater access to a more plentiful supply of energy in the body. Indeed, it appears that increasing fat intake enhances the storage and burning of intramuscular fat as well as improving the ability of the muscles to take up fat from the blood stream (Muoio *et al.*, 1994; Helge *et al.*, 2001; Lambert *et al.*, 1994). However, these effects are observed only in elite or well-conditioned athletes – and the performance advantage only applies at relatively low exercise intensities. For less conditioned athletes or untrained individuals, or those exercising above 65% VO_2max, high fat diets have no performance advantage (Burke *et al.*, 2004). What's more, a high fat intake may increase body fat % (if calorie intake exceeds calorie burning) and, if the diet contains excessive saturated fat, you risk high blood cholesterol levels. US researchers analysed 20 studies that looked at the high fat diets and performance (Erlenbusch *et al.*, 2005). They concluded that high fat diets have no performance advantage for non-elite athletes but all athletes (especially non-elite) benefited from a high carbohydrate diet.

of your training session, you should ensure your pre-exercise glycogen stores are high. This will help to improve your endurance, delay exhaustion and help you exercise longer and harder (Coyle, 1988; Costill & Hargreaves, 1992). Previously, researchers recommended a diet providing 60–70% energy from carbohydrate based on the consensus statement from the International Conference on Foods, Nutrition & Performance in 1991 (Williams & Devlin, 1992).

However, this method is not very user-friendly and can be misleading, as it assumes an optimal energy (calorie) intake. It does not provide optimal carbohydrate for those with very high or low energy intakes. For example, for an athlete consuming 4000–5000 calories daily, 60% energy from carbohydrate (i.e. 600 g +) would exceed their glycogen storage capacity (Coyle, 1995). Conversely, for athletes consuming 2000 calories daily, a diet providing 60% energy from carbohydrate (i.e. 300 g) would not contain enough carbohydrate to maintain muscle glycogen stores.

Scientists recommend calculating your carbohydrate requirement from your body weight and also your training volume (IOC, 2011; ACSM/ ASA/DC, 2009; IAAF, 2007; Burke *et al.*, 2004; IOC, 2004; Burke, 2001; Schokman, 1999), since your glycogen storage capacity is roughly proportional to your muscle mass and body weight – i.e. the heavier you are, the greater your muscle mass and the greater your glycogen storage capacity. The greater your training volume, the more carbohydrate you need to fuel your muscles. It is more flexible because it takes account of different training requirements and can be calculated independently of calorie intake.

Table 3.1 indicates the amount of carbohydrate per kg of body weight needed per day according to your activity level (Burke, 2007). Most athletes training for up to two hours daily require about 5–7 g/ kg body weight, but during periods of heavy training requirements may increase to 7–10 g/ kg BW.

For example, for a 70 kg athlete who trains for 1–2 hours a day:

- Carbohydrate need = 6–7 g /kg of body weight
- Daily carbohydrate need = Between (70 × 6) = 420 g and (70 × 7) = 490 g

i.e. Daily carbohydrate need = 420–490 g

Table 3.1	Guidelines for daily carbohydrate intake
Activity level	**Recommended carbohydrate intake**
Very light training (low intensity or skill based exercise)	3–5 g/ kg BW daily
Moderate intensity training (approx 1 h daily)	5–7 g/ kg BW daily
Moderate – high intensity training (1–3 h daily)	7–12 g / kg BW daily
Very high intensity training (> 4 h daily)	10–12 g / kg BW daily

Source: Burke, 2007

Is a high carbohydrate diet practical?

In practice, eating a high carbohydrate diet can be difficult, particularly for those athletes with high energy needs. Many complex carbohydrate foods, such as bread, potatoes and pasta are quite bulky and the diet quickly becomes very filling, particularly if whole grain and high fibre foods make up most of your carbohydrate intake. Several surveys have found that endurance athletes often fail to consume the recommended carbohydrate levels (Frentsos, 1999; Jacobs & Sherman, 1999). Most get between 45 and 65% of their calories from carbohydrate. This may be partly due to the large number of calories needed and therefore the bulk of their diet, and partly due to lack of awareness of the benefits of a higher carbohydrate intake. It is interesting that most of the studies upon which the carbohydrate recommendations were made, used liquid carbohydrates (i.e. drinks) to supplement meals. Tour de France cyclists and triathletes consume up to one third of their carbohydrate in liquid form. If you are finding a high carbohydrate diet impractical, try eating smaller more frequent meals and supplementing your food with liquid forms of carbohydrate such as meal replacement products (see p. 98) and glucose polymer drinks (see p. 117).

TRAIN LOW, COMPETE HIGH?

The general consensus is that athletes should eat a high carbohydrate diet (7–12 g/ kg body weight/ day) in order to maximise glycogen stores. However, a number of researchers have investigated the possible advantages of eating a low carbohydrate diet during training followed by a high carbohydrate diet prior to competition ('train low, compete high') (Hawley & Burke, 2010). The idea is that training with low muscle glycogen stores forces the muscles to adapt to using fat as a fuel instead of carbohydrate. Indeed, studies have measured increased levels of fat-oxidising enzymes following a period of high intensity training on a low carbohydrate diet (Yeo et al., 2008). In other words, you can 'train' the muscles to better utilise fat for energy production, potentially sparing the limited glycogen stores. However, despite increasing enzyme levels in the muscles, low carbohydrate diets have not been shown to enhance exercise performance (Maughan and Shirreffs, 2012; Hawley et al., 2011; Burke, L.M., 2010; Morton et al., 2009). What's more, athletes training in a glycogen-depleted state tend to choose a lower workload or intensity because the exercise feels harder. To date, there is not enough evidence to support the 'train low, compete high' concept as an effective competitive strategy, and so it remains a theoretical model.

WHICH CARBOHYDRATES ARE BEST?

Carbohydrates are traditionally classified according to their chemical structure. The most simplistic method divides them into two categories: *simple* (sugars) and *complex* (starches and fibres). These terms simply refer to the number of sugar units in the molecule.

Simple carbohydrates are very small molecules consisting of one or two sugar units. They comprise the *monosaccharides* (1-sugar units):

glucose (dextrose), fructose (fruit sugar) and galactose; and the *disaccharides* (2-sugar units): sucrose (table sugar, which comprises a glucose and fructose molecule joined together) and lactose (milk sugar, which comprises a glucose and galactose molecule joined together).

Complex carbohydrates are much larger molecules, consisting of between 10- and several thousand-sugar units (mostly glucose) joined together. They include the starches, amylose and amylopectin, and the non-starch polysaccharides (dietary fibre), such as cellulose, pectin and hemicellulose.

In between simple and complex carbohydrates are glucose polymers and maltodextrin, which comprise between 3- and 10-sugar units. They are made from the partial breakdown of corn starch in food processing, and are widely used as bulking and thickening agents in processed foods, such as sauces, dairy desserts, baby food, puddings and soft drinks. They are popular ingredients in sports drinks and engineered meal-replacement products, owing to their low sweetness and high energy density relative to sucrose.

In practice, many foods contain a mixture of both simple and complex carbohydrates, making the traditional classification of foods into 'simple' and 'complex' very confusing. For example, biscuits and cakes contain flour (complex) and sugar (simple), and bananas contain a mixture of sugars and starches depending on their degree of ripeness.

NOT ALL CARBOHYDRATES ARE EQUAL

It's tempting to think that simple carbohydrates, due to their smaller molecular size, are absorbed more quickly than complex carbohydrates, and produce a large and rapid rise in blood sugar.

Unfortunately, it's not that straightforward. For example, apples (containing simple carbohydrates) produce a small and prolonged rise in blood sugar, despite being high in simple carbohydrates. Many starchy foods (complex carbohydrates), such as potatoes and bread, are digested and absorbed very quickly and give a rapid rise in blood sugar. So the old notion about simple carbohydrates giving fast-released energy and complex carbohydrates giving slow-released energy is incorrect and misleading.

What is more important as far as sports performance is concerned is how rapidly the carbohydrate is absorbed from the small intestine into your bloodstream. The faster this transfer, the more rapidly the carbohydrate can be taken up by muscle cells (or other cells of the body) and make a difference to your training and recovery.

THE GLYCAEMIC INDEX

To describe more accurately the effect different foods have on your blood sugar levels, scientists developed the glycaemic index (GI). While the GI concept was originally developed to help diabetics control their blood sugar levels, it can benefit regular exercisers and athletes too. It is a ranking of foods from 0 to 100 based on their immediate effect on blood sugar levels, a measure of the speed at which you digest food and convert it into glucose. The faster the rise in blood glucose, the higher the rating on the index. To make a fair comparison, all foods are compared with a reference food, such as glucose, and are tested in equivalent carbohydrate amounts. The GI of foods is very useful to know because it tells you how the body responds to them. If you need to get carbohydrates into your bloodstream and muscle cells rapidly – for example, immediately after exercise to kick-start glycogen replenishment – you would choose high GI foods. In 1997 the World Health Organization (WHO) and Food and Agriculture Organization (FOA) of the United Nations endorsed the use of the GI for classifying foods, and recommended that GI values should be used to guide people's food choices.

HOW IS THE GI WORKED OUT?

The GI value of food is measured by feeding 10 or more healthy people a portion of food containing 50 g carbohydrate. For example, to test baked potatoes, you would eat 250 g potatoes, which contain 50 g of carbohydrate. Over the next two hours, a sample of blood is taken every 15 minutes and the blood sugar level measured. The blood sugar level is plotted on a graph and the area under the curve calculated using a computer programme (*see* Fig. 3.2). On another occasion, the same 10 people consume a 50 g portion of glucose (the reference food). Their response to the test food (e.g. potato) is compared with their blood sugar response to 50 g glucose (the reference food). The GI is given as a percentage, which is calculated by dividing the area under the curve after you've eaten potatoes by the area under the curve after you've eaten the glucose. The final GI value for the test food is the average GI value for the 10 people. So, the GI of baked potatoes is 85, which means that eating baked potato produces a rise in blood sugar that is 85% as great as that produced after eating an equivalent amount of glucose.

Appendix 1 ('The glycaemic index and glycaemic load) gives the GI content of many popular foods. Most values lie somewhere between 20 and 100. Sports nutritionists find it useful to classify foods as *high GI* (71–100), *medium GI* (56–70) and *low GI* (0–55). This simply makes it easier to select the appropriate food before, during and after exercise. In a nutshell, the higher the GI, the higher the blood sugar levels after eating that food. In general, refined starchy foods, including potatoes, white rice and white bread, as well as sugary foods, such as soft drinks and biscuits, are high on the glycaemic index. For example, baked potatoes (GI 85) and white rice (GI 87) produce a rise in blood sugar almost the same as eating pure glucose (yes, you read correctly!). Less refined starchy foods – porridge, beans, lentils, muesli – as well as fruit and dairy products are lower on the glycaemic index. They produce a much smaller rise in blood sugar compared with glucose.

Only a few centres around the world provide a legitimate GI testing service. The Human Nutrition Unit at the University of Sydney in Australia has been at the forefront of GI research for over two decades, and has measured the GI of hundreds of foods. International Tables of Glycaemic Index have been published by the American Journal of Clinical Nutrition (Foster-Powell and Brand-Miller, 1995; Foster-Powell *et*

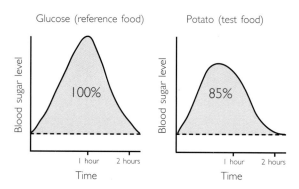

Figure 3.2 Measuring the GI of food

Table 3.2 Factors that influence the GI of a food

Factor	How it works	Examples of foods
Particle size	Processing reduces particle size and makes it easier for digestive enzymes to access the starch. The smaller the particle size (i.e. the more processed the food), the higher the GI.	Most breakfast cereals, e.g. cornflakes and rice crispies have a higher GI than muesli or porridge.
Degree of starch gelatinisation	The more gelatinised (swollen with water) the starch, the greater the surface area for enzymes to attack, the faster the digestion and rise in blood sugar, i.e. higher GI.	Cooked potatoes (high GI); biscuits (lower GI).
Amylose to amylopectin ratio	There are two types of starch: amylose (long straight molecule, difficult access by enzymes) and amylopectin (branched molecule, easier access by enzymes). The more amylose a food contains the slower it is digested, i.e. lower GI.	Beans, lentils, peas and basmati rice have high amylose content, i.e. low GI; wheat flour and products containing it have high amylopectin content, i.e. high GI.
Fat	Fat slows down rate of stomach emptying, slowing down digestion and lowering GI.	Potato crisps have a lower GI than plain boiled potatoes; adding butter or cheese to bread lowers GI.
Sugar (sucrose)	Sucrose is broken down into one molecule of fructose and one molecule of glucose. Fructose is converted into glucose in the liver slowly, giving a smaller rise in blood sugar.	Sweet biscuits, cakes, sweet breakfast cereals, honey.
Soluble fibre	Soluble fibre increases viscosity of food in digestive tract and slows digestion, producing lower blood sugar rise, i.e. lowers GI.	Beans, lentils, peas, oats, porridge, barley, fruit.
Protein	Protein slows stomach emptying and therefore carbohydrate digestion, producing a smaller blood sugar rise, i.e. lowers GI.	Beans, lentils, peas, pasta (all contain protein as well as carbohydrate). Eating chicken with rice lowers the GI.

al., 2002). But new and revised data are constantly being added to the list as commercial foods are reformulated and these are available on the website www.glycemicindex.com (note the US spelling of this website – not to be confused with www.glycaemicindex.com).

WHAT MAKES ONE FOOD HAVE A HIGH GI AND ANOTHER FOOD A LOW GI?

Factors that influence the GI of a food include the size of the food particle, the biochemical make-up of the carbohydrate (the ratio of amylose to amylopectin), the degree of cooking (which affects starch gelatinisation), and the presence of fat, sugar, protein and fibre. How these factors influence the GI of a food is summarised in Table 3.2.

HOW CAN YOU CALCULATE THE GI OF A MEAL?

To date, only the GIs of single foods have been directly measured. In reality, it is more useful to know the GI of a meal, as we are more likely to

Why does pasta have a low GI?

Pasta has a low GI because of the physical entrapment of ungelatinised starch granules in a sponge-like network of protein (gluten) molecules in the pasta dough. Pasta cooked al dente has a slighter lower GI than pasta that has been cooked longer until it is very soft. Pasta is unique in this regard, and as a result, pastas of any shape and size have a fairly low GI (30 to 60).

eat combinations of foods. It is possible to *estimate* the GI of a meal by working out its total carbohydrate content, and then the contribution of each food to the total carbohydrate content. Table 3.3 shows how to calculate the overall GI of a typical breakfast.

For a quick estimate of a simple meal, such as beans on toast, you may assume that half the carbohydrate is coming from the bread and half from the beans. So you can add the GI values

Table 3.3	How to calculate the GI of a meal			
Food	Carbohydrate (g)	% total carbohydrate	GI	Contribution to meal GI
Orange juice (150 ml)	12.5	26	46	26% × 46 = 12
Weetabix (30 g)	21	43	69	43% × 69 = 30
Milk (150 ml)	7	15	27	15% × 27 = 4
1 slice toast	13	27	70	27% × 70 = 19
Total	48	100		Meal GI = 65

Source: Leeds *et al.*, 2000.

of the two foods together and divide by 2: (70 + 48) ÷ 2 = 59.

If you have uneven proportions of two foods, for example 75% milk: 25% muesli, then 75% of the GI of milk can be added to 25% of the GI of muesli.

However, this will give you only a rough guide, not an accurate prediction. Scientists at the University of Otago in New Zealand found that GI values significantly overestimate an individual's blood glucose response to a meal (Dodd *et al.*, 2011).

WHAT ARE THE DRAWBACKS OF THE GI?

The key to efficient glycogen refuelling – and minimal fat storage – is to maintain steady levels of blood glucose and insulin. When glucose levels are high (for example, after consuming high GI foods), large amounts of insulin are produced, which shunts the excess glucose into fat cells. However, it is the combined effect of a large amount of carbohydrate as well as a food's GI value that really matters.

Low GI diet at a glance

In essence, a low GI diet comprises carbohydrate foods with a low GI as well as lean protein foods and healthy fats:

- **Fresh fruit** – the more acidic the fruit the lower the GI. Apples, pears, oranges, grapefruit, peaches, nectarines, plums and apricots have the lowest GI values while tropical fruits such as pineapple, papaya and watermelon have higher values. However, as average portion size is small, the GL would be low.
- **Fresh vegetables** – most vegetables have a very low carbohydrate content and don't have a GI value (you would need to eat enormous amounts to get a significant rise in blood glucose). The exception is potatoes, which have a high GI. Eat them with protein/ healthy fat or replace with low GI starchy vegetables (see below)
- **Low GI starchy vegetables** – these include sweetcorn (GI 46–48), sweet potato (GI 46) and yam (GI 37)
- **Low GI breads** – these include stoneground wholemeal bread (not ordinary wholemeal

bread), fruit or malt loaf, wholegrain bread with lots of grainy bits, breads containing barley, rye, oats, soy and cracked wheat or those containing sunflower seeds or linseeds; chapati and pitta breads (unleavened), pumpernickel (rye kernel) bread, sourdough bread
- **Low GI breakfast cereals** – these include porridge, muesli and other oat or rye based cereals, and high bran cereals (e.g. All Bran)
- **Low GI grains** – these include bulgar wheat, noodles, oats, pasta, basmati (not ordinary brown or white) rice
- **Beans and lentils** – chick peas, red kidney beans, baked beans, cannellini beans, mung beans, black-eyed beans, butter beans, split peas and lentils
- **Nuts and seeds** – almonds, brazils, cashews, hazelnuts, pine nuts, pistachios, peanuts; sunflower, sesame, flax and pumpkin seeds
- **Fish, lean meat, poultry and eggs** – these contain no carbohydrate so have no GI value
- **Low fat dairy products** – milk, cheese and yoghurt are important for their calcium and protein content. Opt for lower fat versions where possible.

The biggest drawback of the GI is that it doesn't take account of the portion size you are eating. For example, watermelon has a GI of 72 – and is therefore classified as a high GI food – which puts it off the menu on a low GI diet. However, an average slice (120g) gives you only 6 g carbohydrate, not enough to raise your blood glucose level significantly. You would need to eat at least 6 slices (720 g) to obtain 50 g carbohydrate – the amount used in the GI test.

Similarly, many vegetables appear to have a high GI, which means they may be excluded on low GI diet. However, their carbohydrate content is low and therefore their effect on blood glucose levels would be small. So despite having a high GI the glycaemic load (GI x g carbohydrate per portion divided by 100) is low.

Another drawback is that some high fat foods have a low GI, which gives a falsely favourable impression of the food. For example, the GI of crisps or chips is lower than that of baked potatoes. Fat reduces the rate at which food is digested but saturated and trans fats (see pp. 135 and 138) can push up heart disease risk. It's important you don't select foods only by their GI – check the type of fat (i.e. saturated or unsaturated) and avoid those that contain large amounts of saturated or trans fats.

WHAT IS THE GLYCAEMIC LOAD?

You can gain a more accurate measure of the rise in your blood glucose (and insulin level) by using the glycaemic load (GL). This concept is derived from a mathematical equation developed by Professor Walter Willett from the Harvard Medical School in the US. It is calculated simply by multiplying the GI of a food by the amount of carbohydrate per portion and dividing by 100. One unit of GL is roughly equivalent to the glycaemic effect of 1 g of glucose. It gives you a good estimate of both the quality (GI) and quantity of carbohydrate:

- GL = (GI x carbohydrate per portion) ÷ 100

So, for watermelon:

- GL = (72 x 6) ÷ 100 = 4.3

	GI value	GL value	Daily GL total
Low	0–55	0–10	0–80
Medium	56–70	11–19	80–120
High	71–100	> 20	> 120

A high glycaemic load can result from eating a small quantity of a high-carbohydrate high GI food (e.g. white bread) or a larger quantity of a low GI food (e.g. pasta). This results in a large surge in blood glucose and insulin.

Conversely, eating smaller amounts of a low-carbohydrate high GI food (e.g. watermelon) or a larger quantity of a low GI food (e.g. beans) produces a low glycaemic 'load'. This results in a smaller and more sustained rise in blood glucose.

To optimise glycogen storage and minimise fat storage, aim to achieve a small or moderate glycaemic load – eat little and often, avoid overloading on carbohydrates, and stick to balanced combinations of carbohydrate, protein and healthy fat.

There's no need to cut out high glycaemic foods. The key is to eat them either in small amounts or combined with protein and/or a little

Glycaemic response in athletes

Scientists say that high GI foods have a smaller effect on blood glucose and insulin in regular exercisers compared with non-exercisers. That's because exercise modifies the glycaemic response. Studies at the University of Sydney in Australia have found that when athletes are fed high GI foods, they produce much less insulin than would be predicted from GI tables. In other words, they don't show the same peaks and troughs in insulin as sedentary people do. Use the GI index only as a rough guide to how various foods are likely to behave in your body.

base their diets on low GI foods in order to prevent chronic diseases.

However, the risk of disease is also predicted by the GL of the overall diet. In other words, GL simply strengthens the relationship, which suggests that the more frequently people eat high GI foods, the greater their health risk.

The downside to GL is that you could end up eating a low carbohydrate diet with a lot of fat and/ or protein. Use the GI table (Appendix One) to compare foods within the same category (e.g. different types of bread) and don't worry about the GI of those foods with a very low carbohydrate content (e.g. watermelon).

healthy fat. This will evoke lower insulin levels and less potential fat storage. For example, have a baked potato (high GI food) with a little margarine and baked beans or tuna (both low GI foods). Both protein and fat put a brake on the digestive process, slowing down the release of glucose.

SHOULD I USE GI OR GL?

GI remains the best-researched and one of the most reliable indicators of health risk. In studies at Harvard University a low GI diet has been correlated with a low risk of chronic diseases like heart disease, type II diabetes and cancer of the bowel, upper gastro-intestinal tract and pancreas. In particular, low GI is linked to high levels of HDL ('good') cholesterol (see p. 139). So if you have a low GI diet the chances are you have a high 'good cholesterol' level and a lower risk of heart disease. In 1999 the World Health Organization (WHO) and Food and Agriculture Organization (FAO) recommended that people

How much fibre?

Dietary fibre is the term used to describe the complex carbohydrates found in plants that are resistant to digestion. It includes cellulose, pectins, glucans, inulin and guar. The Department of Health recommends between 18 g and 24 g a day. The average intake in the UK is 15.2 g/day and 12.6 g/day for men and women respectively. Fibre helps your digestive system work properly and modifies the glycaemic effect of a meal. The soluble kind slows the digestion of carbohydrate, producing a slower blood glucose rise. The richest sources are beans, lentils, oats, rye, fruit and vegetables. Insoluble fibre – found mainly in wholegrain bread, whole grains and wholegrain breakfast cereals, wholewheat pasta, brown rice and vegetables – helps speed the passage of food through the gut, and prevent constipation and bowel problems.

BEFORE EXERCISE

What, when and how much you eat before exercise will effect your performance, strength and endurance. Paradoxically, consuming carbohydrate increases carbohydrate burning in the muscle cells yet still delays the onset of fatigue. Numerous studies have concluded that consuming carbohydrate before exercise results in improved performance when compared with exercising on an empty stomach (Chryssanthopoulos *et al.*, 2002; Neufer *et al.*, 1987; Sherman *et al.*, 1991; Wright *et al.*, 1991).

Does exercise first thing in the morning burn more body fat?

If fat loss is your main goal, exercising on an empty stomach – such as first thing in the morning – may encourage your body to burn slightly more fat for fuel. According to University of Connecticut researchers, insulin levels are at their lowest and glucagen levels are at their highest after an overnight fast. This increases the amount of fat that leaves your fat cells and travels to your muscles, where the fat is burned. On the downside, you may fatigue sooner or drop your exercise intensity and therefore end up burning fewer calories – and less body fat! If performance is your main goal, exercising in a fasted state will almost certainly reduce your endurance. And if strength and muscle mass are important goals, you will be better off exercising after a light meal. After an overnight fast, when muscle glycogen and blood glucose levels are low, your muscles will burn more protein for fuel. So you could end up losing hard-earned muscle!

WHEN IS THE BEST TIME TO EAT BEFORE EXERCISE?

Ideally, you should eat between 2 and 4 hours before training, leaving enough time for your stomach to settle so that you feel comfortable – not too full and not too hungry. This helps increase liver and muscle glycogen levels and enhances your subsequent performance (Hargreaves *et al.*, 2004). Clearly, the exact timing of your pre-exercise meal will depend on your daily schedule and the time of day you plan to train.

Researchers at the University of North Carolina found that performance during moderate to high intensity exercise lasting 35–40 minutes was improved after eating a moderately high carbohydrate, low fat meal 3 hours before exercise (Maffucci & McMurray, 2000). In this study, the volunteers were able to run significantly longer. Researchers asked the athletes to run on treadmills, at a moderate intensity for 30 minutes with high-intensity 30 second intervals and then until they couldn't run any longer, after eating a meal either 6 hours or 3 hours beforehand. The athletes ran significantly longer if they had eaten the meal 3 hours before training compared with 6 hours.

If you leave too long an interval between eating and training, you will be at risk of hypoglycaemia – low blood glucose – and this will certainly compromise your performance. You will fatigue earlier and, if you feel light-headed, risk injury too. On the other hand, training with steady blood glucose levels will allow you to train longer and harder.

HOW MUCH CARBOHYDRATE?

The size and timing of your pre-training meal are inter-related. The closer you are to the start of your training session, the smaller your meal should be (to allow for gastric emptying), whereas larger meals can be consumed when more time is available before training or competition. Intakes between 1–4 g/ kg BW consumed 1–4 hours before exercise have been recommended (Burke, 2007). Most studies suggest 200–300 g carbohydrate or 2.5 g carbohydrate/kg of body weight about 3 hours before exercise (ACSM/ADA/ DC, 2009). Researchers at Loughborough University found that this pre-exercise meal improved endurance running capacity by 9% compared with a no-meal trial (Chryssanthopoulos *et al.*, 2002). So, for example, if you weigh 70 kg, that translates to 175 g carbohydrate. You may need to experiment to find the exact quantity of food or drink and the timing that works best for you. Some athletes can consume a substantial meal in the 2–4 hours before exercise with no ill-effects, while others may experience discomfort and prefer to eat a snack or liquid meal.

WHAT ARE THE BEST FOODS TO EAT BEFORE EXERCISE?

Whether to eat high GI or low GI foods pre-exercise has long been a controversial area. Many experts recommend a low GI meal based on the idea that such a meal would supply sustained energy during exercise. Indeed, a number of well-designed studies carried out at the University of Sydney have supported this recommendation. For example, the researchers found that when a group of cyclists ate a low GI pre-exercise meal of lentils (GI = 29) 1 hour before exercise, they managed to keep going 20 minutes longer than when they consumed high GI foods (glucose drink, GI = 100; or baked potatoes, GI = 85) (Thomas *et al.*, 1991). Lentils were used in this study because they have one of the lowest GI values, but there are, of course, plenty of other low GI foods or food

combinations that you can choose. For example, most fresh fruit, milk or yoghurt would be suitable, or a combination of carbohydrate, protein and healthy fat – for example, cereal with milk, a chicken sandwich or a baked potato with cheese. The box below gives further suggestions for pre-exercise snacks and meals.

In other studies (Thomas *et al.*, 1994; DeMarco *et al.*, 1999), the researchers took blood samples at regular intervals from cyclists and found that low GI meals produce higher blood sugar and fatty acid levels during the latter stages of exercise, which is clearly advantageous for endurance sports. In other words, the low GI meals produce a sustained source of carbohydrate throughout exercise and recovery.

Pre-workout meals
2–4 hours before exercise:
- Sandwich/roll/bagel/wrap filled with chicken, fish, cheese, egg or peanut butter and salad
- Jacket potato with beans, cheese, tuna, coleslaw or chicken
- Pasta with tomato-based pasta sauce and cheese and vegetables
- Chicken with rice and salad
- Vegetable and prawn or tofu stir fry with noodles or rice
- Pilaff or rice salad
- Mixed bean hot pot with potatoes
- Chicken and vegetable casserole with potatoes
- Porridge made with milk
- Wholegrain cereal (e.g. bran or wheat flakes, muesli or Weetabix) with milk or yoghurt
- Fish and potato pie

Pre-workout snacks

1–2 hours before exercise:

- Fresh fruit
- Dried apricots, dates or raisins
- Smoothie (home-made or ready-bought)
- Yoghurt
- Shake (home-made or a meal replacement shake)
- Energy or nutrition bar
- Cereal bar or flapjack
- Toast with honey or jam
- Porridge or wholegrain cereal with milk

A UK study confirmed that athletes burn more fat during exercise following a low GI meal of bran cereal, fruit and milk compared with a high GI meal of cornflakes, white bread, jam and sports drink (Wu *et al.*, 2003). The benefits kick in early during exercise – the difference in fat oxidation is apparent even after 15 minutes.

A 2006 study at the University of Loughborough found that runners who consumed a low GI meal 3 hours before exercise were able to run longer (around 8 minutes) than after a high GI pre-exercise meal (Wu & Williams, 2006). The researchers suggest that the improvements in performance were due to increased fat oxidation following consumption of the low GI meal, which helped compensate for the lower rates of glycogen oxidation during the latter stages of the exercise trial. In other words, the low GI meal allowed the volunteers to burn more fat and less glycogen during exercise, which resulted in increased endurance.

This isn't necessarily a rule of thumb, as other studies have found that the GI of the pre-exercise meal has little effect on performance, with cyclists managing to keep going for the same duration whether they ate lentils (low GI) or potatoes (high GI) (Febbraio & Stewart, 1996). A Greek study also found that ingestion of high GI or low GI foods (containing the same quantity of carbohydrate) 30 minutes before exercise did not result in any differences in exercise performance in a group of 8 cyclists (Jamurtas *et al.*, 2011). It's certainly not a clear-cut case but what you have to consider is the timing of your pre-exercise meal. High GI foods are more 'risky' to your performance, particularly if you are sensitive to blood sugar fluctuations (Burke *et al.*, 1998). Get the timing wrong, and you may be starting exercise with mild hypoglycaemia – remember, they produce a rapid rise in blood sugar and, in some people, a short-lived dip afterwards. The safest strategy may be to stick with low GI pre-exercise and then top up with high GI carbohydrate during exercise if you are training for more than 60 minutes.

DURING EXERCISE

For most activities lasting less than 45 minutes to 1 hour, drinking anything other than water is unnecessary provided your pre-exercise muscle glycogen levels are high, i.e. you have consumed sufficient carbohydrate during the previous few days and eaten a carbohydrate-containing meal 2–4 hours before exercise (Burke *et al.*, 2011; IOC, 2011; Desbrow *et al.*, 2004).

It is well-established that consuming carbohydrate during prolonged exercise (more than 1–2 hours) can enhance performance but research since the late 1990s has suggested that very small amounts of carbohydrate may be beneficial for high intensity exercise (> 75% VO_2max) lasting 45–60 minutes (Carter *et al.*, 2004; Below,

1995; Jeukendrup *et al.*, 1997). The reasons are quite different.

Exercise lasting 45–75 minutes

In the first scenario, the performance enhancing effect is mediated by the central nervous system (the brain), and not by any increase in carbohydrate uptake. Researchers have found that simply rinsing the mouth with a carbohydrate drink improves performance even when you do not swallow the drink (Carter, 2004; Burke *et al.*, 2011). This is thought to be due to carbohydrate receptors in the mouth signalling to the brain that food is on its way. This somehow overrides the perception of effort and fatigue so you are able to continue exercising despite not actually consuming any carbohydrate. In practice, then, for exercise lasting 45 minutes to 1 hour, you don't have to consume any carbohydrate – simply swilling or rinsing a carbohydrate drink, or sucking a sweet, will be enough to give you a performance boost.

Exercise lasting more than 1–2 hours

In the second scenario, consuming carbohydrate during your workout can help maintain blood glucose levels, delay fatigue and enable you to perform longer at a higher intensity. It may also help you to continue exercising when your muscle glycogen stores are depleted.

During that first hour of exercise, most of your carbohydrate energy comes from muscle glycogen. After that, muscle glycogen stores deplete significantly, so the exercising muscles must use carbohydrate from some other source. That's where blood sugar (glucose) comes into its own. As you continue exercising hard, the muscles take up more and more glucose from the bloodstream.

Eventually, after 2–3 hours, your muscles will be fuelled entirely by blood glucose and fat.

Sounds handy, but, alas, you cannot keep going indefinitely because blood glucose supplies eventually dwindle. Some of this blood glucose is derived from certain amino acids and some comes from liver glycogen. When liver glycogen stores run low, your blood glucose levels will fall, and you will be unable to carry on exercising at the same intensity. That's why temporary hypoglycaemia is common after 2–3 hours of exercise without consuming carbohydrate. In this state, you would feel very fatigued and light-headed, your muscles would feel very heavy and the exercise would feel very hard indeed. In other words, the depletion of muscle and liver glycogen together with low blood sugar levels would cause you to reduce exercise intensity or stop completely. This is sometimes called 'hitting the wall' in marathon running.

Clearly, then, consuming additional carbohydrate would maintain your blood sugar levels and allow you to exercise longer (Coggan & Coyle, 1991; Coyle, 2004; Jeukendrup, 2004).

HOW MUCH CARBOHYDRATE?

For exercise longer than one hour, the consensus recommendation is an intake of between 30–60 g carbohydrate/hour (IOC, 2011; Burke *et al.*, 2011; ACSM/ADA/DC, 2009; Coggan and Coyle, 1991). This matches the maximum amount of a single type of carbohydrate (e.g. glucose) that can be oxidised by the muscles during aerobic exercise because the transporter responsible for carbohydrate absorption in the intestine becomes saturated. Consuming more than 60 g carbohydrate per hour would not improve your energy output nor reduce fatigue.

However, for intense exercise lasting more than 3 hours, it would be beneficial to consume greater amounts of carbohydrate. Research at the University of Birmingham has found that this can be achieved by consuming a mixture of carbohydrates ('multiple transportable carbohydrates') – glucose + fructose, or maltodextrin + fructose in a 2:1 ratio – which increases the uptake of carbohydrates from the intestines and also the oxidation rate in the muscles (IOC, 2010; Jeukendrup, 2008). It may also increase fluid uptake. It is possible to make up these drinks yourself although commercial sports drinks and gels with this formulation are becoming available at the time of going to press.

You should experiment with different drinks and foods during training to develop your own fuelling strategy.

It is important to begin consuming carbohydrate *before* fatigue sets in. Coggan and Coyle stress that it takes at least 30 minutes for the carbohydrate to be absorbed into the bloodstream. The best strategy is to begin consuming carbohydrate soon after the start of your workout, certainly within the first 30 minutes.

While consuming carbohydrate during exercise can delay fatigue, perhaps by up to 45 minutes, it will not allow you to keep exercising hard indefinitely. Eventually, factors other than carbohydrate supply will cause fatigue.

WHICH FOODS OR DRINKS SHOULD I CONSUME DURING EXERCISE?

It makes sense that the carbohydrate you consume during exercise should be easily digested and absorbed. You need it to raise your blood sugar level and reach your exercising muscles rapidly. Thus, high or moderate GI carbohydrates are generally the best choices (*see* Table 3.5). Whether you choose solid or liquid carbohydrate makes little difference to your performance, provided you drink water with solid carbohydrate (Kennerley *et al.*, 2011; Mason *et al.*, 1993). Most athletes find liquid forms of carbohydrate (i.e. sports drinks) more convenient. Carbohydrate-containing drinks have a dual benefit because they provide fluid

Table 3.4	Summary of recommendations for carbohydrate intake during exercise

Exercise duration	Recommended amount of carbohydrate	Type of carbohydrate
< 45 minutes	None	None
45–75 minutes	v. small amounts (mouth rinse)	Any
1–2 hours	Up to 30 g/h	Any
2–3 hours	Up to 60 g/h	Glucose, maltodextrins
3 hours	Up to 90 g/h	Multiple transportable carbohydrates (glucose + fructose, or maltodextrin + fructose in 2:1 ratio)

Table 3.5	Suitable foods and drinks to consume during exercise	
Food or drink	Portion size providing 30 g carbohydrate	Portion size providing 60 g carbohydrate
Isotonic sports drink (6 g/100 ml)	500 ml	1000 ml
Glucose polymer drink (12 g/100 ml)	250 ml	500 ml
Energy bar	½–1 bar	1–2 bars
Diluted fruit juice (1:1)	500 ml	1000 ml
Raisins or sultanas	1 handful (40 g)	2 handfuls (80 g)
Cereal or breakfast bar	1 bar	2 bars
Energy gel	1 sachet	2 sachets
Bananas	1–2 bananas	2–3 bananas

as well as fuel, which reduces dehydration and fatigue. Obviously, you do not have to consume a commercial drink; you can make your own from fruit juice, or sugar, or squash, and water (*see* Chapter 7).

If you prefer to consume food as well as drinks during exercise, energy or 'sports nutrition' bars, sports gels, ripe bananas, raisins or fruit bars are all suitable. Have a drink of water at the same time. In one study at Apalachian State University, there was no difference in exercise performance when cyclists were given equal amounts of carbohydrate either in the form of a banana or a 6% carbohydrate sports drink (Kennerly *et al.*, 2011). Whether you choose liquid or solid carbohydrate, aim to consume at least 1 litre of fluid per hour.

CARBOHYDRATE PLUS PROTEIN DURING EXERCISE?

Some studies have suggested that consuming a drink containing protein as well as carbohydrate during exercise improves endurance to a greater extent than carbohydrate alone. It may also minimise protein breakdown following exercise and improve recovery. A study at the University of Texas found that cyclists were able to exercise 36% longer when they consumed a carbohydrate-protein drink immediately before, and then every 20 minutes, during exercise, compared with a carbohydrate-only drink (Ivy *et al.*, 2003). Researchers at James Madison University, Vancouver, measured a 29% increase in endurance when cyclists consumed a carbohydrate-protein drink every 15 minutes compared with a carbohydrate-only drink (Saunders *et al.*, 2004). A number of studies also suggest that consuming protein plus carbohydrate during exercise improves recovery from exercise and results in less muscle damage (Berardi *et al.*, 2008; Saunders, 2007; Luden *et al.*, 2007; Romano-Ely *et al.*, 2006). This would most likely help improve your subsequent performance. The exact amount of each ingredient is not clear, but most of the trials used drinks containing a carbohydrate to protein ratio of approximately 4:1 (e.g. 80 g carbohydrate: 20 g whey protein).

AFTER EXERCISE

The length of time that it takes to refuel depends on four main factors:

- how depleted your glycogen stores are after exercise
- the extent of muscle damage
- the amount and the timing of carbohydrate you eat
- your training experience and fitness level.

Depletion

The more depleted your glycogen stores, the longer it will take you to refuel, just as it takes longer to refill an empty fuel tank than one that is half-full. This, in turn, depends on the intensity and duration of your workout.

The higher the *intensity*, the more glycogen you use. For example, if you concentrate on fast, explosive activities (e.g. sprints, jumps or lifts) or high-intensity aerobic activities (e.g. running), you will deplete your glycogen stores far more than for low-intensity activities (e.g. walking or slow swimming) of equal duration. The minimum time it would take to refill muscle glycogen stores is 20 hours (Coyle, 1991). After prolonged and exhaustive exercise (e.g. marathon), it may take up to 7 days.

The *duration* of your workout also has a bearing on the amount of glycogen you use. For example, if you run for one hour, you will use up more glycogen than if you run at the same speed for half an hour. If you complete 10 sets of shoulder exercises in the gym, you will use more glycogen from your shoulder muscles than if you had completed only 5 sets using the same weight. Therefore, you need to allow more time to refuel after high intensity or long workouts.

Muscle damage

Certain activities that involve eccentric exercise (e.g. heavy weight training, plyometric training or hard running) can cause muscle fibre damage. Eccentric exercise is defined as the forced lengthening of active muscle. Muscle damage, in turn, delays glycogen storage and complete glycogen replenishment could take as long as 7–10 days.

Carbohydrate intake

The higher your carbohydrate intake, the faster you can refuel your glycogen stores. Figure 3.3(a) shows how glycogen storage increases with carbohydrate intake.

This is particularly important if you train on a daily basis. For example, cyclists who consumed a low-carbohydrate diet (250–350 g/day) failed to replenish fully their muscle glycogen stores

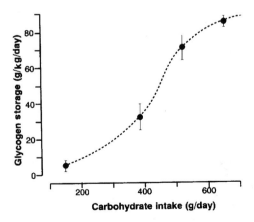

Figure 3.3(a) Glycogen depends on carbohydrate intake

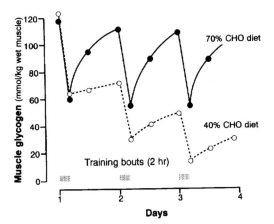

Figure 3.3(b) A low carbohydrate intake results in poor refuelling

(Costill *et al.*, 1971). Over successive days of training, their glycogen stores became progressively lower. However, in a further study, cyclists who consumed a high-carbohydrate diet (550–600 g/day) fully replaced their glycogen stores in the 22 hours between training sessions (Costill, 1985) (*see* Fig. 3.3(b)).

Therefore, if you wish to train daily or every other day, make sure that you consume enough carbohydrate. If not, you will be unable to train as hard or as long, you will suffer fatigue sooner and achieve smaller training gains.

Training experience

Efficiency in refuelling improves automatically with training experience and raised fitness levels. Thus, it takes a beginner longer to replace his glycogen stores than an experienced athlete eating the same amount of carbohydrate. That's why elite sportspeople are able to train almost every day while beginners cannot and should not!

Another adaptation to training is an increase in your glycogen storing capacity, perhaps by as much as 20%. This is an obvious advantage for training and competition. It is like upgrading from a 1-litre saloon car to a 3-litre sports car.

HOW SOON SHOULD I EAT AFTER EXERCISE?

The best time to start refuelling is as soon as possible after exercise, as glycogen storage is faster during this post-exercise 'window' than at any other time. Research has shown that glycogen storage following exercise takes place in three distinct stages. During the first 2 hours, replenishment is most rapid – at approximately 150% (or one-and-a-half times) the normal rate (Ivy *et al.*, 1988). During the subsequent 4 hours the rate slows but remains higher than normal; after this period glycogen manufacture returns to the normal rate. Therefore, eating carbohydrate during this time speeds glycogen recovery. This is most important for those athletes who train twice a day.

There are two reasons why glycogen replenishment is faster during the post-exercise period. Firstly, eating carbohydrate stimulates insulin release, which, in turn, increases the amount of glucose taken up by your muscle cells from the bloodstream, and stimulates the action of the glycogen-manufacturing enzymes. Secondly, post-exercise, the muscle cell membranes are more permeable to glucose, so they can take up more glucose than normal.

HOW MUCH CARBOHYDRATE?

Most researchers recommend consuming 1 g/kg body weight during the 2-hour post-exercise period (IAAF, 2007; Ivy *et al.*, 1988). So, for example, if you weigh 70 kg you need to consume 70 g carbohydrate within 2 hours of exercise. Even if you finish training late in the evening,

> ## Post-exercise snack box
> Each of the following provides 60–90g carbo-
> hydrate and 15–25g protein
> - 500 ml flavoured milk; one cereal bar, one banana
> - Two bananas; 500 ml of semi-skimmed milk
> - A wholemeal tuna sandwich (two slices of bread, 50 g tuna); one pot (150 g) yogurt
> - Recovery milkshake – mix 300 ml low fat milk; one pot (150 g) fruit yogurt, one banana; 100 g strawberries and two heaped teaspoons (30 g) honey in a blender
> - A wholemeal cheese sandwich (two slices bread; 40 g cheese); 100 g dried apricots
> - 200 g baked beans on two slices wholemeal toast
> - Two cereal bars plus 500 ml skimmed milk
> - 60 g raisins and 50 g nuts
> - Two weetabix; 300 ml low-fat milk; one pot (150 g) fruit yogurt; 30 g sultanas
> - A jacket potato (200 g) with 200 g baked beans and 40 g cheese
> - Cooked pasta (85 g uncooked weight) with 130 g chicken breast
> - Three oatcakes; 60 g hummus; 500 g low-fat milk

you still need to start the refuelling process, so do not go to bed on an empty stomach! For efficient glycogen refuelling, you should continue to eat at least 50 g carbohydrate every 2 hours until your next main meal. Therefore, plan your meals and snacks at regular intervals. If you leave long gaps without eating, glycogen storage and recovery will be slower.

ARE HIGH GI OR LOW GI CARBOHYDRATES BEST FOR RECOVERY?

Since high GI foods cause a rapid increase in blood glucose levels, it seems logical that foods with a high GI would increase glycogen replenishment during the initial post-exercise period. Indeed, a number of studies have shown that you get faster glycogen replenishment during the first 6 hours after exercise (and, in particular, the first 2 hours) with moderate and high GI carbohydrates compared with low GI (Burke *et al.*, 2004; Burke *et al.*, 1993). When the recovery period between training sessions is less than 8 hours, you should

eat as soon as practical after the first workout to maximise recovery. It may be more effective to consume several smaller high-carbohydrate snacks than larger meals during the early recovery phase, according to researchers at the Australian Institute of Sport (Burke *et al.*, 2004). It makes no difference to the glycogen storage rate whether you consume liquid or solid forms of carbohydrate (Keizer *et al.*, 1986).

However, Danish researchers discovered that, after 24 hours, muscle glycogen storage is about the same on a high GI as on a low GI diet (Kiens *et al.*, 1990). In other words, high GI foods post-exercise get your glycogen recovery off to a quick start, but low GI foods will result in the same level of recovery 24 hours after exercise.

But there are other performance benefits of a low GI recovery diet – it may improve your endurance the next day. Researchers at Loughborough University found that when athletes consumed low GI meals during the 24-hour period following exercise, they were able to exercise longer before exhaustion compared with those who had consumed high GI meals (Stevenson *et al.*, 2005). Further tests showed that they used a greater amount of fat to fuel their muscles during exercise. In other words, a low GI diet encourages greater fat burning, which not only benefits your performance but may also help you achieve faster weight (body fat) loss.

The bottom line is that if you are training intensely every day or twice a day, make sure you consume high GI foods during the first 2 hours after exercise. However, if you train once a day (or less frequently), low GI meals increase your endurance and performance during your subsequent workout.

DOES PROTEIN COMBINED WITH CARBOHYDRATE IMPROVE RECOVERY?

Combining protein with carbohydrate has been shown to be more effective in promoting glycogen recovery than carbohydrate alone. This is because protein-carbohydrate mixtures stimulate a greater output of insulin, which, in turn, speeds the uptake of glucose and amino acids from the bloodstream into the muscle cells – thereby promoting glycogen and protein synthesis – and blunts the rise in cortisol that would otherwise follow exercise. Cortisol suppresses the rate of protein synthesis and stimulates protein catabolism.

Consuming protein stimulates muscle synthesis, inhibits protein breakdown and promotes positive protein balance in the muscle after both resistance and endurance exercise (Howarth *et al.*, 2009).

One of the first studies to demonstrate the advantages of consuming a carbohydrate-protein drink after exercise was carried out at the University of Texas at Austin in 1992 (Zawadski *et al.*,

1992). Researchers found that a carbohydrate-protein drink (112 g carbohydrate, 40 g protein) increased glycogen storage by 38% compared with a carbohydrate-only drink. Other studies subsequently have noted similar results (Ready *et al.*, 1999; Tarnopolsky *et al.*, 1997; Beelan *et al.*, 2008; Bellan *et al.*, 2010).

Researchers at the University of Texas at Austin measured significantly greater muscle glycogen levels 4 hours after 2.5 hours intense cycling when cyclists consumed a protein-carbohydrate drink (80 g carbohydrate, 28 g protein, 6 g fat) compared with a carbohydrate-only drink (80 g carbohydrate, 6 g fat) (Ivy *et al.*, 2002).

A joint study by researchers at the University of Bath and Loughborough University found that subsequent exercise performance after a carbohydrate-protein recovery drink was greater compared with consumption of a carbohydrate-only drink (Betts *et al.*, 2007). The runners in the study were able to run longer following a four-hour recovery period during which they consumed a drink containing 0.8 g carbohydrate and 0.3 g protein/ kg body weight/ hour.

Consuming a protein-carbohydrate drink also appears to enhance recovery and muscle protein synthesis following resistance exercise compared with carbohydrate alone. Researchers at the University of Texas Medical Branch measured higher levels of protein retention in athletes after consuming a recovery drink containing a mixture of carbohydrate, protein and amino acids, compared with a carbohydrate-only drink that provided the same number of calories (Borsheim *et al.*, 2004). According to researchers at Ithaca College, New York, consuming a protein-carbohydrate drink immediately after resistance exercise promotes more efficient muscle tissue growth as well as faster glycogen refuelling, compared with a carbohydrate-only drink or a placebo (Bloomer *et al.*, 2000). In this study, the researchers measured higher levels of anabolic hormones such as testosterone and lower levels of catabolic hormones such as cortisol for 24 hours after a weights workout when the volunteers consumed a protein-carbohydrate drink. Canadian researchers measured an increased protein uptake in the muscles after volunteers drank a protein-carbohydrate drink following resistance exercise (Gibala, 2000). A review of studies from Maastrict University in the Netherlands, concluded that consuming a protein-carbohydrate drink following resistance exercise helps increase glycogen storage, stimulate protein synthesis and inhibit protein breakdown (Van Loon, 2007).

Researchers at James Madison University have shown that a carbohydrate-protein drink also reduces post-exercise muscle damage and muscle soreness (Luden *et al.*, 2007). Cyclists who consumed a recovery drink containing a mixture of protein, carbohydrate and antioxidants immediately after exercise had lower levels of creatine kinase in their urine (an enzyme that indicates muscle breakdown) compared with those who consumed a carbohydrate-only drink. This speeds recovery and, the authors suggest, could lead to performance improvements.

HOW MUCH AND WHAT TYPE OF PROTEIN SHOULD BE CONSUMED AFTER EXERCISE?

The optimal post-workout meal or drink, it seems, should include 15–25 g protein in order to maximise muscle repair and promote a more anabolic hormonal environment (Moore *et al.*, 2009; IOC, 2010; ACSM/ASA/DC, 2009). It should also include carbohydrate in a ratio of about 1:4. Ideally, you should consume this amount of protein at each meal or snack, so your protein intake is distributed evenly throughout the day.

In terms of types of protein, milk-based proteins (whey and casein) have been shown to promote greater protein uptake in the muscle as well as greater muscle building compared with soy protein (Wilkinson *et al.*, 2007; Tipton *et al.*, 2004; Tipton *et al*, 2007). A study at McMaster University found that those who consumed milk after resistance training gained more muscle mass than those who consumed soy drinks (Phillips *et al.*, 2005).

MILK AS A RECOVERY DRINK?

Milk is a near-perfect recovery drink, in terms both of glycogen and muscle replenishment and of rehydration. Researchers at the University of Connecticut were among the first to demonstrate that skimmed milk produces a more favourable hormonal environment immediately following exercise compared with a carbohydrate sports drink (Miller *et al.*, 2002). This, they suggest, may spare body protein and encourage protein anabolism during recovery. Since then, milk as a recovery drink has been extensively investigated. University of Texas researchers found that drinking milk (any type: whole, semi-skimmed and skimmed) after resistance training resulted in muscle synthesis (Elliot, 2006). Several studies have shown that milk promotes muscle manufacture and muscle gains more effectively than soy drinks (Wilkinson, 2007; Phillips, 2005).

Milk appears to have a favourable effect on body composition. Canadian researchers found that when novice male weight trainers consumed skimmed milk as part of a 12-week resistance training programme, it promoted greater hypertrophy than isoenergetic soy or carbohydrate drinks (Hartman *et al*, 2007). A similar study with women found that drinking skimmed milk after resistance exercise for 12 weeks reduced body fat levels, increased lean mass and strength (Josse *et al.*, 2010). It is thought that milk somehow changes the metabolism of proteins in muscle and thus enhances muscle adaptation to exercise.

What's more, milk has been proven to be an effective rehydration drink. In 2007, researchers at Loughborough University showed that skimmed milk resulted in better post-exercise rehydration than either sports drinks or water (Shireffs *et al.*, 2007). Studies have also shown that consuming milk after training can help alleviate symptoms of exercise-induced muscle damage, including delayed-onset muscle soreness and reductions in muscle performance. The original benefits were demonstrated based on drinking quite a large volume of milk (1 l) but recently, a smaller volume (500 ml) of milk was to found to have similar effects on muscle performance, blood measures and muscle soreness in comparison to the larger volume of milk (Cockburn *et al.*, 2012). In this study, twenty-four men consumed either 500 ml semi-skimmed milk, 1 l semi-skimmed milk or 1 l water after performing leg exercises. Those drinking either 500 ml or 1 l milk experienced less muscle damage than those drinking water with no difference between the two milk-drinking groups.

Many studies have highlighted the benefits of chocolate milk as a recovery drink, particularly after endurance exercise. Flavoured milk and plain milk have the advantage of additional nutrients not found in sports drinks; and are therefore good options for a recovery drink.

A 2008 study by researchers at Northumbria University found that athletes who drank 500 ml of semi-skimmed milk or chocolate milk immediately after training had less muscle soreness and more rapid muscle recovery compared with commercial sports drinks or water (Cockburn *et al.*, 2008).

A 2009 study from James Madison University, US, found that chocolate milk promoted better muscle recovery compared with a commercial sports drink (Gilson *et al.*, 2009). Football players who drank chocolate milk after training had less muscle damage and faster muscle recovery compared with those who consumed a sports drink with the same amount of calories.

University of Texas researchers found that chocolate milk not only promotes muscle glycogen recovery but also results in greater aerobic capacity, lean body mass and reduced body fat compared with carbohydrate (sports) drinks (Ferguson-Stegall *et al.*, 2011). The exact mechanism is not clear, but it is thought that the peptides released during the digestion of milk protein are responsible for alterations in protein metabolism and increasing training adaptations.

For longer, harder training sessions, extra carbohydrate may be needed to refuel energy stores. Researchers at the University of Texas at Austin found that consuming a bowl of wholegrain cereal plus milk was as effective at refuelling glycogen stores as sports drinks after two hours of moderate exercise (Kammer *et al.*, 2009). It also promoted greater muscle protein synthesis compared with the sports drink.

WHICH FOODS ARE BEST BETWEEN WORKOUTS?

After you have taken advantage of the 6-hour post-exercise window, when and which carbohydrates you eat for the rest of the day are still important for glycogen recovery. To optimise glycogen replenishment, you should ensure a relatively steady supply of carbohydrates into the bloodstream. In practice, this means eating carbohydrates in small meals throughout the day. Researchers at the Human Performance Laboratory of Ball State University have shown that slowly digested carbohydrate – that is, meals with a low GI – cause much smaller rises and falls in blood sugar and insulin and create the ideal environment for the replenishment of steady glycogen stores (Costill, 1988). Avoid consuming large, infrequent meals or lots of high GI meals, as they will produce large fluctuations in blood sugar and insulin. This means there will be periods of time when blood sugar levels are low, so glycogen storage will be minimal. Surges of blood sugar and insulin are more likely to result in fat gain.

ARE THERE ANY OTHER BENEFITS OF A LOW GI DAILY DIET?

While a low GI diet is important for regular exercisers for promoting glycogen recovery, it also has numerous health benefits and is widely promoted to the general population for weight loss. Reducing the GI of the diet increases satiety (feelings of satisfaction after eating), improves appetite control and makes it easier to achieve a healthy body weight (Brand-Miller *et al.*, 2005; Warren *et al.*, 2003). Studies have shown that the lower the GI of a meal, the more satisfied and less hungry you are likely to be during the following 3 hours (Holt, 1992). A low GI diet has also been shown to increase the resting metabolic rate, which increases daily energy expenditure and increases the rate of weight loss (Pereira *et al.* 2004). What's more, low GI diets can help reduce the risk of cardiovascular disease by lowering total and LDL ('bad')

cholesterol levels (Sloth *et al.*, 2004). This is due to the lower insulin levels associated with low GI eating – high insulin levels stimulate cholesterol manufacture in the liver (Rizkalla *et al.*, 2004). Total cholesterol may drop by as much as 15% on a low GI diet (Jenkins *et al.*, 1987).

A low GI diet is also promoted for the management of type 2 diabetes. Studies have found that it can improve blood glucose control as well as lower levels of total and LDL ('bad') cholesterol, typically associated with type 2 diabetes (Rizkalla, 2004; Brand-Miller *et al*, 2003). There is mounting evidence, too, that a low GI diet can help prevent and manage the metabolic syndrome – the concurrent existence of raised blood glucose, high blood pressure, obesity and insulin resistance – and also polycystic ovary syndrome.

CARBOHYDRATE LOADING

Carbohydrate loading is a technique originally devised in the 1960s to increase the muscles' glycogen stores above normal levels. With more glycogen available, you may be able to exercise longer before fatigue sets in. This is potentially advantageous in endurance events lasting longer than 90 minutes (e.g. long distance running or cycling) or for events that involve several heats or matches over a short period (e.g. tennis tournaments or swimming galas). It is unlikely to benefit you if your event lasts less than 90 minutes because muscle glycogen depletion would not be a limiting factor to your performance. Carbohydrate loading increases time to exhaustion by about 20% and improves performance by about 2–3% (Hawley *et al.*, 1997). The classical 6-day regimen involved 2 bouts of glycogen-depleting exercise separated by 3 days of low-carbohydrate intake and followed by

Table 3.6	Carbohydrate loading (classical regimen)							
Normal training	Exhaustive prolonged exercise	Taper training	Taper training	Taper training	Taper training	Taper training		
Day 1	**Day 2**	**Day 3**	**Day 4**	**Day 5**	**Day 6**	**Day 7**		**Competition**
Normal diet	Low-carbohydrate diet	Low-carbohydrate diet	Low-carbohydrate diet	High-carbohydrate diet	High-carbohydrate diet	High-carbohydrate diet		

Table 3.7	Carbohydrate loading (modified regimen)							
Endurance training	Taper training	Taper training	Taper training	Taper training	Taper training	Taper training		
Day 1	**Day 2**	**Day 3**	**Day 4**	**Day 5**	**Day 6**	**Day 7**		**Competition**
Normal diet	Moderate-carbohydrate diet	Moderate-carbohydrate diet	Moderate-carbohydrate diet	High-carbohydrate diet	High-carbohydrate diet	High-carbohydrate diet		

3 days of high-carbohydrate intake and minimal exercise (Ahlborg *et al.*, 1967; Karlsson & Saltin, 1971) (Table 3.6). The theory behind this 2-phase regimen is that glycogen depletion stimulates the activity of glycogen synthetase, the key enzyme involved in glycogen storage, resulting in above-normal levels of muscle glycogen.

But this regimen had a number of drawbacks. Not only did it interfere with exercise tapering, but the low-carbohydrate diet left athletes weak, irritable and tired. Worse, many failed to achieve high glycogen levels even after 3 days of high carbohydrate intake.

Researchers at Ohio State University, Ohio, US developed a 6-day carbohydrate loading regimen that resulted in similar increases in glycogen levels but without the disadvantages described above (Sherman *et al.*, 1981). This required tapering training on 6 consecutive days while following a normal diet during the first 3 days followed by a carbohydrate-rich diet during the next 3 days (Table 3.7).

More recently, researchers at the University of Western Australia, have found that equally high levels of glycogen can be achieved by taking in 10 g of carbohydrate per kilogram of bodyweight over the course of a single day following a 3 minute bout of high-intensity exercise (Fairchild *et al.*, 2002; Bussau, *et al.*, 2002). It appears that the rate of glycogen storage is greatly increased following such a workout. The advantage of this new regimen is that only one instead of 6 days is needed to achieve high glycogen levels, and very little change to your usual training programme needs to be made.

Table 3.8 shows a recommended programme for carbohydrate loading. On Day 1, carry out endurance training for about 1 hour to reduce the amount of glycogen in your liver and muscles. For the following 3 days, taper your training and eat a moderate-carbohydrate diet (5–7 g carbohydrate /kg body weight). For the final 3 days, continue your exercise taper, or rest, and increase your carbohydrate intake to 8–10 g/ kg body weight.

Table 3.8	Carbohydrate loading (1 day regimen)						
Taper training	Taper training	Taper training	Taper training	Taper training	Taper training	Warm-up & 3 min high intensity exercise (sustained sprint)	
Day 1	**Day 2**	**Day 3**	**Day 4**	**Day 5**	**Day 6**	**Day 7**	**Competition**
Normal diet	Low-carbohydrate diet	Low-carbohydrate diet	Low-carbohydrate diet	High-carbohydrate diet	High-carbohydrate diet	High-carbohydrate diet 10 g carbohydrate/ kg bodyweight	

Since glycogen storage is associated with approximately 3 g water for each 1 g of glycogen, carbohydrate loading can produce a weight increase of 1–2 kg. This may or may not affect your performance.

If you decide to try carbohydrate loading, rehearse it during training to find out what works best for you. Never try anything new before an important competition. You may need to try the technique more than once, adjusting the types and amounts of foods you eat.

PUTTING IT TOGETHER: WHAT, WHEN AND HOW MUCH

Table 3.9 summarises the recommendations on carbohydrate intake covered in this chapter. The simplest way to plan your daily food intake is to divide the day into four 'windows': before, during, and after exercise, and between training sessions. You can then work out how much and what type of carbohydrate to consume during each 'window' to optimise your performance and recovery.

SUMMARY OF KEY POINTS

- A carbohydrate intake of 5–7 g/kg body weight/ day is recommended for most regular exercisers,

and 7–10 g/kg body weight/day is recommended during periods of intense training.

- The glycaemic index (GI) is a more useful way of categorising carbohydrates for athletes than the traditional 'complex' versus 'simple' classification.

- The GI is a ranking of carbohydrates based on their immediate effect on blood glucose (blood sugar) levels. Carbohydrates with a high GI produce a rapid rise in blood sugar; those with a low GI produce a slow rise in blood sugar.

- The glycaemic load (GL) takes into account the GI as well as the amount of carbohydrate (serving size) consumed and thus provides a measure of the total glycaemic response to a food or meal. GL = GI (%) × grams of carbohydrate per serving.

- Low GI foods consumed 2–4 hours before exercise may help improve endurance and delay fatigue. High GI foods consumed pre-exercise benefit some athletes but may produce temporary hypoglycaemia at the start of exercise in those athletes sensitive to blood sugar fluctuations.

- The pre-exercise meal should contain approx. 2.5 g carbohydrate/kg body weight.

- For moderate–high intensity exercise lasting more than 60 minutes, consuming 30–60 g

Table 3.9	Summary – what, when, and how much carbohydrate?			
	Before exercise	**During exercise lasting > 60 min**	**After exercise**	**Between workouts**
How much	2.5 g/kg of body weight	30–60 g/hour	1 g/kg body weight	5–10 g/kg body weight, or 60% of energy
Time period	2–4 hours before exercise	Begin after 30 min; regular intervals	Up to 2 hours; then every 2 hours	4–6 meals/snacks
GI	Low	High	High or low	Low
Examples	• Jacket potato with beans, chicken or cheese • Pasta with tomato based sauce and salad • Porridge • Rice with chicken and vegetables	• 500–1000 ml isotonic drink or diluted fruit juice (6 g/100 ml) • Energy bar with water • 1–2 handfuls of raisins (40–80 g) • 1–2 bananas	• Meal replacement shake • Fresh fruit with milk or yoghurt • Sports bar • Tuna or cottage cheese sandwich	• Pasta or rice with beans/chicken/fish • Noodles with tofu/poultry/seafood • Beans on toast • Jacket potato with cottage cheese/tuna

moderate or high GI carbohydrate (in solid or liquid form) during exercise can help maintain exercise intensity for longer and delay fatigue.

- Glycogen recovery takes, on average, 20 hours but depends on the severity of glycogen depletion, extent of muscle damage and the amount, type and timing of carbohydrate intake.
- Glycogen replenishment is faster than normal during the 2-hour post-exercise period. To kick-start recovery, it is recommended to consume 1 g moderate–high GI carbohydrate/kg body weight during this period.
- High or moderate GI carbohydrates produce faster glycogen replenishment for the first 6 hours post-exercise, which is most important for athletes who train twice a day.

- A low GI recovery diet may improve endurance the next day, and increase fat utilisation during subsequent exercise.
- Combining carbohydrate with protein has been shown to be more effective in promoting muscle glycogen recovery and muscle tissue growth compared with carbohydrate alone.
- A low GI daily diet comprising 4–6 small meals and supplying 5–10 g/kg body weight (depending on training hours and intensity) will promote efficient muscle glycogen recovery as well as improve satiety and appetite control, reduce cardiovascular risk factors and improve the management of type 2 diabetes.
- A modified form of carbohydrate loading may improve endurance capacity by 20% and performance by 2–3%.

PROTEIN REQUIREMENTS FOR SPORT

4

The importance of protein – and the question of whether extra protein is necessary – for sports performance is one of the most hotly debated topics among sports scientists, coaches and athletes and has been contended ever since the time of the Ancient Greeks. Protein has long been associated with power and strength, and as the major constituent of muscle, it would seem logical that an increased protein intake would increase muscle size and strength.

Traditionally, scientists have held the view that athletes do not need to consume more than the RDA for protein and that consuming anything greater than this amount would produce no further benefit. However, research since the 1980s has cast doubt on this view. There is considerable evidence that the protein needs of active individuals are consistently higher than those of the general population.

This chapter will help to give you a fuller understanding of the role of protein during exercise, and enable you to work out how much you need. It will show how individual requirements depend on the sport concerned and the training programme, and also how they are related to carbohydrate intake. An example of a daily menu is given to show how to meet your own protein requirements, and to provide a basis for developing your own menu. As more athletes are giving up meat and choosing a vegetarian diet, this chapter explains how you can obtain sufficient protein and other nutrients for peak performance on a meat-free diet.

Protein supplementation is discussed in detail in Chapter 6.

WHY DO I NEED PROTEIN?

Protein makes up part of the structure of every cell and tissue in your body, including your muscle tissue, internal organs, tendons, skin, hair and nails. On average, it comprises about 20% of your total body weight. Protein is needed for the growth and formation of new tissue, for tissue repair and for regulating many metabolic pathways, and can also be used as a fuel for energy production. It is also needed to make almost all of the body enzymes as well as various hormones (such as adrenaline and insulin) and neurotransmitters. Protein has a role in maintaining optimal fluid balance in tissues, transporting nutrients in and out of cells, carrying oxygen and regulating blood clotting.

WHAT ARE AMINO ACIDS?

The 20 amino acids are the building blocks of proteins. They can be combined in various ways to form hundreds of different proteins in the body. When you eat protein, it is broken down in your digestive tract into smaller molecular units – single amino acids and dipeptides (two amino acids linked together).

Twelve of the amino acids can be made in the body from other amino acids, carbohydrate and nitrogen. These are called dispensable, or non-essential, amino acids (NEAAs). The other eight are termed indispensable, or essential, amino acids (EAAs) meaning they must be supplied in the diet. All 20 amino acids are listed in Table 4.1. Branched-chain amino acids (BCAAs) include the three EAAs with a branched molecular configuration: valine, leucine and isoleucine. They make up one-third of muscle protein and are a vital substrate for two other amino acids, glutamine and alanine, which are released in large

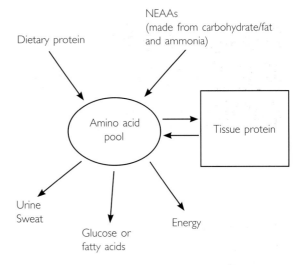

Figure 4.1 Protein metabolism

quantities during intense aerobic exercise. Also they can be used directly as fuel by the muscles, particularly when muscle glycogen is depleted. Strictly speaking, the body's requirement is for amino acids rather than protein.

Table 4.1	Essential and non-essential amino acids
Essential amino acids (EAAs)	**Non-essential amino acids (NEAAs)**
Isoleucine	Alanine
Leucine	Arginine
Lysine	Asparagine
Methionine	Aspartic acid
Phenylalanine	Cysteine
Threonine	Glutamic acid
Tryptophan	Glutamine
Valine	Glycine
	Histidine*
	Proline
	Serine
	Tyrosine

* Histidine is essential for babies (not for adults)

Protein metabolism

Tissue proteins are continually broken down (catabolised), releasing their constituent amino acids into the 'free pool', which is located in body tissues and the blood. For example, half of your total body protein is broken down and replaced every 150 days. Amino acids absorbed from food and non-essential amino acids made in the body from nitrogen and carbohydrate can also enter the free pool. Once in the pool, amino acids have four fates. They can be used to build new proteins, they can be oxidised to produce energy and they can be converted in glucose via gluconeogenesis or they can be converted into fatty acids. During energy production, the nitrogen part of the protein molecule is excreted in urine, or possibly in sweat.

These are then re-assembled into new proteins containing hundreds or even thousands of amino acids linked together.

PROTEIN AND EXERCISE
HOW DOES EXERCISE AFFECT MY PROTEIN REQUIREMENT?

Numerous studies involving both endurance and strength exercise have shown that the current recommended protein intake of 0.75 g/ kg BW/ day is inadequate for people who participate in regular exercise or sport (IOC, 2011; Phillips & Van Loon, 2011). Additional protein is needed to compensate for the increased breakdown of protein during and immediately after exercise, and to facilitate repair and growth. Exercise triggers the activation of an enzyme that oxidises key amino acids in the muscle, which are then used as a fuel source. The greater the exercise intensity and the longer the duration of exercise, the more protein is broken down for fuel.

Your exact protein needs depend on the type, intensity and duration of your training. How these needs differ for endurance athletes and strength and power athletes are discussed in detail below.

Endurance training

Prolonged and intense endurance training increases your protein requirements for two reasons. Firstly, you will need more protein to compensate for the increased breakdown of protein during training. When your muscle glycogen stores are low – which typically occurs after 60–90 minutes of endurance exercise – certain amino acids, namely, glutamate and the BCAAs valine, leucine and isoleucine (*see* page 80) can be used for energy. One of the BCAAs, leucine, is converted into another amino acid, alanine, which is converted in the liver into glucose. This glucose is released back into the bloodstream and transported to the exercising muscles, where it is used for energy. In fact, protein may contribute up to 15% of your energy production when glycogen stores are low. This is quite a substantial increase, as protein contributes less than 5% of energy needs when muscle glycogen stores are high. Secondly, additional protein is needed for the repair and recovery of muscle tissue after intense endurance training.

Strength and power training

Strength and power athletes have additional protein needs compared with endurance athletes. After resistance training, the rate of protein breakdown and synthesis (building) increases,

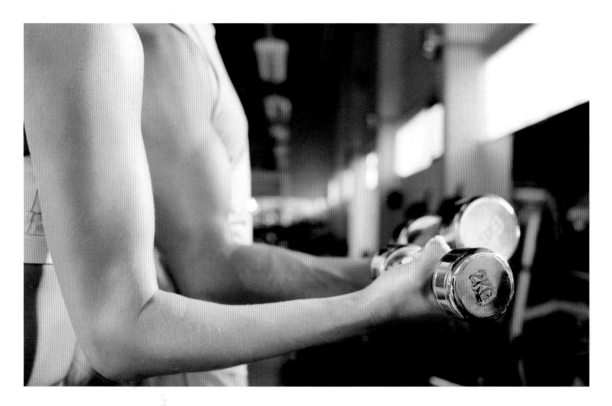

although for the first few hours the rate of break-down exceeds the rate of synthesis (Phillips *et al.*, 1997; Phillips *et al.*, 1999).

In addition, dietary protein provides an enhanced stimulus for muscle growth. To build muscle, you must be in 'positive nitrogen balance'. This means the body is retaining more dietary protein than is excreted or used as fuel. A sub-optimal intake of protein will result in slower gains in strength, size and mass, or even muscle loss, despite hard training. In practice the body is capable of adapting to slight variations in protein intake. It becomes more efficient in recycling amino acids during protein metabolism if your intake falls over a period of time. The body can also adapt to a consistently high protein intake by oxidising surplus amino acids for energy.

It is important to understand that a high-protein diet *al*one will not result in increased strength or muscle size. These goals can be achieved only when an optimal protein intake is combined with heavy resistance (strength) training.

DO BEGINNERS NEED MORE OR LESS PROTEIN THAN EXPERIENCED ATHLETES?

Contrary to popular belief, studies have shown that beginners have slightly higher requirements for protein per kg body weight compared with more experienced athletes (Phillips & Van Loon, 2011). When you begin a training programme your protein needs rise due to increases in protein turnover (Gontzea *et al.*, 1975). After about 3 weeks of training, the body adapts to the exercise and becomes more efficient at recycling protein. Broken down protein can be built up again from amino acids released into the amino acid pool. The body also becomes more efficient in conserving protein. One study has shown that the requirements per kg body weight of novice bodybuilders can be up to 40% higher than those of experienced bodybuilders (Tarnopolsky, 1988).

CAN I MINIMISE PROTEIN BREAKDOWN DURING EXERCISE?

Protein is broken down in increased quantities when muscle glycogen stores are low. Thus, during high-intensity exercise lasting longer than 1 hour, protein can make a substantial contribution to your energy needs (up to 15%). Clearly, it is advantageous to start your training session with high muscle-glycogen stores. This will reduce the contribution protein makes to your energy needs at any given point during training.

If you are on a weight/fat loss programme, make sure you do not reduce your carbohydrate too drastically, otherwise protein will be used as an energy source, making it unavailable for tissue growth. Aim to maintain 60% of your calorie intake from carbohydrate by reducing your calorie intake from carbohydrate in proportion to your calorie reduction (see Chapter 9 on weight loss).

HOW MUCH PROTEIN DO I NEED FOR MAXIMUM PERFORMANCE?

Table 4.2 summarises the daily protein requirements for different types of athletes.

At low–moderate exercise intensities (<50% VO_2max), it appears there is no significant increase in protein requirements (Hargreaves & Snow, 2001).

For higher intensities, the protein requirements are greater. Most experts recommend an intake in the range 1.2–1.8 g/ kg BW/ day. The 2010 International Olympic Committee (IOC) Consensus statement recommends between 1.3 and 1.8 g protein/ kg BW/ day for athletes (IOC, 2011; Phillips and Van Loon, 2011); the American College of Sports Medicine, American Dietetic Association and Dietitians of Canada (ACSM/ADA/DC) consensus statement, and the International Association of Athletic Federations (IAAF) both recommend 1.2–1.7 g protein/ kg BW/ day (ACSM/AD/DC, 2009; IAAF, 2007; Tipton & Wolfe, 2007). That's equivalent to 84–119 g daily for a 70 kg person.

Table 4.2 Protein requirements of athletes	
Type of athlete	**Daily protein requirements per kg body weight (g)**
Endurance athlete – moderate or heavy training	1.2–1.4
Strength and power athlete	1.4–1.8
Athlete on fat-loss programme	1.6–2.0
Athlete on weight-gain programme	1.8–2.0

Source: William & Devlin, 1992; Williams, 1998; Tarnopolsky *et al.*, 1992; Lemon *et al.*, 1992

Protein plus exercise equals greater weight loss for dieters

A study at the University of Illinois in the US suggests that a protein-rich diet boosts the weight loss benefits of exercise (Layman *et al.*, 2005). Women who ate a protein-rich diet lost significantly more body fat when they exercised regularly (5 x 30 minute walking sessions; 2 x 30 minute weight training sessions per week) compared with those who ate a high carbohydrate diet containing the same number of calories. What's more, almost 100% of the weight loss in the high protein dieters was fat, and much of that was from the abdominal region. In contrast, in the high-carbohydrate group, up to a third of the weight loss was muscle. Researchers suggest that the protein diet worked better because it contained a high level of leucine, which works with insulin to stimulate fat-burning while preserving muscle.

A sedentary person requires 0.75 g protein per kg body weight daily.

For an endurance athlete, most studies recommend an intake at the lower end of the range, around 1.2–1.4 g/ kg body weight/ day (ACSM/ ADA/DC, 2009; Phillips *et al.*, 2007; Tipton *et al*, 2007; Lemon, 1998; Williams & Devlin, 1992; Williams, 1998; ACSM, 2000).

It is generally agreed that strength and power athletes have a greater daily requirement for protein than most endurance athletes, with researchers recommending an intake at the higher end of the range: between 1.4 and 1.7 g/ kg body weight/ day (Phillips *et al*, 2007; Tipton *et al.*, 2007; Williams, 1998; Tarnopolsky *et al.*, 1992;

Lemon *et al.*, 1992). So, for example, a distance runner weighing 70 kg would need 84–98 g/day. A sprinter or bodybuilder with the same body weight would need 98–126 g/ day.

IS THE TIMING OF PROTEIN INTAKE IMPORTANT?

The timing of protein intake appears to be important too. A review of studies on protein needs by researchers at McMaster University, Canada, concluded that protein should be consumed early in the post-exercise recovery phase, ideally within the first hour after exercise, and combined with carbohydrate in a ratio of 1:4 (Phillips *et al.*, 2007). Consuming 15–25 g protein with carbohydrate enhances recovery and promotes muscle building (*see* p. 47, Chapter 3 'Does protein combined with carbohydrate improve recovery?'). Studies suggest that the muscles are most 'sensitive' or receptive to amino acid uptake in the 2-hour post-exercise period, but this may extend to 24 hours. This is the time when muscle synthesis takes place at the fastest rate, so it is important to consume protein throughout the day at regular intervals.

Aim to distribute your protein intake evenly between meals. This may mean re-thinking your breakfast options, as most people focus on carbohydrates (e.g. cereal, toast) at this meal. Try including extra milk, a milk-based drink, eggs or yoghurt.

Experts recommend consuming 15–25 g protein with each main meal as well as immediately after exercise (IOC, 2011; Phillips & Van Loon, 2011). Most studies have involved athletes weighing more than 80 kg, so it is likely that intakes at the higher end of this range, 20–25 g, are more appropriate for heavier athletes while lower intakes, say 15–20 g, would be more appropriate for lighter athletes (Phillips *et al.*, 2011).

Consuming some of your protein before sleep may give you additional benefits. A study at Maastrict University in the Netherlands found that protein synthesis was 22% higher in volunteers who consumed 40 g of protein (in the form of a casein drink) before sleep (Res *et al*, 2012).

WHAT TYPE OF PROTEIN IS BEST AFTER EXERCISE?

Most studies suggest that 'high quality' milk proteins (and in particular whey) are the best type of protein to consume after exercise (Phillips *et al*, 2011). Whey is a 'fast' protein, which means it is digested and absorbed faster than 'slow' proteins such as casein and soy (Boirie *et al.*, 1997; Dangin *et al.*, 2001). It results in greater muscle synthesis, which is thought to be due to its higher content of leucine. This amino acid is an important trigger for protein synthesis (Burd *et al.*, 2009; Tang *et al.*, 2009). Although the exact mechanism isn't clear, whey seems to be the most effective protein in stimulating muscle growth because it produces the most rapid rise in blood leucine levels (Phillips *et al*, 2011).

ARE PROTEIN SUPPLEMENTS BETTER THAN FOOD SOURCES?

While many studies have used protein or amino acid supplements, experts maintain that protein requirements can be met from diet alone without the use of protein or amino acid supplements (ACSM/ ADA/ DC, 2009).

Indeed, food sources of protein, such as milk, have been found to be just as effective as supplements (Wilkinson, 2007; Phillips, 2005). A US study found that consuming 237 ml of either whole milk or skimmed milk within an hour following resistance training resulted in greater protein synthesis (Elliot *et al.*, 2006). A Canadian study found that adding protein to a sports drink did not make any difference to the performance of cyclists in a 80 km time trial (Van Essen & Gibala, 2006). Milk also appears to be a good post-training option for those wishing to increase mass. Those who consumed skimmed milk immediately after and then 1 hour after resistance training for 12 weeks experienced greater muscle gains than those consuming isoenergetic soy or carbohydrate drinks (Hartman *et al.*, 2007). Similarly, a study with women found that drinking skimmed milk after resistance exercise for 12 weeks reduced body fat levels, increased lean mass and strength (Josse *et al.*, 2010). It is thought that milk somehow changes the metabolism of proteins in muscle and thus enhances muscle adaptation to exercise.

HOW CAN I MEET MY PROTEIN NEEDS?

In practice, protein intakes generally reflect total calorie intake, so provided you are meeting your calorie needs from a wide variety of foods, you are likely to be getting enough protein. Dietary surveys show that most athletes already consume diets providing protein intakes above the maximum recommended level without the use of protein supplements. So the debate over the precise protein needs of athletes is largely unnecessary (IAAF, 2007).

But if you severely reduce your calorie intake or cut out entire food groups (for example, if you eat a vegan diet or you have a dairy allergy), you may find it more difficult to meet your protein needs. An adequate calorie intake is important for promoting protein balance or increasing protein retention in the body. Table 4.3 lists a wide range

Table 4.3   Good sources of protein

Food	Portion size	Protein (g)	Kcal
Meat and Fish			
Beef, fillet steak, grilled, lean	2 slices 105 g	31	197
Chicken breast, grilled meat only	1 breast 130 g	39	191
Turkey, light meat, roasted	2 slices 140 g	47	214
Cod, poached	1 fillet 120 g	25	113
Mackerel, grilled	1 fillet 150 g	31	359
Tuna, canned in brine	1 small tin (100 g)	24	99
Dairy products and eggs			
Cheese, cheddar	1 thick slice (40 g)	10	165
Cottage cheese	1 small carton (112 g)	15	110
Skimmed milk	1 glass (200 ml)	7	66
Low-fat yoghurt, plain	1 carton (150 g)	8	84
Low-fat yoghurt, fruit	1 carton (150 g)	6	135
Fromage frais, fruit	1 small carton (100 g)	7	131
Eggs	1, size 2	8	90
Nuts and seeds			
Peanuts, roasted and salted	1 handful (50 g)	12	301
Peanut butter	on 1 slice bread (20 g)	5	125
Cashew nuts, roasted and salted	1 handful (50 g)	10	306
Walnuts	1 handful (50 g)	7	344
Sunflower seeds	2 tbsp (32 g)	6	186
Sesame seeds	2 tbsp (24 g)	4	144
Pulses			
Baked beans	1 small tin (205 g)	10	166
Red lentils, boiled	3 tbsp (120 g)	9	120
Red kidney beans, boiled	3 tbsp (120 g)	10	124
Chickpeas, boiled	3 tbsp (140 g)	12	169
Soya products			
Soya milk, plain	1 glass (200 ml)	6	64
Soya mince	2 tbsp dry weight (30 g)	13	79
Tofu	Half a pack (100 g)	8	73
Tofu burger	1 burger 60 g	5	71
Quorn products			
Quorn mince	4 tbsp (100 g)	12	86
Quorn chilli	1 bowl (200 g)	9	163
Quorn korma	1 bowl (200 g)	8	280

Table 4.3	Good sources of protein (continued)		
Food	**Portion size**	**Protein (g)**	**Kcal**
Grains and cereals			
Wholemeal bread	2 slices (76 g)	6	164
White bread	2 slices (72 g)	6	156
Pasta, boiled	1 bowl (230 g)	7	198
Brown rice, boiled	1 bowl (180 g)	5	254
White rice, boiled	1 bowl (180 g)	5	248

of foods containing protein. Animal sources generally provide higher levels of essential amino acids, but some foods (such as meat and cheese) are high in saturated fat. Keep these to a minimum and choose lean and low-fat versions. Use the table to estimate your current intake of protein and use the eating plans detailed in Chapter 15 as a basis for developing your personal nutrition programme.

You can estimate your protein requirements from your body weight using the guidelines in Table 4.2.

EXAMPLES:

(a) For an endurance athlete weighing 70 kg

$70 \times 1.2 = 84$ g

$70 \times 1.4 = 98$ g

i.e. between 84–98 g/day

(b) For a strength or power athlete weighing 70 kg

$70 \times 1.4 = 98$ g

$70 \times 1.8 = 126$ g

i.e. between 98–126 g/day

IS MORE PROTEIN BETTER?

Although some strength athletes and bodybuilders consume as much as 2–3 g/ kg BW/ day, there is no evidence that these high daily intakes result in further muscle mass and strength gains (Tipton & Wolfe, 2007; IOC, 2003). In a study carried out at McMaster University, Ontario, strength athletes were given either a low-protein diet (0.86 g/ kg body weight/ day – similar to the RDA), a medium-protein diet (1.4 g/ kg body weight/ day) or a high-protein diet (2.3 g/ kg body weight/ day) for 13 days (Tarnopolsky et al., 1992). The low-protein diet, which was close to the RDA for sedentary people, caused the athletes to lose muscle mass. Both the medium- and high-protein diets resulted in an increased muscle mass, but the amount of the increase was the same for the two groups. In other words, no further benefits were gained by increasing the protein intake from 1.4 g to 2.4 g/kg body weight/ day.

Similar findings were reported at Kent State University, Ohio. Researchers gave 12 young volunteers either a protein supplement (total daily protein was 2.62 g/ kg body weight) or a carbohydrate supplement (total daily protein was 1.35 g/ kg body weight) for 1 month, during which time they performed intense weight training 6 days a week (Lemon et al., 1992). Nitrogen balance measurements were carried out after each diet and the researchers found that an intake of 1.4–1.5 g/ kg body weight/ day was needed to maintain nitrogen balance, although strength, muscle mass and size were the same with either

What is bioavailability?

Bioavailability refers to the 'usefulness' of the protein food or supplement. Foods that contain all eight EAAs are traditionally called 'complete' proteins. These include dairy products, eggs, meat, fish, poultry and soya. Various plant foods, such as cereals and pulses, contain high amounts of several EAAs, but only very small amounts (or none) of the others. The EAA that is missing or in short supply is called the limiting amino acid.

The ratio of EAAs to NEAAs and the amounts of specific amino acids is what determines the bioavailability of the protein food or supplement. For example, the content of glutamine and the BCAAs (leucine, isoleucine and valine) determine the extent the protein is absorbed and utilised for tissue growth.

The bioavailability of a particular protein is often measured by its biological value (BV), which indicates how closely matched the proportion of amino acids are in relation to the body's requirements. It is a measure of the percentage of protein that is retained by the body for use in growth and tissue maintenance. In other words, how much of what is consumed is actually used for its intended purpose.

An egg has a BV of 100, which means, out of all foods, it contains the most closely matched ratio of EAAs and NEAAs to the body's needs. Therefore a high percentage of the egg protein can be used for making new body proteins. Dairy products, meat, fish, poultry, quorn and soya have a relatively high BV (70–100); nuts, seeds, pulses and grains have a relatively low BV (less than 70).

level of protein intake. The researchers concluded two main points. First, strength training approximately doubles your protein needs (compared with sedentary people). Secondly, increasing your protein intake does not enhance your strength, mass or size in a linear fashion. Once your optimal intake has been reached, additional protein is not converted into muscle.

IS TOO MUCH PROTEIN HARMFUL?

Consuming more protein than you need certainly offers no advantage in terms of health or physical performance. Once your requirements have been met, additional protein will not be converted into muscle, nor will it further increase muscle size, strength or stamina.

The nitrogen-containing amino group of the protein is converted into a substance called urea in the liver. This is then passed to the kidneys and excreted in the urine. The remainder of the protein is converted into glucose and used as an energy substrate. It may either be used as fuel immediately or stored, usually as glycogen. If you are already eating enough carbohydrate to refill your glycogen stores, excess glucose may be converted into fat. However, in practice this does not occur to a great extent. Fat gain is usually the result of excessive calorie consumption, in particular of fats. Recent studies have shown that eating protein increases the metabolic rate, so a significant proportion of the protein calories are oxidised and given off as heat (*see* Chapter 9). Thus, a slight excess of protein is unlikely to be converted into fat.

It was once thought that excess protein may cause liver or kidney damage and place excessive stress on these organs. But this has never been demonstrated in healthy people, so it remains only a theoretical possibility (Tipton & Wolfe, 2007). Those with liver or kidney problems, however, are advised to consume a low-protein diet.

It has also been claimed that eating too much protein leads to dehydration because extra water is drawn from the body's fluids to dilute and excrete the increased quantities of urea. The only evidence for this comes from a study reported at the 2002 Experimental Biology meeting in New Orleans, which found that a high protein diet (246 g daily) consumed for 4 weeks caused dehydration in trained athletes. Their blood urea nitrogen – a clinical test for proper kidney function – reached abnormal levels and they produced more concentrated urine. According to the researchers at the University of Connecticut, this could have been avoided by increasing their fluid intake. This is unlikely to be a problem if you drink enough fluids.

Fears that high-protein diets cause an excessive excretion of calcium, increasing the risk of osteoporosis, are largely unfounded too. A study at the University of Maastrict, Belgium, found that a 21% protein diet produced no negative effect on calcium status compared with a 12% protein diet (Pannemans *et al.*, 1997).

In conclusion, while eating too much protein is unlikely to be harmful in the short term, it certainly offers no advantages.

SHOULD I CONSUME MORE PROTEIN IF I AM ON A FAT-LOSS PROGRAMME?

When cutting calories to lose body fat, you risk losing muscle mass as well. A higher protein intake can offset some of the muscle-wasting effects associated with any weight-reducing programme. Researchers recommend increasing your protein intake to 1.8–2.0 g/ kg BW/ day in order to prevent lean mass losses (Phillips &

Van Loon, 2011). For example, a 70 kg athlete would need to consume 126–140 g protein/ day.

SUMMARY OF KEY POINTS

- Protein is needed for the maintenance, replacement and growth of body tissue. It is used to make the enzymes and hormones that regulate the metabolism, maintain fluid balance, and transport nutrients in and out of cells.
- Athletes require more than the current RDA for protein of 0.75 g/ kg body weight/ day for the general population.
- Additional protein is needed to compensate for the increased breakdown of protein during intense training and for the repair and recovery of muscle tissue after training.
- Strength and power athletes have additional needs to facilitate muscle growth.
- For endurance athletes, the recommended intake is 1.2–1.4 g /kg body weight/ day. For strength and power athletes, the recommended intake is 1.4–1.7 g / kg body weight/ day.
- Protein breakdown is increased when muscle glycogen stores are low, e.g. during intense exercise lasting more than 1 hour, or during a calorie/carbohydrate-restricted programme.
- Protein intake above your optimal requirement will not result in further muscle mass or strength gains.
- Athletes should be able to meet their protein needs from a well-planned diet that matches their calorie needs. Low-fat protein sources are advised.
- Vegetarian athletes can meet their protein needs from low-fat dairy products and protein-rich plant sources eaten in the right combinations so that protein complementation is achieved.

VITAMINS AND MINERALS

5

Vitamins and minerals are often equated with vitality, energy and strength. Many people think of them as health enhancers, a plentiful supply being the secret to a long and healthy life.

In fact, vitamins and minerals do not in themselves provide energy. Nor does an abundant supply automatically guarantee bounce and vigour or optimal health.

The truth is that vitamins and minerals are needed in certain quantities for good health, as well as for peak physical performance. However, it is the *balance* of vitamins and minerals in the diet that is most important.

For sportspeople, it is tempting to think that extra vitamins lead to better performance. Because a small amount is 'good for us', more would surely be better. Or would it?

This chapter explains what vitamins and minerals do, where they come from, and how exercise affects requirements. Do athletes need extra amounts; and should they take supplements?

The functions, sources, requirements and upper safety levels of vitamins and minerals are given in the Glossary of Vitamins and Minerals (Appendix Two). The table also examines the claims made for supplementation of vitamins and minerals and whether they could benefit athletic performance.

WHAT ARE VITAMINS?

Vitamins are required in tiny amounts for growth, health and physical well-being. Many form the essential parts of enzyme systems that are involved in energy production and exercise performance. Others are involved in the functioning of the immune system, the hormonal system and the nervous system.

Our bodies are unable to make vitamins, so they must be supplied in our diet.

WHAT ARE MINERALS?

Minerals are inorganic elements that have many regulatory and structural roles in the body. Some (such as calcium and phosphorus) form part of the structure of bones and teeth. Others are involved in controlling the fluid balance in tissues, muscle contraction, nerve function, enzyme secretion and the formation of red blood cells. Like vitamins, they cannot be made in the body and must be obtained in the diet.

HOW MUCH DO I NEED?

Everyone has different nutritional requirements. These vary according to age, size, level of physical activity and individual body chemistry. It is, therefore, impossible to state an intake that would be right for everyone. To find out your exact requirements, you would have to undergo a series of biochemical and physiological tests.

However, scientists have studied groups of people with similar characteristics, such as age and physical activity, and have come up with some estimates of requirements. The Reference Nutrient Intake (RNI) is the measure used in the UK, but the RNI value for a nutrient can vary from country to country. European Union (EU) regulations require Recommended Daily Amounts (RDAs) to be shown on food and supplement labels. RDAs are said to apply to 'average adults' and are only very rough guides.

RNI values are derived from studies of the physiological requirements of healthy people. For example, the RNI for a vitamin may be the amount needed to maintain a certain blood concentration of that vitamin. The RNI is not the amount of a nutrient recommended for optimum nutrition or for athletic performance. Some guidelines for optimal intakes have been produced by reputable scientists but none have yet been adopted by the government.

WHAT ARE DIETARY REFERENCE VALUES (DRVS)?

In 1991 the Department of Health published *Dietary Reference Values for Food Energy and Nutrients for the United Kingdom*. A Dietary Reference Value (DRV) is a generic term for various daily dietary recommendations and covers three values that have been set for each nutrient:

1. the **Estimated Average Requirement (EAR)** is the amount of a nutrient needed by an average person, so many people will need more or less.

2. the **Reference Nutrient Intake (RNI)** is the amount of a nutrient that should cover the needs of 97% of the population. It is more than most people require, and only a very few people (3%) will exceed it.

3. the **Lower Reference Nutrient Intake (LRNI)** is for a small number of people who have low needs (about 3% of the population). Most people will need more than this amount.

In practice, the majority of the general population are somewhere in the middle. Athletes and sportspeople may exceed the upper limits because they have the highest requirements.

How are DRVs set?

It is not easy to set a DRV. First of all, scientists have to work out what is the minimum amount of a particular nutrient that a person needs to be healthy. Once this has been established, scientists usually add on a safety margin, to take account of individual variations. No two people will have exactly the same requirement. Next, a storage requirement is assessed. This allows for a small reserve of the nutrient to be kept in the body.

Unfortunately, scientific evidence of human vitamin and mineral requirements is fairly scanty and contradictory. A lot of scientific guesswork is inevitably involved, and results are often extrapolated from animal studies.

In practice, DRVs are arrived at through a compromise between selected scientific data and good judgement. They vary from country to country and are always open to debate.

SHOULD I PLAN MY DIET AROUND RNI?

The RNI is not a target intake to aim for – it is only a guideline. It should cover the needs of most people but, of course, it is possible that some athletes may need more than the RNI, due to their higher energy expenditure.

In practice, if you are eating consistently less than the RNI, you may be lacking in that nutrient.

CAN A BALANCED DIET PROVIDE ALL THE VITAMINS AND MINERALS I NEED?

Most athletes eat more food than the average sedentary person. With the right food choices, this means you should automatically achieve a higher vitamin and mineral intake. However, in practice many athletes do not plan their diets well enough, or they restrict their calorie intake so it can be difficult to obtain sufficient amounts of vitamins and minerals from food. Vitamin losses also occur during food processing, preparation and cooking, thus further reducing your actual intake. Intensive farming practices have resulted in crops with a lower nutrient content. For example, the use of agro-chemicals has depleted the mineral content of the soil so plants have a smaller mineral content. EU pricing policy, which keeps prices artificially high, has resulted in mountains of cauliflowers, cabbages and many other produce, which remain

in storage for up to a year before being sold in supermarkets. Obviously, considerable vitamin losses may have occurred during that time. See 'How does exercise increase my requirements for vitamins and minerals?' (p. 68) for more details.

The best sort of diet is one that provides enough vitamins and minerals to meet your needs. They should come from a wide variety of foods. In the UK, the Department of Health has produced a guide describing a balanced diet centred around the five main food groups (*see* Table 5.1).

WHEN MAY VITAMIN AND MINERAL SUPPLEMENTS BE USEFUL?

Eating a balanced diet may not always be easy in practice, particularly if you travel a lot, work shifts or long hours, train at irregular times, eat on the run or are unable to purchase and prepare your own meals. Planning and eating a well-balanced diet requires considerably more effort under these circumstances, so you may not be getting all the vitamins and minerals you need. A deficient intake is also likely if you are on a restricted diet (e.g. eating less than 1500 calories a day for a period of time or excluding a food group from your regular diet).

Table 5.1 Achieving a balanced diet	
Foods	**Portions/day**
Cereals and starchy vegetables	5–11
Fruit and vegetables	> 5
Milk and dairy products	2–3
Meat, fish and vegetarian alternatives	2–3
Oils and fats	0–3

Source: Department of Health, 1994.

A number of surveys have shown that many sportspeople do not achieve an adequate intake of vitamins and minerals from their diet (Short & Short, 1983; Steen & McKinney, 1986; Bazzare *et al.*, 1986). Low intakes of certain minerals and vitamins are more common among female athletes compared with males. A study of 60 female athletes found that calcium, iron and zinc intakes were less than 100% of the RDA (Cupista *et al.*, 2002). US researchers also measured low intakes of vitamin E, calcium, iron, magnesium, zinc and phosphorus in US national figure skaters (Ziegler, 1999). This was correlated with lower than recommended intakes of fruit, vegetables, dairy and high-protein foods. Study of US elite female heptathletes by researchers at the University of Arizona found that while average nutrient intakes were greater than 67% of the RDA, vitamin E intakes fell below this minimum level (Mullins, 2001). However, more than half of the athletes were taking vitamin and mineral supplements, which would boost their overall intake. A study of 58 swimmers found that 71% of males and 93% of females did not meet the recommended intakes for at least one of the anti-oxidant vitamins (Farajian *et al.*, 2004).

All these results suggest that athletes do not consume a well balanced diet, with not enough fruit and vegetables in particular.

WHO MAY BENEFIT FROM TAKING SUPPLEMENTS?

Research shows that one in three people take some form of vitamin supplement – the most popular being multivitamins (Gallup, 2000). A study of 411 university athletes found that over half routinely took supplements (Krumbach, 1999). The most common reasons were to 'improve performance' and 'build muscle'. Obviously, supplements are not a substitute for poor, or lazy, eating habits. If you think you may be lacking in vitamins and minerals, try to adjust your diet to include more vitamin- and mineral-rich foods.

As a temporary measure, you may benefit from taking supplements if:

- you have erratic eating habits
- you eat less than 1500 kcal a day
- you are pregnant (folic acid)
- you eat out a lot/rely on fast foods
- you are a vegan (vitamin B12 and possibly other nutrients)
- you are anaemic (iron)
- you have a major food allergy or intolerance (e.g. milk)
- you are a heavy smoker or drinker
- you are ill or convalescing.

HOW DOES EXERCISE INCREASE MY REQUIREMENTS OF VITAMINS AND MINERALS?

Regular, intense exercise increases your requirements for a number of vitamins and minerals, particularly those involved in energy metabolism, tissue growth and repair, red blood cell manufacture and free radical defence.

Vitamin E

Vitamin E is a powerful antioxidant (*see* p. 74), which prevents the oxidation of fatty acids in cell membranes and protects the cell from damage. Indeed, a study with elite cyclists showed that vitamin E supplementation reduced the amount of free radical (*see* p. 74) damage following prolonged intense cycling to exhaustion, compared with a placebo (Rokitzki *et al.*, 1994).

Vitamin C

Vitamin C has several exercise-related functions. It is required for the formation of connective tissue and certain hormones (e.g. adrenaline), which are produced during exercise; it is involved in the formation of red blood cells, which enhances iron absorption; it is a powerful antioxidant, which, like vitamin E, can also protect against exercise-related cell damage.

A vitamin C supplement may be useful if you are involved in prolonged high-intensity training because it may stabilise cell membranes and protect against viral attack. One study (Peters *et al.*, 1993) found a reduced incidence in upper respiratory tract infections in ultra-marathon runners after taking 600 mg vitamin C for 21 days prior to the race. Another study at the University of North Carolina, US found that vitamin C supplementation before and after resistance exercise reduced post-exercise muscle soreness and muscle damage and promoted recovery (Bryer & Goldfarb, 2006).

B vitamins

The B vitamins thiamin (B_1), riboflavin (B_2) and niacin (B_3), are involved in releasing energy from food. Since requirements for these are based on the amount of carbohydrate and calories consumed, athletes do need more than sedentary people. In general, it is easy to obtain these vitamins from wholegrain carbohydrate-rich foods such as bread, breakfast cereals, oatmeal and brown rice. However, if you use carbohydrate supplements, such as glucose polymer drinks and bars, you may need to take supplements. If you are restricting your calorie intake (e.g. on a fat-loss programme) or you eat lots of refined carbohydrates, you may also be missing out on B vitamins. To compensate for any shortfall, you should take a multivitamin supplement that contains at least 100% of the RDA of the B vitamins.

Vitamin B_6 is involved in protein and amino acid metabolism. It is needed for making red blood cells and new proteins, so getting the right amount of vitamin B_6 is very important to athletes.

Pantothenic acid (vitamin B_5) is necessary for making glucose and fatty acids from other metabolites in the body. It is also used in the manufacture of steroid hormones and brain chemicals. Obviously, a deficiency would be detrimental to health and athletic performance.

Folic acid and vitamin B12

These are both involved with red blood cell production in the bone marrow. They are also needed for cell division, and protein and DNA manufacture. Clearly, exercise increases all of these processes and therefore your requirements for folic acid and vitamin B_{12}. Vegans, who eat no animal products, must obtain vitamin B_{12} from fortified foods such as Marmite and breakfast cereals or fermented foods such as tempeh and miso. Taking a multivitamin supplement is a good insurance.

Beta-carotene

Beta-carotene is one of 600 carotenoid pigments that give fruit and vegetables their yellow, orange and red colours. They are not vitamins but act as antioxidants by protecting cells from free radical damage. Beta-carotene enhances the antioxidant function of vitamin E, helping to regenerate it after it has disarmed free radicals. However, carotenoids function most effectively together, so it is best to take these nutrients packaged together, in a supplement or in food.

Vitamin D

Vitamin D has been under the nutritional spotlight since the publication of the 6th edition of this book. The role of this vitamin in maintaining bone health is well recognised, but recent research in sports nutrition has focused on its role in muscle structure and function. Several studies suggest that vitamin D deficiency is widespread among athletes, particularly those in northern latitudes who train mainly indoors or get little sun exposure, or who do not consume vitamin D-rich foods (Larson-Meyer & Willis, 2010; Lovell, 2008; Meier *et al.*, 2004). This is an area of concern because there is increasing evidence that a deficiency reduces muscle function, strength and performance (Hamilton, 2011). Potentially vitamin D deficiency may also increase the risk of injury and illness risk, and have a detrimental effect on your training and performance (Halliday 2011).

Several studies have observed a correlation between vitamin D status and athletic performance (Larson-Meyer & Willis, 2010). Low levels are associated with reduced performance while high levels may enhance performance. A review of studies has highlighted a seasonal variation in performance (Cannell, 2009). The latter found that performance peaks in the summer months (when vitamin D levels peak), declines in winter months (when vitamin D levels decline), and reaches its lowest point when vitamin D levels are at their lowest. Peak athletic performance seems to occur when vitamin D levels approach those obtained by natural, full-body, summer sun exposure, which is around 50 ng/ ml. An adequate vitamin D status may also help protect against acute and chronic medical conditions, such as stress fractures, muscle weakness, impaired muscle function and reduced performance. Getting adequate levels of vitamin D whether from sun exposure or diet is, therefore, important for optimal performance.

Supplementation is a controversial area and scientific opinion is divided. Some believe that it would be a good idea for those who get little sun exposure or perhaps during the winter months when levels of vitamin D are low (IOC, 2011; Halliday, 2011). Others say that vitamin D supplements may not benefit athletic performance (Powers *et al*, 2011). If you think you may be at risk of vitamin D deficiency, you should consult your doctor and/or sports nutritionist who may recommend a simple blood test to determine whether you would benefit from vitamin D supplements. Researchers recommend a blood concentration above 32–40 ng/ ml (Larson-Meyer & Willis, 2010). Supplementation with vitamin D at the EU and US RDA level (5 ug/ day) should be sufficient (ACSM/ASA/DC, 2009).

Calcium

Calcium is an important mineral in bone formation, but it also plays an important role in muscle growth, muscle contraction and nerve transmission. While the body is able to increase or decrease the absorption of this mineral according to its needs, extra calcium is recommended for female athletes with low oestrogen levels (*see* p. 179). Weight-bearing exercise, such as running and weight training, increases bone mass and calcium absorption so it is important to get enough calcium in your diet.

Iron

Iron is important for athletes. Its major function is in the formation of haemoglobin (which transports oxygen in the blood) and myoglobin (which transports oxygen in the muscle cells).

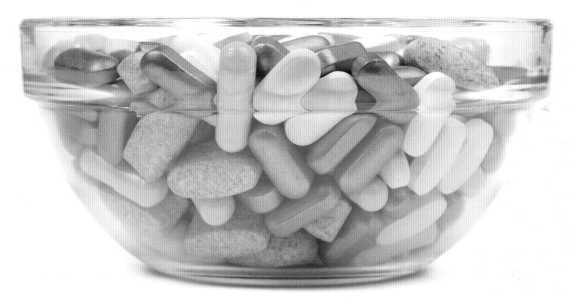

Many muscle enzymes involved in energy metabolism require iron. Clearly, athletes have higher requirements for iron compared with sedentary people. Furthermore, iron losses may occur during exercise that involves pounding of the feet, such as running, aerobics and step aerobics. Also at risk of iron-deficiency are women who have been pregnant in the last year (lower iron stores) and athletes who eat less than about 2000 kcal a day. Athletes who tend to avoid red meat, a rich source of iron, need to ensure they get iron from other sources or supplements. Iron deficiency and sports anaemia are discussed in detail in Chapter 11 (*see* pp. 179–182).

CAN VITAMIN AND MINERAL SUPPLEMENTS IMPROVE YOUR PERFORMANCE?

Many studies have been carried out over the years using varying doses of supplements. In the vast majority of cases, scientists have been unable to measure significant improvements in the performance of healthy athletes. Where a beneficial effect has been observed – for example, increased endurance – this has tended to be in athletes who started with a sub-optimal vitamin or mineral status. Taking supplements simply restored the athletes' nutrient stores to 'normal' levels.

In other words, low body stores or deficient intakes can adversely affect your performance, but vitamin and mineral supplements taken in excess of your requirements will not necessarily produce a further improvement in performance. More does not mean better!

The scientific consensus is that vitamin and mineral supplements are unnecessary for those consuming a varied diet that provides enough energy to maintain your body weight (ACSM/ADA/DC, 2009).

To find out if your diet is deficient in any nutrient, you should consult a registered nutritionist or sports dietician (look for the initials BSc or SRD, see useful addresses and online resources on pp. 325–326) for a dietary analysis. He or she will then be able to advise you about your diet and supplementation.

CAN HIGH DOSES OF SUPPLEMENTS BE HARMFUL?

Except perhaps in the case of vitamin A from liver (owing to modern animal feeding practices), it is almost impossible to overdose on vitamins and minerals from food. Problems are more likely to arise from the indiscriminate use of supplements, so always follow the guidelines on the label or the advice of a nutritionist. As a rule of thumb, never take more than 10 times the RDA of the fat-soluble vitamins A and D, and no more than the RDA for any mineral.

Certain vitamins and minerals taken in high doses can be harmful. The Food Standards Agency in the UK have published safe upper levels for vitamins and minerals (Food Standards Agency, 2003). In particular, it warns against high doses of:

- Chromium in the form of chromium picolinate – may cause cancer although up to 10 mg/ day of other forms of chromium is unlikely to be harmful.
- Vitamin C – although excess vitamin C is excreted in the urine, levels above 1000 mg/ day may result in stomach cramps, diarrhoea and nausea.
- Iron – levels above 17 mg/ day may result in constipation and discomfort through an upset or bloated stomach.
- Vitamin D – large doses can cause weakness, thirst, increased urination and, if taken for a long period result in high blood pressure and kidney stones.
- Vitamin A – large doses over a prolonged period can cause nausea, skin changes such as flakiness, liver damage and birth defects in unborn babies. Pregnant women are advised

Vitamin Controls in Europe

Under the EU Food Supplements Directive, which came into effect in August 2005, supplements will only be able to include vitamins and minerals taken from an approved list. This means that certain vitamin and mineral supplements may have to be reformulated, banned or have big drops in the doses of certain ingredients. The aim is to ensure that all vitamin and mineral products on sale in the EU are approved by the European Food Safety Authority as safe, that they contain forms of vitamins and minerals that offer some benefit, and that they are clearly labelled.

to avoid vitamin A supplements, fish liver oils and concentrated food sources of vitamin A such as liver and liver paté.
- Vitamin B_6 – doses over 10 mg/ day taken for a long period may lead to numbness, persistent pins and needles and unsteadiness (a type of neuropathy).

CAN SUPPLEMENTS CAUSE IMBALANCES?

Taking single vitamins or minerals can easily lead to imbalances and deficiencies. Many interact with each other, competing for absorption, or enhancing or impairing each other's functions. For example, iron, zinc and calcium share the same absorption and transport system, so taking large doses of iron can reduce the uptake of zinc and calcium. For healthy bones, a finely tuned balance of vitamin D, calcium, phosphorus, magnesium, zinc, manganese, fluoride, chloride, copper and boron is required. Vitamin C enhances the absorption of iron, converting it from its inactive ferric form to the active ferrous form. Most of the B vitamins are involved in energy metabolism, so a short-term shortage of one may be compensated for by a larger than normal use of another.

If in doubt about supplements, it is safest to choose a multivitamin and mineral formulation rather than individual supplements. Single supplements should be taken only upon the advice of your doctor or nutritionist.

ARE 'NATURAL' VITAMIN SUPPLEMENTS BETTER THAN SYNTHETIC?

There is no proof that so-called 'natural' or 'food state' vitamin supplements are better absorbed than synthetic vitamins. The majority have an identical chemical structure. In other words, they are the same thing and such terms on supplement labels are meaningless. Tests have shown that a relatively new type of supplement called 'food form' vitamins and minerals are more readily absorbed than synthetic vitamins. 'Food form' vitamins and minerals are micronutrients that are grown from food-based (yeast) cultures in the lab and are therefore intricately bound to protein, in a similar way as naturally occurring vitamins in food. That means you need to take lower doses for maximum effect.

ARE TIME-RELEASE SUPPLEMENTS BETTER THAN NORMAL SYNTHETIC SUPPLEMENTS?

Time-release vitamins are coated with protein and embedded in micropellets within the supplement. In theory, the supplement should take longer to dissolve, with the protein coating slowing down vitamin absorption. However, there is little evidence that this is the case or that they are better for you. Some may not even dissolve fully and end up passing straight through the digestive tract. If you take any supplement with a meal, the absorption of the vitamins and minerals is retarded anyway by the carbohydrate/fat/protein in the food. So, it is not worth paying extra money for time-release supplements.

HOW SHOULD I CHOOSE A MULTI-VITAMIN/MINERAL SUPPLEMENT?

Here are some basic guidelines.

- Choose a multivitamin/mineral supplement that highlights its antioxidant content.
- Check it contains at least 23 vitamins and minerals.
- The amounts of each vitamin should be between 100 and 1000% of the RDA stated on the label, but below the safe upper limit (see Appendix Two).
- Avoid supplements containing more than the RDA of any mineral as these nutrients compete for absorption and can be harmful in doses that are higher than the RDA.
- Choose beta-carotene rather than vitamin A – it is a more powerful antioxidant and has no harmful side effects in high doses.
- Avoid supplements with unnecessary ingredients such as sweeteners, colours, artificial flavours and talc (a bulking agent).
- Choose 'food form' if possible – the supplement is better absorbed.
- Choose low-dose supplements, designed to be taken in 2 or more doses daily, rather than mega-doses.
- Take with food and water.

ANTIOXIDANTS
WHAT ARE ANTIOXIDANTS?

Antioxidants are enzymes and nutrients in the blood that 'disarm' free radicals (*see* below) and render them harmless. They work as free radical scavengers by donating one of their own electrons to 'neutralise' the free radicals. Fortunately, your body has a number of natural defences against free radicals. They include various enzymes (e.g. superoxide dismutase, glutathione, peroxidase) which have minerals such as manganese, selenium and zinc incorporated in their structure; vitamins C and E, as well as hundreds of other natural substances in plants, called phytochemicals. These include carotenoids (such as beta-carotene), plant pigments, bioflavanoids and tannins.

WHAT ARE FREE RADICALS?

Free radicals are atoms or molecules with an unpaired electron and are produced all the time in our bodies as a result of normal metabolism and energy production. They can easily generate other free radicals by snatching an electron from any nearby molecule, and exposure to cigarette smoke, pollution, exhaust fumes, UV light and stress can increase their formation.

In large numbers, free radicals have the potential to wreak havoc in the body. Free radical damage is thought to be responsible for heart disease, many cancers, ageing and post-exercise muscle soreness, as unchecked free radicals can damage cell membranes and genetic material (DNA), destroy enzymes, disrupt red blood cell membranes, and oxidise LDL cholesterol in the bloodstream, thus also increasing the risk of atherosclerosis or the furring of arteries – the first stage of heart disease. Recent studies have demonstrated increased levels of free radicals following exercise and these have been held responsible for muscle soreness, pain, discomfort, oedema (fluid retention) and tenderness post-exercise (Halliwell & Gutteridge, 1985).

HOW DOES EXERCISE AFFECT FREE RADICAL LEVELS?

Because exercise increases oxygen consumption, there is an increased generation of free radicals. No one knows exactly how or why exercise does this, but it is thought to be connected to energy metabolism. During the final steps of ATP production (from carbohydrates or fats), electrons (the negative particles of atoms) sometimes get off course and collide with other molecules, creating free radicals. Exercise increases ATP production and so creates more free radicals.

Another source is the damage done to muscle cell membranes during high-intensity eccentric exercise, such as heavy weight training or plyometrics exercise, causing minor tears and injury to the muscles that results in the production of free radicals.

Other factors such as increased lactic acid production, increased haemoglobin breakdown, and heat generation may be involved too. In essence, the more you exercise, the more free radicals you generate.

The good side of free radicals

Not all free radicals are damaging. Some help to kill germs, fight bacteria and heal cuts. The problem arises when too many are formed and they cannot be controlled by the body's defence system.

WHAT ARE THE BEST SOURCES OF ANTIOXIDANTS?

The best source of antioxidants is the natural one: food! There are hundreds of natural substances in food called phytochemicals. These substances, which are found in plant foods, have antioxidant properties that are not present in supplements. Each appears to have a slightly different effect and to protect against different types of cancer and other degenerative diseases. For example, the phytochemicals in soya beans may prevent the development of hormone dependent cancers, such as breast, ovarian and prostate cancer, while those in garlic can slow down tumour development. It is therefore wise to obtain as wide a range of phytochemicals from food as possible.

Table 5.2 lists the food sources for the various types of antioxidants. Tables 5.3 and 5.4 list the food sources of antioxidants that assist in protecting against cancer and heart disease.

HOW MUCH DO YOU NEED?

There are few official guidelines for daily intakes of antioxidants, and debate between scientists about optimal intakes for athletes. See Chapter 6, pages 80–83 for further details.

SUMMARY OF KEY POINTS

- Vitamin and mineral requirements depend on age, body size, activity level and individual metabolism.

Table 5.2	Good sources of antioxidants
Antioxidant	**Source**
Vitamins	
Vitamin C	Most fruit and vegetables, especially blackcurrants, strawberries, oranges, tomatoes, broccoli, green peppers, baked potatoes
Vitamin E	Sunflower/safflower/corn oil, sunflower seeds, sesame seeds, almonds, peanuts, peanut butter, avocado, oily fish, egg yolk
Minerals	
Selenium	Wholegrains, vegetables, meat
Copper	Wholegrains, nuts, liver
Manganese	Wheatgerm, bread, cereals, nuts
Zinc	Bread, wholegrain pasta, grains, nuts, seeds, eggs
Carotenoids	
Beta-carotene	Carrots, red peppers, spinach, spring greens, sweet potatoes, mango, cantaloupe melon, dried apricots
Alpha- and gamma-carotene	Red coloured fruit, red and green coloured vegetables
Canthaxanthin and lycopene	Tomatoes, watermelon
Flavanoids	
Flavanols and polyphenols	Fruit, vegetables, tea, coffee, red wine, garlic, onions

Table 5.3 Anti-cancer phytochemicals

Antioxidant	Food source
Beta-carotene	Carrots, red peppers, spinach, spring greens, mangoes, apricots
Alpha- and gamma-carotene	Red coloured fruit, red and green coloured vegetables
Canthaxanthin	Tomatoes, watermelon
Coumaric acid	Green peppers, tomatoes, carrots
Allicin saponins	Onions, garlic, leeks
Glucosinolates	Broccoli, cabbage, cauliflower, brussel sprouts
Sulphoramine	Broccoli
Lycopene	Tomatoes
Lutein	Green vegetables
D-limonene	Pith of citrus fruits
Ellagic acid	Grapes, strawberries, cherries

Table 5.4 Heart disease protection

Antioxidant	Food source
Folate	Spinach, broccoli, curly kale, green cabbage and other green leavy vegetables
Quercetin	Onions, garlic, apples, grapes
Phenols	Grapes
Resveratrol	Grape skins, red wine

- DVRs should be used as a guide for the general population; they are not targets and do not take account of the needs of athletes.
- Regular and intense exercise increases the requirements for a number of vitamins and minerals. However, there are no official recommendations for athletes.
- Low intakes can adversely affect health and performance. However, high intakes exceeding requirements will not necessarily improve performance.
- Vitamins A, D and B_6 and a number of minerals may be toxic in high doses (more than 10 × RNI). Indiscriminate supplementation may lead to nutritional imbalances and deficiencies.
- Due to an erratic lifestyle or restricted food intake, many athletes consume sub-optimal amounts of vitamins and minerals. Therefore a supplement containing a broad spectrum of vitamins and minerals would benefit their long-term health and performance.
- A well-formulated supplement should contain between 100–1000% of the RDA for vitamins (but below the safe upper limit); and no more than 100% of the RDA for minerals.
- Optimal doses of certain antioxidants have been suggested by scientists but have not yet been adopted by the UK government.

SPORTS SUPPLEMENTS

6

The most effective way to develop your natural sports ability and achieve your fitness goals is through efficient training combined with optimal nutrition. But there is a huge variety of sports supplements marketed to athletes, including pills, powders, drinks and bars, which claim to increase muscle and strength, or burn fat. Can these products really speed your progress and give you the competitive edge?

Many athletes believe supplements are an essential component for sports success and it has been estimated that the majority of elite athletes are using some form of performance-enhancing agent. A study of Canadian varsity athletes found that 99% took supplements (Kritiansen *et al.*, 2005). A US study of collegiate varsity athletes found that 65% used some type of supplement regularly (Herbold *et al.*, 2004). The most commonly used supplements in the studies were vitamin/minerals, carbohydrate supplements, creatine and protein supplements. Creatine and ephedra are more popular among bodybuilders than other athletes, according to a study at Long Island University, New York, US (Morrison *et al.*, 2004). Most athletes in the studies said they took supplements to improve their health and athletic performance, reduce body fat or increase muscle mass.

Sifting through the multitude of products on offer can be an overwhelming task for athletes. It can be hard to pinpoint which ones work, especially when advertising claims sound so persuasive. Scientific research may be exaggerated or used selectively by manufacturers trying to sell a product. Testimonials from well-known athletes are also a common ploy that is used to hype products. Over the page guidelines are given for evaluating the claims of supplements. But you need to be wary of all ergogenic products because of the risk of contamination with prohibited substances not listed on the label. Some supplements, such as ephedrine, are sold through the internet, but are banned in sport and could result in a positive doping test.

This chapter examines the evidence for some of the most popular supplements and provides an expert rating on their effectiveness and safety.

ARE SPORTS SUPPLEMENTS SAFE?

There is currently no specific European or national legislation governing the safety of sports supplements. As they are classified as foods, supplements are not subject to the same strict manufacturing, safety testing or labelling requirements as licensed medicines. This means that there is no guarantee that a supplement lives up to its claims. At the time of going to print, the European Union (EU) is reviewing the situation with a view to introducing stricter labelling requirements in the future. However, there is stricter legislation covering vitamin and mineral supplements (the EU Food Supplements Directive, 2002, amended August 2005). Manufacturers can only use nutrients and ingredients from a 'permitted' list, and then within maximum limits. Each ingredient must undergo extensive safety tests before it is allowed on the permitted list and, therefore, into a supplement. Manufacturers must also provide scientific proof to support a product's claims and ensure that it is clearly labelled.

However, as many supplements are sold through the internet, it is difficult to regulate the market and there remains the risk of purchasing contaminated products.

Guidelines for evaluating the claims of sports supplements*

1 How valid is the claim?

- Does the claim made by the manufacturer of the product match the science of nutrition and exercise, as you know it? If it sounds too good to be true, then it probably isn't valid.
- Does the amount and form of the active ingredient claimed to be present in the supplement match that used in the scientific studies on this ergogenic aid?
- Does the claim make sense for the sport for which the claim is made?

2 How good is the supportive evidence?

- Is the evidence presented based on testimonials or scientific studies?
- What is the quality of the science? Check the credentials of the researchers (look for University-based or independent) and the journal in which the research was published (look for a peer-reviewed journal reference). Did the manufacturer sponsor the research?
- Read the study to find out whether it was properly designed and carried out. Check that it contains phrases such as 'double-blind placebo controlled', i.e. that a 'control group' was included in the study and that a realistic amount of the ergogenic substance/placebo was used.
- The results should be clearly presented in an unbiased manner with appropriate statistical procedures. Check that the results seem feasible and the conclusions follow from the data.

3 Is the supplement safe and legal?

- Are there any adverse effects?
- Does the supplement contain toxic or unknown substances?
- Is the substance contraindicated in people with a particular health problem?
- Is the product illegal or banned by any athletic organisations?

*Adapted from ACSM/ADA/DC (2000), Butterfield (1996), Clark (1995).

Beware of contamination of supplements

Contaminants – anabolic androgenic steroids and other prohibited stimulants – have been found in many different supplements. The largest survey was from the International Olympic Committee-accredited laboratory in Cologne. They looked for steroids in 634 supplements and found 15% contained substances – including nandrolone – that would lead to a failed drugs test. Nineteen per cent of UK samples were contaminated. In another study, researchers from the Olympic Analytical Laboratory at the University of California found that some brands of androstenedione are grossly mislabelled and contain the illegal anabolic steroid, testosterone (Catlin et al., 2000). Men who took either 100 mg or 30 mg of androstenedione for one week tested positive for 10-norandrostenrone, a metabolic by-product of nandrolone. In another report, Swiss researchers found different substances than those declared on the labels, including testosterone, in seven out of 17 pro-hormone supplements, i.e. 41% of the supplements! (Kamber, 2001)

The following substances may be found in supplements but they are banned by the IOC and may cause a positive drugs test:

- Ephedrine
- Strychnine
- Androstenedione
- Androstenediol
- Dehydroepiandrosterone (DHEA)
- 19-Norandrostenedione
- 19-Norandrostenediol

Advice to UK athletes on the use of supplements

In light of concerns about contamination and poor labelling of supplements, UK Sport, the British Olympic Association, the British Paralympic Association, National Sports Medicine Institute and the Home Country Sports Councils have issued a position statement on supplements. They advise UK athletes to be 'extremely cautious' about the use of any supplement. No guarantee can be given that any particular supplement, including vitamins and minerals and ergogenic aids, and herbal remedies, is free from prohibited substances as these products are not licensed and are not subject to the same strict manufacturing and labelling requirements as licensed medicines. Anti-doping rules are based on the principle of strict liability and therefore supplements are taken at an athlete's risk. Athletes sign a code of conduct agreeing that they are responsible for what they take. Athletes are advised to consult a medical practitioner, accredited sports dietitian or registered nutritionist before taking supplements. For more information about drugs in sports, see The Global Drug Information Database www.globaldro.com.

AMINO ACID SUPPLEMENTS
WHAT ARE THEY?

The most popular amino acid supplement comprises the branched-chain amino acids (BCAAs): valine, leucine and isoleucine. These three essential amino acids make up one-third of muscle proteins.

WHAT DO THEY DO?

The theory behind BCAA supplements is that they can help prevent the breakdown of muscle tissue during intense exercise. They are converted into two other amino acids – glutamine and alanine – which are released in large quantities during intense aerobic exercise. Also they can be used directly as fuel by the muscles, particularly when muscle glycogen is depleted.

WHAT IS THE EVIDENCE?

Studies at the University of Guelph, Ontario, suggest that taking 4 g BCAA supplements during and after exercise can reduce muscle breakdown (MacLean et al., 1994). They may help preserve muscle in athletes on a low-carbohydrate diet (Williams, 1998) and, taken before resistance training, reduce delayed onset muscle soreness (Nosaka et al., 2006; Shimomura et al., 2006). A study by researchers at Florida State University found that BCAA supplementation before and during prolonged endurance exercise reduced muscle damage (Greer et al., 2007). However, similar benefits were obtained following consumption of a carbohydrate drink and it is not clear whether chronic BCAA supplementation benefits performance. Studies with long distance cyclists at the University of Virginia found that supplements taken before and during a 100 km bike performance test did not improve performance compared with a carbohydrate drink (Madsen et al., 1996). In other words, BCAAs may not offer any advantage over carbohydrate drinks taken during exercise.

DO I NEED THEM?

They probably won't improve your endurance but doses of 6–15 g may help improve your recovery during hard training periods by reducing muscle protein breakdown and post-exercise injuries. Given that many recovery drinks contain a mixture of carbohydrate, protein and amino acids, there is little point taking a separate BCAA supplement.

ARE THERE ANY SIDE EFFECTS?

BCAAs are relatively safe becuase they are normally found in protein in the diet. Excessive intake may reduce the absorption of other amino acids.

ANTIOXIDANT SUPPLEMENTS
WHAT ARE THEY?

Antioxidant supplements contain various combinations of antioxidant nutrients and plant extracts, including beta-carotene, vitamin C, vitamin E, zinc, magnesium, copper, lycopene (pigment found in tomatoes), selenium, co-enzyme Q10, catechins (found in green tea), methionine (an amino acid) and anthocyanidins (pigments found in purple or red fruit).

WHAT DO THEY DO?

Intense exercise increases oxygen consumption and the generation of free radicals. This may result in a drop in the body's antioxidant levels and increase your susceptibility to free radical damage. Left unchecked, free radicals can harm

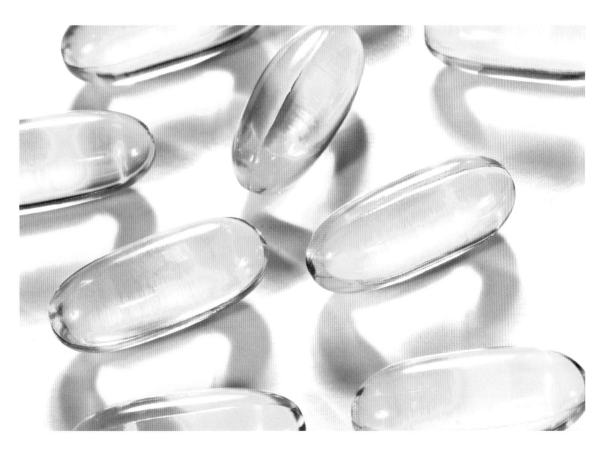

cell membranes, disrupt DNA, destroy enzymes and increase the risk of atherosclerosis and cancer. High levels of free radicals are also associated with post-exercise muscle soreness. While researchers have found that regular exercise enhances athletes' natural antioxidant defences (Robertson *et al.*, 2001; Ji, 1999) it has also been proposed that supplements of antioxidant nutrients may boost your natural antioxidant defences.

WHAT IS THE EVIDENCE?

There is considerable evidence that antioxidant supplements protect against age-related diseases such as heart disease, certain forms of cancer and cataracts. But the evidence for supplementation for sports performance is less clear (Goldfarb, 1999). Researchers at Loughborough University found that daily vitamin C supplementation (200 mg) for 2 weeks reduced muscle soreness and improved recovery following intense exercise (Thompson *et al.*, 2001). A US study found that women who took an antioxidant supplement (vitamin E, vitamin C and selenium) before and after weight training had significantly less muscle damage (Bloomer *et al.*, 2004). Researchers at the University of North Carolina, US found that vitamin C supplementation before and after resistance exercise reduced post-exercise muscle soreness and muscle damage and promoted recovery (Bryer & Goldfarb, 2006). Sports scientists in South Africa measured enhanced levels of immune cells (neutrophils) in runners who had taken an antioxidant supplement (vitamin C, vitamin E and beta-carotene) following a strenuous 2 hour run compared with runners who had been given a placebo (Robson *et al.*, 2003). A study by German researchers looked at the effects of vitamin E on the performance of 30 top racing cyclists (Rokitzki *et al.*, 1994). The researchers concluded that vitamin E helped to protect the cells from free radical damage although it had no immediate effect on their performance.

But a review of studies presented at the 2003 IOC Consensus Conference on Sports Nutrition concluded that there is limited evidence that antioxidant supplements improve performance (Powers, *et al.*, 2004). Similarly, the consensus statement by the ASCM, ADA and DC cautions against the use of antioxidant supplements (ACSM/ADA/DC, 2009). High doses could be pro-oxidative with potential negative effects. The reason for these conflicting results may be that different studies used different antioxidant combinations and doses, making it difficult to draw clear conclusions.

DO I NEED THEM?

On balance, athletes may gain health benefits from antioxidant supplements but the benefits on performance are less clear (Sen, 2001; Faff, 2001; Kanter M. M. & Eddy D. M. (1992); Kanter M. M. *et al.*, 1993). Broad-spectrum antioxidant supplements (rather than single nutrients) may be worth taking, as some research suggests they help promote recovery after intense exercise and reduce post-exercise muscle soreness.

But antioxidant supplements should not be a substitute for a healthy diet. Aim to eat at least five portions of fruit and vegetables daily – the more intense the colour, the higher the antioxidant content – as well as foods rich in essential fats (such as avocados, oily fish and pure vegetable oils) for their vitamin E content. Scientists at the American Institute for Cancer Research say that eating at least five portions of fruit and vegetables each day can prevent 20% of all cancers. The Department of Health in the UK and the World Health Organisation advise a minimum of 400 g or five portions of fruit and vegetables a day. The EU recommended daily amount for vitamin C is 60 mg and for vitamin E 10 mg. These are levels judged sufficient to support health; they are not optimal amounts for athletic performance or heart disease prevention. A number of scientists believe the UK and US recommended intakes are too low. Professor Mel Williams, of the Department of Exercise Science, Physical Education and Recreation at Old Dominion University, Virginia, US, advises 500–1000 mg vitamin C, 250–500 mg vitamin E and 50–100 mg selenium (Williams, 1998).

ARE THERE ANY SIDE EFFECTS?

No toxic effects have been found for the antioxidant vitamins. Large doses of carotenoids consumed in the form of food or supplements can turn your skin orange, but this effect is harmless and will gradually go away. Large doses of vitamin C (over 2000 mg) can cause diarrhoea and flatulence but can obviously be corrected by reducing your supplement dose. Vitamin E, despite being a fat-soluble vitamin and capable of being stored, appears safe even at levels 50 times higher than the RDA. However, you should be careful with selenium supplements because the margin of safety between a healthy dose of selenium (up

Training and immunity

During periods of intense training or immediately following endurance race events, many athletes find that they become more susceptible to minor respiratory illness, such as colds and sore throats. While moderate training boosts your immune system, prolonged periods of intense training appears to depress immune cell functions. Such changes create an 'open window' of decreased protection, during which viruses and bacteria can gain a foothold, increasing the risk of developing an infection. It is thought that the increased levels of stress hormones, such as adrenaline and cortisol, associated with intense exercise, inhibit the immune system. Other factors such as stress, lack of sleep and poor nutrition can also depress immunity.

A healthy diet that meets your energy needs and provides adequate micronutrients required for immune cell function (iron, zinc, magnesium, manganese, vitamins A, C, D, E, B6, B12 and folic acid) is important for maintaining immune defences. Even short-term dieting during periods of hard training can result in a loss of immune function and make you more prone to infections.

Here are some practical ways of combating exercise-related suppression of immunity.

- Match your calorie intake and expenditure – under-eating will increase cortisol levels.
- Ensure you're consuming plenty of foods rich in immunity-boosting nutrients – vitamins A, C, and E, vitamin B6, zinc, iron and magnesium. Best sources are fresh fruit, vegetables, whole grains, beans, lentils, nuts and seeds.
- Avoid low carbohydrate diets. Low glycogen stores are associated with bigger increases in cortisol levels and bigger suppression of your immune cells.
- Consume a sports drink (approximately 6 g carbohydrate/100 ml, providing 30–60 g carbohydrate per hour) during intense exercise lasting longer than 1 hour. This can reduce stress hormone levels and the associated drop in immunity following exercise (Bishop, 2002).
- Drink plenty of fluid. This increases your saliva production, which contains anti-bacterial proteins that can fight off airborne germs.
- A modest antioxidant supplement or a vitamin C supplement may help to reduce the risk of upper respiratory tract infection during periods of intense training (Gleeson, 2011). In one study of ultra-marathon runners, those who took daily vitamin C supplements (1500 mg) seven days prior to a race had lower levels of stress hormones following the race, which suggests greater protection against infection (Peters et al., 2001).
- Glutamine supplements may reduce the risk of infections. Glutamine levels can fall by up to 20% following intense exercise (Antonio, 1999), putting the immune system under greater strain.
- Echinacea taken for up to four weeks during a period of hard training may boost immunity and reduce the risk of catching a cold by stimulating the body's own production of immune cells.
- Quercetin supplements (1000 mg/day) taken during periods of intense training may reduce the risk of upper respiratory illness (Nieman et al, 2009).
- Probiotic supplements may help reduce the severity and duration of respiratory illness and benefit immunity (Gleeson, 2008).

to 200 mg a day) and a toxic dose (as little as 900 mg) is very small. Toxic symptoms include nausea, vomiting, hair loss and loss of fingernails.

The other antioxidant minerals – zinc, magnesium and copper – may produce toxic symptoms in high doses, so stick to the upper safe limits given in Appendix 2.

BETA-ALANINE (β-ALANINE)
WHAT IS IT?

β-alanine is an amino acid that is used to make carnitine (a dipeptide formed from β-alanine and histidine). Carnitine is an important buffer in muscles – it buffers the acidity (hydrogen ions) produced during high intensity exercise.

WHAT DOES IT DO?

Taking β-alanine supplements increases muscle carnitine levels. Taking 5–6 g/day increases muscle carnitine content by 60% after 4 weeks and 80% after 10 weeks (Harris *et al*, 2006). This raises the buffering capacity of the muscles, increasing the ability of muscles to tolerate high intensity exercise for longer. Normally, a build-up of acidity results in fatigue.

WHAT IS THE EVIDENCE?

Studies carried out since 2006 have found that β-alanine supplementation may improve performance in high intensity events lasting between 1 and 7 minutes. It may also be beneficial in events involving repeated sprints or lifts. However, the research has involved only small numbers of volunteers and not all studies have found significant benefits. In a study at Ghent University, Belgiam, β-alanine supplements reduced fatigue when performing a set of knee extensions

(Derave *et al*, 2007). This is thought to be due to the increased buffer capacity of the muscles. Another study at the College of New Jersey found that β-alanine supplements resulted in increased training volume and reduced subjective feelings of fatigue in football players (Hoffman *et al*, 2008).

DO I NEED IT?

β-alanine supplements may be beneficial if you are competing in high intensity events such as swimming, rowing, cycling and running lasting between 1 and 7 minutes; or sports such as football and tennis that involve repeated sprints. They may also be advantageous for bodybuilders and those following a strength training programme. Typical doses used in studies are 3.2–6.4 g/day for 6–10 weeks.

ARE THERE ANY SIDE EFFECTS?

There have been reports of parathesia (skin tingling), although this appears to be harmless, and is associated mainly with higher doses. Smaller doses or sustained-release formulations are less likely to cause side effects. Importantly, the long-term effects of β-alanine supplements are not known.

BEETROOT JUICE (NITRATE)
WHAT IS IT?

Beetroot juice (and beetroot) is a rich source of nitrate. Nitrate is also found in smaller amounts in other vegetables, such as spincach, rocket, celeriac, cabbage, endive, leeks and broccoli. And it may also be taken in the form of sodium nitrate supplements.

WHAT DOES IT DO?

Beetroot juice increases the amount of nitrate in the blood. Nitrate is then converted into nitric oxide (NO) in the body. This gas plays an important role in vasodilation and regulating blood pressure. Increasing NO levels prior to exercise could be an advantage, as it means blood vessels become more dilated, aiding the delivery of oxygen and nutrients to muscles during exercise.

WHAT IS THE EVIDENCE?

Nitrate appears to be a very potent ergogenic aid. A number of studies have shown that nitrate in the form of beetroot juice enhances stamina and performance. It also reduces resting blood pressure and the oxygen cost of exercise, meaning that athletes can tolerate higher intensity levels for longer. For example, researchers at the University of Exeter, UK, found that drinking 500 ml beetroot juice a day for a week enabled volunteers to run 15% longer before experiencing fatigue (Lansley *et al*, 2011). This was due to the higher levels of nitrate measured in the blood, which reduced muscle uptake of oxygen and made them more fuel-efficient. A further study by the same researchers found that cyclists given 500 ml beetroot juice 2½ hours before a time trial race improved their performance by 2.8% in a 4 km race and 2.7% in a 16.1 km race (Lansley *et al.*, 2011). University of Maastricht researchers found that 170 ml beetroot juice concentrate over 6 days improved 10 km time trial performance and power output in cyclists (Cermak *et al.*, 2012). But whole beetroot works equally well. Athletes who consumed 200 g cooked beetroot an hour before exercise were able to run faster in the latter stages of a 5 km run (Murphy *et al.*, 2012). These results suggest that the nitrates in beetroot juice reduce maximal oxygen uptake, improve exercise economy and allow athletes to exercise longer.

DO I NEED IT?

Beetroot may help improve your performance time in cycling or running events lasting between 4 and 30 minutes. Typical doses used in studies are around 500 ml beetroot juice or 170 ml beetroot juice concentrate or 200 g cooked beetroot (equivalent to 300 mg nitrate). This may be taken daily for a week or between 1 and 2½ hours before exercise.

ARE THERE ANY SIDE EFFECTS?

No side effects of beetroot have been reported to date although the safety of sodium nitrate supplements has not been investigated. There have been questions whether beetroot juice could theoretically increase cancer risk (dietary nitrates can be converted to nitrite in the body and then go on to react with amino acids to produce carcinogenic compounds called nitrosamines). However, research has shown that the opposite is true, that high intakes of fruit and vegetables (naturally containing high levels of nitrate/nitrite) actually decrease the risk of these harmful compounds being produced in the body, probably due to the high levels of protective antioxidants they contain.

Beetroot juice may cause a harmless, temporary pink colouration of urine and stools.

BICARBONATE
WHAT IS IT?

Sodium bicarbonate, sometimes marketed as a 'pH buffer', is an extracellular anion that helps maintain pH gradients between the cells and blood. It is also a raising agent and a main ingredient of baking powder. Other buffers include sodium citrate.

WHAT DO THEY DO?

Bicarbonate is already found in the blood, but consuming supplements ('bicarbonate loading') will increase the concentration further. Both bicarbonate and citrate act as pH buffers, increasing the pH of the blood and making it more alkaline. During high intensity (anaerobic) exercise, hydrogen ions are produced, which gradually accumulate and and result in fatigue ('the burn'!). However, by raising the pH of the blood, hydrogen ions can pass more easily from the muscle cells to the blood, where they can be removed (buffered), which allows you to continue exercising at a high intensity a little longer. It also means lactate is removed faster so you can recover faster.

WHAT IS THE EVIDENCE?

Research has shown improvement in high intensity events lasting 1–7 minutes. One meta analysis found an improvement of 1.7% for events lasting about 1 minute with a bicarbonate dose of 0.3 g/ kg body mass BM) although no improvement with sodium citrate (Carr *et al.*, 2011).

DO I NEED THEM?

You may benefit from bicarbonate if you are competing in high intensity events lasting 1–7 minutes – for example, sprint and middle distance swimming, running and rowing events – or in events that involve multiple sprints, e.g. tennis, football, rugby. The most common dose for bicarbonate loading is 0.3 g/ kg 90 minutes before the start of exercise. However, the side effects may cancel out any potential improvement.

ARE THERE ANY SIDE EFFECTS?

Typical side effects include gastrointestinal upset, nausea, stomach pain, diarrhoea and vomiting. Bicarbonate loading may also cause water retention, which may be a disadvantage in many events. These side effects could negate any possible performance advantage. Symptoms may be reduced by taking the loading dose in divided doses over a 2–2½ hour period before the event, along with a small carbohydrate-rich meal and plenty of water. Alternatively, if you will be competing in several events over a few days, you could try taking 0.5 g/ kg/ day over the course of 1–3 days and then stop 12–24 hours before the event. Theoretically, the benefits will persist but with less risk of side effects.

CAFFEINE
WHAT IS IT?

Caffeine is a stimulant and has a pharmacological action on the body so is classed as a drug rather than a nutrient. It was once classed as a banned substance but was removed from the World Anti-Doping Agency (WADA) Prohibited List in 2004. This change was based on the recognition that caffeine enhances performance at doses that are indistinguishable from everyday caffeine use, and that the previous practice of monitoring caffeine use via urinary caffeine concentrations is not reliable.

It is found in everyday drinks and foods such as coffee, tea and cola, herbs such as guarana, and chocolate. It is also added to a number of energy drinks and sports drinks and gels. Table 6.1 lists the caffeine content of popular drinks and foods. The amounts used in research range from 3–15 mg/ kg BW, which is equivalent to 210–1050 mg for a 70 kg athlete. Studies normally used caffeine pills rather than drinks.

WHAT DOES IT DO?

Caffeine acts on the central nervous system, increasing alertness and concentration, which could be considered advantageous in many sports. Indeed, the performance benefits of caffeine appear to be achieved by central nervous system effects. These effects reduce the perception of fatigue and allow exercise to be maintained at a higher intensity for a longer period.

It was once believed that caffeine enhances endurance performance because it promotes an increase in the utilisation of fat as an exercise fuel and 'spares' the use of glycogen. In fact, studies now show that the effect of caffeine on 'glycogen sparing' during sub-maximal exercise is short-lived and inconsistent – not all athletes respond in this way. Therefore, it is unlikely to explain the enhancement of exercise capacity and performance seen in many studies.

WHAT IS THE EVIDENCE?

Most studies of caffeine and performance have been carried out in laboratories rather than during real-life sports events. Nevertheless, there is sound evidence that caffeine may enhance the performance of a range of sports:

- Endurance sports (> 60 min)
- High-intensity sports (1–60 min)
- Team and intermittent sports

There is a huge amount of research evidence suggesting that caffeine improves endurance (Dodd, 1993; Graham & Spriet, 1991; Spriet, 1995). An analysis by UK researchers of 40

Table 6.1	The caffeine content of popular drinks and foods
Product	Caffeine content, mg/cup
Instant coffee	60 mg
Espresso	45–100 mg
Cafetiere/filter	60–120 mg
Tea	40 mg
Green tea	40 mg
Energy drinks	100 mg
Cola	40 mg
Energy gel (1 sachet)	25 mg
Dark chocolate (50 g)	40 mg
Milk chocolate (50 g)	12 mg

studies on caffeine and performance concluded that it significantly improves endurance, on average by 12% (Doherty & Smith, 2004).

One study with swimmers showed a 23 second improvement in a 21-minute swim (MacIntosh, 1995). Researchers at RMIT University, Victoria, Australia found that caffeine improved performance by 4–6 seconds in competitive rowers during a 2000 metre row (Anderson et al., 2000). However, not all studies have shown positive results. Researchers at the University of Stirling, UK, and the University of Cape Town, South Africa found that caffeine had no effect on performance during a 100 km cycling time trial (Hunter et al., 2002). But the benefits for short-term high-intensity activities, such as sprinting, are less clear with roughly half the studies suggesting an improvement in performance; half suggesting no benefit.

DO I NEED IT?

A large number of studies now show that caffeine intake can enhance performance at doses of 1–3 mg/kg, which is considerably less than once believed (6 mg/kg). There appears to be little increase in performance above 3 mg/kg. For a 70 kg person, this would be 210 mg, equivalent to about 2 cups of coffee or 2 cans of caffeinated energy drink.

Performance benefits occur soon after consumption, so caffeine may be consumed just before exercise, spread throughout exercise, or late in exercise as fatigue is beginning to occur. As individual responses vary, you should experiment during training to find the dose and protocol that suits you.

Australian researchers have found that 1.5 mg/kg (105 mg for a 70 kg athlete) taken in divided doses (e.g. 4 caffeine-containing energy gels over 2 hours) throughout an intense workout benefits performance in serious athletes (Armstrong, 2002). It was once thought that cutting down on caffeine for several days before competition results in a more marked ergogenic effect. However, studies show that there is no difference in the performance response to caffeine between non-

Does caffeine promote dehydration?

Although caffeine is a diuretic, a daily intake of less than 300 mg caffeine results in no larger urine output than water. At this level, caffeine is considered safe and unlikely to have any detrimental effect on performance or health (Armstrong, 2002). Taking caffeine regularly (e.g. drinking coffee) builds up your caffeine tolerance so you experience smaller diuretic effects.

According to a study from Ohio State University, caffeine taken immediately before exercise does not promote dehydration (Wemple, 1997). Six cyclists consumed a sports drink with or without caffeine over a 3-hour cycle ride. Researchers found that there was no difference in performance or urine volume during exercise. Only at rest was there an increase in urine output.

In another study, when 18 healthy men consumed 1.75 litres of three different fluids at rest, the caffeine-containing drink did not change their hydration status (Grandjean, 2000).

Researchers at the University of Maastricht found that cyclists were able to rehydrate after a long cycle equally well with water or a caffeine-containing cola drink (Brouns, 1998). Urine output was the same after both drinks. However, large doses of caffeine – over 600 mg, enough to cause a marked ergogenic effect – may result in a larger fluid loss. A study at the University of Connecticut, US, found that both caffeine-containing cola and caffeine-free cola maintained hydration in athletes (during the non-exercise periods) over three successive days of training (Fiala et al., 2004). The athletes drank water during training sessions but rehydrated with either caffeinated or caffeine-free drinks. A further study by the same researchers confirmed that moderate caffeine intakes (up to 452 mg caffeine/kg body weight/day) did not increase urine output compared with a placebo and concluded that caffeine does not cause a fluid electrolyte balance in the body (Armstrong et al., 2005).

users and users of caffeine, and that withdrawing from caffeine does not increase the improvement in performance.

ARE THERE ANY SIDE EFFECTS?

The effects of an acute intake of caffeine follow a U-shaped curve. Low-moderate doses produce positive effects and a sense of well-being, but higher doses of caffeine can have negative effects. It may increase the heart rate, impair fine motor control and technique, and cause anxiety or over-arousal, trembling and sleeplessness. Some people are more susceptible to these than others. If you are sensitive to caffeine, it is best to avoid it.

Scientific research shows, on balance, no link between long-term caffeine use and health problems, such as hypertension and bone mineral loss. The connection between raised cholesterol levels and heavy coffee consumption is now known to be caused by certain fats in coffee, which are more pronounced in boiled coffee than instant or filter coffee.

CONJUGATED LINOLEIC ACID (CLA)
WHAT IS IT?

CLA is an unsaturated fatty acid (in fact, it is a mixture of linoleic acid isomers) found naturally in small amounts in full fat milk, meat and cheese. Supplements are made from sunflower and safflower oils.

WHAT DOES IT DO?

It is marketed as a fat loss supplement. It is thought that CLA works by stimulating the enzyme hormone sensitive lipase (which releases fat from fat cells) and suppressing the hormone lipoprotein lipase (which transports fat into fat cells).

WHAT IS THE EVIDENCE?

Most of the initial research on CLA has been done using animal studies. Studies with humans have produced mixed results. Some have found that CLA supplements reduce fat levels (Gaullier et al., 2005, Thom et al., 2001) while others found no change in body composition (Ferreira et al., 1998). For example, Norwegian researchers observed a 20% reduction in body fat after volunteers took 3 g per day for 3 months (Thom et al., 2001). When combined with resistance training, CLA may also enhance mass and strength. University of Memphis researchers gave CLA supplements to experienced weight-lifters and found that, compared with a placebo, CLA improved strength (Ferreira et al., 1998). A study with 24 novice bodybuilders at Kent State University, US, found that 6 weeks of supplementation resulted in increased arm circumference, total muscle mass and overall strength compared with a placebo group (Lowery et al., 1997).

DO I NEED IT?

CLA may help reduce your body fat while maintaining or increasing muscle mass. Most researchers recommend 2–5 g per day (divided into 3 doses).

ARE THERE ANY SIDE EFFECTS?

None have been reported to date.

COLOSTRUM
WHAT IS IT?

Colostrum supplements are derived from bovine colostrum, the milk produced in the first few days after the birth of a calf. It has a high concentration of immune and growth compounds, such as immunoglobulins and antimicrobial proteins.

WHAT DOES IT DO?

It is claimed that bovine colostrum supplements enhance immunity, improve performance, recovery and body composition.

WHAT IS THE EVIDENCE?

It is unclear whether supplements help reduce the suppression of the immune system associated with prolonged intense exercise. Some studies found a reduction in self-reported upper respiratory tract infections (Brinkworth & Buckley, 2003), but others have found no effect (Crooks et al., 2006). University of Queensland researchers measured an increase in immunoglobulins but no significant difference in incidence of upper respiratory infection among a group of cyclists during high intensity training (Shing et al., 2007). There is inconclusive evidence that colostrum supplements improve performance, strength and power. One study at the University of South Australia suggests supplements improve anaerobic power after 8 weeks (Buckley et al, 2003). But another study by the same researchers found that supplements had no effect on body composition after 8 weeks of weight training (Brinkworth, 2004).

DO I NEED IT?

While supplements may help boost your immunity during periods of high intensity training, it is not certain whether they will reduce your risk of upper respiratory tract infection. It is unlikely that supplements have any benefit on your athletic performance.

ARE THERE ANY SIDE EFFECTS?

There are no known side effects.

CREATINE
WHAT IS IT?

Creatine is a protein that is made naturally in the body from three amino acids (arginine, glycine and methionine), but can also be found in meat and fish or taken in higher doses as a supplement. It is available as a single supplement, but it is often an ingredient in 'all-in-one' meal replacement drinks and supplement 'stacks'.

WHAT DOES IT DO?

Creatine combines with phosphorus to form phosphocreatine (PC) in your muscle cells. This is an energy-rich compound that fuels your muscles during high intensity activities, such as lifting weights or sprinting. Creatine supplementation raises PC levels typically around 2% (Hultman et al., 1996). This enables you to sustain all-out effort longer than usual and recover faster between sets so it would be beneficial for training that involves repeated high-intensity sets. Creatine supplements also help promote protein manufacture and muscle hypertrophy (by drawing water into the cells), increasing lean body mass; reduce muscle acidity (it buffers excess hydrogen ions), thus allowing more lactic acid to be produced before fatigue sets in; and reduces muscle protein breakdown following intense exercise, resulting in greater strength and improved ability to do repeated sets.

WHAT IS THE EVIDENCE?

Hundreds of studies have measured the effects of creatine supplements on anaerobic performance. Just over half of these report a positive effect on performance; the remainder show no real effect (Volek & Kraemer, 1996; Volek et al., 1997). Studies reviewed in the Journal of Strength and

Conditioning Research (Volek & Kraemer, 1996) found creatine supplements improved strength (such as the 1 rep-max bench press), the number of repetitions (70% of 1 rep-max) performed to fatigue, jump-squat peak power and the ability to perform repeated sprints. Creatine appears to enhance performance in both men and women. Researchers at McMaster University, Ontario gave 12 male and 12 female volunteers either creatine supplements or a placebo before a high intensity sprint cycling test (Tarnopolsky & McLennan, 2000). Creatine improved the performance equally in both sexes.

Researchers at the Australian Institute of Sport found that creatine improved sprint times and agility run times in football players (Cox *et al.*, 2002). A study in former Yugoslavia found that creatine supplementation improved sprint power, dribbling and vertical jump performance in young football players, but had no effect on endurance (Ostojic, 2004). Another study found that creatine supplements improved performance in events lasting 90–300 seconds in elite kayakers (McNaughton *et al.*, 1998).

If creatine improves the quality of resistance training over time, this would lead to faster gains in mass, strength and power. The vast majority of studies indeed show that short-term creatine supplementation increases body mass. Professor Kreider of the University of Memphis estimates athletes can gain up to 1.5 kg during the first week of a loading dose and up to 4.5 kg after 6 weeks. Dozens of studies show significant increases in lean mass and total mass, typically between 1–3% lean body weight (approx. 0.8–3 kg) after a 5-day loading dose, compared with controls.

However, not all studies have demonstrated positive results with creatine. Creatine supplements

How does creatine work?

The observed gains in weight are due partly to an increase in cell volume and partly to muscle synthesis. Creatine causes water to move across cell membranes. When muscle cell creatine concentration goes up, water is drawn into the cell, an effect that boosts the thickness of muscle fibres by around 15%. The water content of muscle fibres stretches the cells' outer sheaths – a mechanical force that can trigger anabolic reactions. This may stimulate protein synthesis and result in increased lean tissue (Haussinger *et al.*, 1996).

Creatine may have a direct effect on protein synthesis. In studies at the University of Memphis, athletes taking creatine gained more body mass than those taking the placebo, yet both groups ended up with the same body water content (Kreider *et al.*, 1996; Clark, 1997.)

There is less evidence for the use of creatine with aerobic-based sports – only a few laboratory studies have shown an improvement in performance. This is probably due to the fact that the PC energy system is less important during endurance activities. However, one study at Louisiana State University suggests creatine supplements may be able to boost athletes' lactate threshold and therefore prove beneficial for certain aerobic-based sports (Nelson *et al.*, 1997).

failed to improve sprint swim performance in a group of 20 competitive swimmers (Mujika *et al.*, 1996). Also there is less evidence to show that creatine supplementation is beneficial to endurance athletes. This is probably due to the fact that the

PC energy system is less important during endurance activities. However, one study at Louisiana State University, Kentucky, US, suggests creatine supplements may be able to boost athletes' lactate threshold and, therefore, prove beneficial for certain aerobic-based sports.

DO I NEED IT?

If you train with weights or do any sport that includes repeated high-intensity movements, such as sprints, jumps or throws (as in, say, rugby and football), creatine supplements may help increase your performance, strength and muscle mass. In some people (approx. 2 out of every 10), muscle creatine concentrations increase only very slightly. It may be partly due to differences in muscle fibre types. Fast-twitch (FT) fibres tend to build up higher concentrations of creatine than slow-

What is the best form of creatine?

Creatine monohydrate is the most widely available form of creatine. It is a white powder that dissolves readily in water and is virtually tasteless. It is the most concentrated form available commercially and the least expensive. Creatine monohydrate comprises a molecule of creatine with a molecule of water attached to it so it is more stable.

Although other forms of creatine such as creatine serum, creatine citrate and creatine phosphate are available, there is no evidence that they are better absorbed, produce higher levels of phosphocreatine in the muscle cells or result in greater increases in performance or muscle mass (Jager et al., 2011).

Will I lose strength when I stop taking creatine supplements?

When you stop taking supplements, elevated muscle creatine stores will drop very slowly to normal levels over a period of 4 weeks (Greenhaff, 1997). During supplementation your body's own synthesis of creatine is depressed but this is reversible. In other words, you automatically step up creatine manufacture once you stop supplementation. Certainly, fears that your body permanently shuts down normal creatine manufacture are unfounded. You may experience weight loss and there are anecdotal reports about athletes experiencing small reductions in strength and power, although not back to pre-supplementation levels.

It has been proposed that creatine is best taken in cycles, such as 3–5 months followed by a 1-month break.

twitch (ST) fibres. This means that athletes with a naturally low FT fibre composition may experience smaller gains from creatine supplements. Taking creatine with carbohydrate may help solve the problem as carbohydrate raises insulin, which, in turn, helps creatine uptake by muscle cells.

HOW MUCH CREATINE?

The most common creatine-loading protocol is 4 x 5–7 g doses per day over a period of 5 days, i.e. 20–25 g daily. It works, but that doesn't mean it's the best way to load up. In fact, it's a pretty inefficient and costly way of getting creatine into your muscles and is more likely to produce side effects such as water retention. Around two-thirds of this

Can muscle creatine levels be enhanced further?

Studies have shown that insulin helps shunt creatine faster in to the muscle cells (Green et al., 1996; Steenge et al., 1998). Taking creatine along with carbohydrate – which stimulates insulin release – will increase the uptake of creatine by the muscle cells and raise levels of PC. The exact amount of carbohydrate needed to produce an insulin spike is debatable but estimates range from 35 g to around 100 g. Some scientists recommend taking creatine with or shortly after eating a meal. The idea is to take advantage of the post-meal rise in insulin to get more creatine into the muscle cells. Taking plain creatine monohydrate is the least expensive way to achieve this. Creatine drinks and supplements containing carbohydrate are expensive and may add a lot of unwanted calories to your diet.

Creatine uptake is also greater immediately after exercise so adding creatine to the post-exercise meal will help to boost muscle creatine levels.

Canadian researchers have suggested that muscle creatine levels may be enhanced when alpha-lipoic acid (an antioxidant) is given at the same time (Burke et al., 2001a). And researchers at St Francis Xavier University, Nova Scotia found that those who supplemented with whey protein and creatine achieved greater increases in strength (bench press) and muscle mass compared with those who took only whey protein or placebo (Burke et al., 2001b).

creatine ends up in your urine and only one-third ends up in your cells. The key to efficient creatine supplementation is to take small quantities at a time – and to slow down the speed of absorption from the gut. That gives the maximum chance of all the creatine consumed ending up in your muscle cells and not your urine.

According to a Canadian study, relatively low doses of creatine supplementation can significantly improve weight-training performance to the same extent as higher doses (Burke et al., 2000). Volunteers who took 7.7 g creatine daily for 21 days were able to perform more repetitions on the bench press and maintain maximum power longer than those who took a placebo. They also gained significantly more muscle mass (2.3% versus a 1.4% increase with placebo).

Some researchers recommend taking 6 daily doses of 0.5–1 g (i.e. 6 x 1 g doses) and sprinkling it on your food to increase the absorption rate (Harris, 1998). Over a 5- or 6-day period, that will produce results equivalent to taking 20 g a day. After that, a maintenance dose of 2 g a day will maintain muscle creatine levels. Alternatively, you can load up with 3 g a day over 30 days. This technique also results in saturation of your muscles with creatine, and should produce the least water retention (Hultman et al., 1996).

ARE THERE ANY SIDE EFFECTS?

The main side effect is weight gain. This is due partly to extra water in the muscle cells and partly to increased muscle tissue. While this is desirable for bodybuilders and people who work out with weights, it could be disadvantageous in sports where there is a critical ratio of body weight and speed (e.g. running) or in weight-category sports. In swimmers, a heavier body weight may cause more drag and reduce swim efficiency. It's a matter of weighing up the potential advantage of increased maximal power and/or lean mass against the possible disadvantage of increased weight.

There have been anecdotal reports about muscle cramping, gastrointestinal discomfort, dehydration, muscle injury, and kidney and muscle damage. However, there is no clinical data to support these statements (Williams *et al.*, 1999; Robinson *et al.*, 2000; Mihic *et al.*, 2000; Kreider, 2000; Greenwood *et al.*, 2003; Mayhew *et al.*, 2002; Poortmans & Francaux, 1999). But, while short-term and low-dose creatine supplementation appears to be safe, the effects of long-term and/or high-dose creatine supplementation, alone or in combination with other supplements, remain unknown.

ENERGY GELS
WHAT ARE THEY?

Energy gels come in small squeezy sachets and have a jelly-like texture. They consist of simple sugars (such as fructose and glucose) and malto-dextrin (a carbohydrate derived from corn starch, consisting of 4–20 glucose units). They may also contain sodium, potassium and, sometimes, caffeine. Most contain between 18 and 25 g of carbohydrate per sachet.

WHAT DO THEY DO?

Gels provide a concentrated source of calories and carbohydrate and are designed to be consumed during endurance exercise.

WHAT IS THE EVIDENCE?

Studies show that consuming 30–60 g of carbohydrate per hour during prolonged exercise delays fatigue and improves endurance. This translates into 1–2 sachets per hour. A 2007 study from Napier University, Edinburgh showed that gels have a similar effect on blood sugar levels and performance as sports drinks (Patterson & Gray, 2007). Soccer players who consumed an energy gel (with water) immediately before and during high-intensity interval training increased their endurance by 45% compared with a placebo.

DO I NEED THEM?

Energy gels provide a convenient way of consuming carbohydrate during intense endurance exercise lasting longer than an hour. But you need to drink around 350 ml of water with each (25 g carb) gel to dilute it to a 7% carb solution in your stomach. Try half a gel with 175 ml (6 big gulps) every 15–30 minutes. On the downside, some people dislike their texture, sweetness and intensity of flavour – it's really down to personal preference – and they don't do away with the need for carrying a water bottle with you.

ARE THERE ANY SIDE EFFECTS?

Energy gels don't hydrate you so you must drink plenty of water with them. If you don't drink enough, you'll end up with a gelatinous goo in your stomach. This drags water from your bloodstream into your stomach, increasing the risk of dehydration.

EPHEDRINE/'FAT BURNERS'/THERMOGENIC SUPPLEMENTS
WHAT IS IT?

The main ingredient in 'fat burners' or thermogenics is ephedrine, a synthetic version of the

Chinese herb Ephedra or ma huang. Ephedrine is, strictly, a drug rather than a nutritional supplement. It is also used at low concentrations in cold and flu remedies (pseudoephedrine).

WHAT DOES IT DO?

Ephedrine is chemically similar to amphetamines, which act on the brain and the central nervous system. Athletes use it because it increases arousal, physical activity and the potential for neuromuscular performance. It is often combined with caffeine, which enhances the effects of ephedrine.

WHAT IS THE EVIDENCE?

Ephedrine is a proven stimulant. However, research studies generally show it has little effect on strength and endurance. This is probably because relatively low doses were used. What is more likely is that these products have a 'speed-like' effect; they make you feel more awake and alert, more motivated to train hard and more confident.

There is some evidence that ephedrine helps fat loss: partly due to an increase in thermogenesis (heat production), partly because it suppresses your appetite and partly because it makes you more active.

When taken as a 'caffeine–ephedrine stack', or a 'caffeine–ephedrine–aspirin stack', it is thought that ephedrine has a greater effect in terms of thermogenesis and weight loss. In one study, volunteers who took a combination of caffeine and ephedrine before a cycle sprint (anaerobic exercise) achieved a better performance than those who took caffeine only, ephedrine only or a placebo (Bell, 2001). However, the fat-burning effect of ephedrine seems to decrease over time, i.e. weight loss slows or stops after 12 weeks.

DO I NEED IT?

It is an addictive drug and I would strongly recommend avoiding any fat-burner containing ephedrine or ma huang because of the significant health risks. The International Olympic Committee (IOC) bans ephedrine, whether in cold remedies or in supplements. Exercise and good nutrition are the safest methods for burning fat.

ARE THERE ANY SIDE EFFECTS?

Ephedrine is judged to be safe in doses containing around 18–25 mg; that's the amount used in decongestants and cold remedies. Taking too much can have serious side effects. These include increased heart rate, increased blood pressure, palpitations, anxiety, nervousness, insomnia, nausea, vomiting and dizziness. Very high doses (around 3000 mg) cause heart attacks and can even be fatal. Caffeine–ephedrine stacks produce adverse effects at even lower doses. A case of a sportsman who suffered an extensive stroke after taking high doses of 'energy pills' (caffeine–ephedrine) has been reported in the *Journal of Neurology, Neurosurgery and Psychiatry* (Vahedi, 2000).

In 2002, the American Medical Association called for a ban on ephedrine due to concerns over its side effects. Since 1997 the FDA in the US has documented at least 70 deaths and more than 1400 'adverse effects' involving supplements containing ephedrine. These included heart attacks, strokes and seizures. Ephedrine's risks far outweigh its potential benefits. It is addictive and people can develop a tolerance to it (you need to keep taking more and more to get the same effects).

FAT BURNERS (EPHEDRINE-FREE)
WHAT ARE THEY?

Certain fat-burning and weight loss supplements claim to mimic the effects of ephedrine, boost the metabolism and enhance fat loss but without harmful side effects. The main ingredients in these products include *citrus aurantium* (synephrine or bitter orange extract); green tea extract and *Coleus forskohlii* extract (a herb, similar to mint).

WHAT DO THEY DO?

Citrus aurantium is a weak stimulant, chemically similar to ephedrine and caffeine. It contains a compound called synephrine which, according to manufacturers, reduces appetite, increases the metabolic rate and promotes fat-burning. However, despite the hype, there is no sound scientific evidence to back up the weight loss claims.

The active constituents in green tea are a family of polyphenols called catechins (the main type is epigallocatechin gallate, EGCG) and flavanols, which possess potent antioxidant activity. Apart from the clear benefits of green tea as an antioxidant, initial research suggests that it may also stimulate thermogenesis, increasing calorie expenditure, promoting fat burning and weight loss (Dulloo *et al.*, 1999).

The theory behind *Coleus forskohlii* as a dietary supplement is that its content of forskolin can be used to stimulate adenyl cyclase activity, which will increase cAMP (cyclic adenosine monophosphate) levels in the fat cell, which will in turn activate another enzyme (hormone sensitive lipase) to start breaking down fat stores. But there are no published trials showing that *Coleus forskohlii* extract promotes weight loss.

DO I NEED THEM?

The research on ephedrine-free fat burners is not robust and any fat-burning boost they provide would be relatively small or none. The doses used in some brands may be too small to provide a measurable effect. A careful calorie intake and exercise are likely to produce better weight loss results in the long term. The only positive data is for green tea, but you would need to drink at least six cups daily (equivalent to 100–300 mg EGCG) to achieve a significant fat-burning effect.

ARE THERE ANY SIDE EFFECTS?

While the herbal alternatives to ephedrine are generally safer, you may get side effects with high doses. *Citrus aurantium* can increase blood pressure as much, if not more, than ephedrine. High doses of forskolin may cause heart disturbances.

GLUTAMINE
WHAT IS IT?

Glutamine is a nonessential amino acid. It can be made in the muscle cells from other amino acids (glutamic acid, valine and isoleucine) and is the most abundant free amino acid in muscle cells. It is essential for cell growth and a critical source of energy for immune cells called lymphocytes.

WHAT DOES IT DO?

Glutamine is needed for cell growth, as well as serving as a fuel for the immune system. During periods of heavy training or stress, blood levels of glutamine fall, weakening your immune system and putting you at risk of infection. Muscle levels of glutamine also fall, which results in a loss of muscle tissue, despite continued training.

Manufacturers claim that glutamine has a protein-sparing effect during intense training. This is based on the theory that glutamine helps draw water into the muscle cells, increasing the cell volume. This inhibits enzymes from breaking down muscle proteins and also counteracts the effects of stress hormones (such as cortisol), which are increased after intense exercise.

WHAT IS THE EVIDENCE?

The evidence for glutamine is divided. Some studies have suggested that supplements may reduce the risk of infection and promote muscle growth (Parry-Bollings *et al.*, 1992; Rowbottom *et al.*, 1996). Researchers at Oxford University have shown that glutamine supplements taken immediately after running and again two hours later appeared to lower the risk of infection and boost immune cell activity in marathon runners (Castell & Newsholme, 1997). Only 19% of those taking glutamine became ill during the week following the run while 51% of those taking a placebo became ill. However, not all studies have managed to replicate these findings.

Glutamine does not improve performance, body composition or muscle breakdown (Haub, 1998). According to a Canadian study, glutamine produces no increase in strength or muscle mass compared with a placebo (Candow *et al.*, 2001). After 6 weeks of weight training, those taking glutamine achieved the same gains in strength and muscle mass as those taking a placebo.

DO I NEED IT?

The case for glutamine is not clear. Studies have used doses of around 100 mg glutamine per kg body weight during the 2 hours following a strenuous workout or competition (Bledsoe, 1999).

That's equivalent to a 7 g dose in a 70 kg athlete. But that doesn't mean you will get any benefit. Many protein and meal replacement supplements contain glutamine.

ARE THERE ANY SIDE EFFECTS?

No side effects have been found so far.

HMB
WHAT IS IT?

HMB (beta-hydroxy beta-methylbutyrate) is made in the body from the BCAA, leucine. You can also obtain it from a few foods such as grapefruit, alfalfa and catfish.

WHAT DOES IT DO?

No one knows exactly how HMB works, but it is thought to be involved in cellular repair. HMB is a precursor to an important component of cell membranes that helps with growth and repair of muscle tissue. HMB supplements claim to protect muscles from excessive breakdown during exercise, accelerate repair and build muscle.

WHAT IS THE EVIDENCE?

The evidence for HMB is divided. A number of studies suggest that HMB may increase strength and muscle mass and reduce muscle damage after resistance exercise (Nissen *et al.*, 1996; Panton *et al.*, 2000). For example, researchers at Iowa State University have shown muscle mass gains of 1.2 kg and strength gains of 18% after three weeks with HMB, compared with 0.45 kg muscle gain and 8% strength gain from a placebo (Nissen *et al.*, 1996; Nissen *et al.*, 1997). One study suggests HMB may boost muscle mass more effectively when taken together with creatine (Jowko *et al.*, 2001).

However, this degree of improvement hasn't been found in all HMB studies. It appears to have little effect in experienced athletes (Kreider *et al.*, 2000). One study at the Australian Institute of Sport failed to find strength or mass improvements in 22 athletes taking 3 g per day for 6 weeks (Slater *et al.*, 2001). Researchers at the University of Queensland in Australia found no beneficial effect on reducing muscle damage or muscle soreness following resistance exercise (Paddon-Jones *et al.*, 2001).

There is some evidence that HMB combined with alpha-ketoisocaproic acid may reduce signs and symptoms of exercise-induced muscle damage in novice weight trainers (van Someren *et al.*, 2005).

DO I NEED IT?

If you're new to lifting weights, HMB may help to boost your strength and build muscle, but probably for only the first 2 months of training. No long-term studies have been carried out to date – it is unlikely to benefit more experienced athletes.

ARE THERE ANY SIDE EFFECTS?

No side effects have yet been found.

MEAL REPLACEMENT PRODUCTS (MRPS)
WHAT ARE THEY?

MRPs are available as powders as well as ready-to-drink shakes and bars. They contain a mixture of milk proteins (usually whey protein and/or casein), carbohydrate (maltodextrin and/or sugars), vitamins and minerals. Some brands also contain small amounts of unsaturated fatty acids and other nutrients that claim to boost performance. Weight gain products are very similar to MRPs but usually contain more calories in the form of carbohydrates and good fats to help promote growth.

MRPs differ from protein shakes in that they often contain carbohydrates, fats and additional vitamins etc.

WHAT DO THEY DO?

MRPs provide a nutritionally balanced and convenient alternative to solid food. They are tailored towards aiding muscular growth and recovery.

DO I NEED THEM?

They will not necessarily improve your performance, but can be a helpful and convenient addition (rather than replacement) to your diet if you struggle to eat enough real food, you need to eat on the move or you need the extra nutrients they provide.

ARE THERE ANY SIDE EFFECTS?

Side effects are unlikely.

NITRIC OXIDE SUPPLEMENTS
WHAT ARE THEY?

The active ingredient in nitric oxide (NO) supplements is L-arginine, a non-essential amino acid, made naturally in the body. It is usually sold as arginine alpha keto-glutarate (A-AKG) and arginine keto iso-caproate (A-KIC). Supplements are marketed to bodybuilders for promoting and prolonging muscle pumps and increasing lean body mass and strength.

WHAT DO THEY DO?

Arginine is an amino acid that is readily converted to NO in the body. NO is a gas that is involved in vasodilation, which is the process that increases blood flow to muscles, allowing better delivery of nutrients and oxygen. The idea behind the NO-boosting supplements is to use L-arginine, A-AKG and A-KIC to increase the production of NO to bring a greater influx of nutrients and oxygen to the muscles, causing a better pump when lifting weights, and increased recovery and muscle growth.

WHAT IS THE EVIDENCE?

Little research supports these assertions directly. An analysis of several studies concludes that NO supplements may produce a small benefit for beginners, but not for more highly trained athletes and not for females (Bescos et al, 2012)

DO I NEED THEM?

It's certainly plausible that these NO supplements may improve muscle pump when lifting weights. However, more research needs to be done to confirm whether they increase muscle mass and strength in humans.

ARE THERE ANY SIDE EFFECTS?

Side effects are unlikely from the doses recommended on the supplement label. Arginine supplements have been used safely with heart disease patients in doses of up to 20 g a day.

PROTEIN SUPPLEMENTS
WHAT'S IN THEM?

Protein supplements can be divided into three main categories: protein powders (which you mix with milk or water into a shake); ready-to-drink shakes; and high-protein bars. They may contain whey protein, casein, soy protein or a mixture of these.

WHAT DO THEY DO?

They provide a concentrated source of protein to supplement your usual food intake. Whey protein is derived from milk and contains high levels of the essential amino acids, which are readily digested, absorbed and retained by the body for muscle repair. Whey protein may also help enhance the immune function. Casein, also derived from milk, provides a slower-digested protein, as well as high levels of amino acids. It may help protect against muscle breakdown during intense training. Soy protein is less widely used in supplements but is a good option for vegans and people with high cholesterol levels – 25 g of soya protein daily (as part of a diet low in saturated fat) can help reduce cholesterol levels.

WHAT IS THE EVIDENCE?

It is undisputed that resistance training increases muscle protein turnover and therefore the daily protein requirement. But it remains controversial whether protein supplements actually increase muscle mass and strength. Some studies have shown positive effects of protein supplements (Candow, 2006; Burke et al., 2001b; Brown et al., 2004). For example, male volunteers who consumed a whey protein supplement (1.2 g/ kg BW/ day) during 6 weeks of resistance training achieved greater muscle mass and strength gains compared with those who took a placebo (Candow et al., 2006), but others have reported no or minimal effects (Cambell et al., 1995; Haub, 2002).

DO I NEED THEM?

Most athletes can get enough protein from 2–4 daily portions of meat, chicken, fish, dairy products, eggs and pulses. Vegetarians can meet their protein needs by eating a variety of plant proteins, such as tofu, Quorn, beans, lentils, and nuts, each day. However, protein supplements may benefit you if you have particularly high protein requirements (e.g. through strength and power training), you are on a calorie-restricted diet or you cannot consume enough protein from food alone (e.g. through a vegetarian or vegan diet). Estimate your daily protein intake from food and compare that with your protein requirement. Experts recommend an intake between 1.2 and 1.4 g per kg of body weight per day for endurance athletes and 1.4 and 1.8 g per kg body weight per day for strength athletes. For example, a strength athlete weighing 80 kg may need as much as 144 g protein a day. This may be difficult to get from food alone. If there is a consistent shortfall, consider adding a supplement.

ARE THERE ANY SIDE EFFECTS?

An excessive intake of protein, whether from food or supplements, is not harmful but offers no health or performance advantage. Concerns about excess protein harming the liver and kidneys or causing calcium loss from the bones have been disproved.

Whey vs casein supplements

Most of the research on whey vs casein shows there is no difference in muscle mass and strength gains between those taking whey or casein proteins (Dangin, 2000; Kreider, 2003; Candow et al., 2004; Brown et al., 2004), although some studies have suggested that whey produces greater gains in strength and muscle mass compared with casein (Cribb et al., 2006).

Whey protein, the most popular protein ingredient, is derived from milk using either a process called micro-filtration (the whey proteins are physically extracted by a microscopic filter) or by ion-exchange (the whey proteins are extracted by taking advantage of their electrical charges). It has a higher BV than milk (and other protein sources) and is digested and absorbed relatively rapidly, making it useful for promoting post-exercise recovery. It has a higher concentration of Essential Amino Acids (around 50%) than whole milk, about half of which are BCAAs (23–25%), which may help minimise muscle protein breakdown during and immediately after high-intensity exercise. Research at McGill University in Canada suggests that the amino acids in whey protein also stimulate glutathione production in the body (Bounous & Gold, 1991). Glutathione is a powerful antioxidant and also helps support the immune system. This is particularly useful during periods of intense training when the immune system is suppressed. Whey protein may also help to stimulate muscle growth, by increasing insulin-like growth factor-1 (IGF-1) production – a powerful anabolic hormone made in the liver that enhances protein manufacture in muscles.

Casein, also derived from milk, comprises larger protein molecules which are digested and absorbed more slowly than whey. It also has high biological value and a high content of the amino acid gluta-mine (around 20%) – a high glutamine intake may help spare muscle mass during intense exercise and prevent exercise-induced suppression of the immune system.

PRE-HORMONES/ PRO-HORMONES/ STEROID PRECURSORS/ TESTOSTERONE BOOSTERS

WHAT ARE THEY?

Pre-hormone supplements include dehydroepiandrosterone (DHEA), androstenedione ('andro') and norandrostenedione, weak androgenic steroid compounds. They are produced naturally in the body and converted into testosterone. Supplements are marketed to bodybuilders and other athletes for increased strength and muscle mass.

WHAT DO THEY DO?

Manufacturers claim the supplements will increase testosterone levels in the body and produce similar muscle-building effects to anabolic steroids, but without the side effects.

WHAT IS THE EVIDENCE?

Current research does not support supplement manufacturers' claims. Studies show that andro supplements and DHEA have no significant testosterone-raising effects, and no effect on muscle mass or strength (King *et al.*, 1999; Broeder *et al.*, 2000; Powers, 2002; Maughan *et al.*, 2004). A study at Iowa State University found that 8 weeks of supplementation with andro, DHEA, saw palmetto, *Tribulus terrestris* and chrysin combined with a weight training programme failed to raise testosterone levels or increase muscle strength or mass – in spite of increased levels of androstenedione – compared with a placebo (Brown *et al.*, 2000).

DO I NEED THEM?

It is unlikely that pro-hormones work and they may produce unwanted side effects (see below). Most

athletic associations, including the International Olympic Committee (IOC), ban pre-hormones. What's more, their contents cannot always be guaranteed. In tests carried out by the IOC laboratory in Cologne, Germany, 15% of the supplements contained substances that would lead to a failed drugs test, including nandrolone, despite them not being listed on the label. Pre-hormones are highly controversial supplements and, despite the rigorous marketing, there is no research to prove the testosterone-building claims.

ARE THERE ANY SIDE EFFECTS?

Studies have found that pre-hormones increase oestrogen (which can lead to gynecomastia, male breast development) and decrease HDL (high density lipoproteins or good cholesterol) levels (King *et al.*, 1999). Reduced HDL carries a greater heart disease risk. Other side effects include acne, enlarged prostate and water retention.

Some supplements include anti-oestrogen substances, such as chrysin (dihydroxyflavone), to counteract the side effects, but there is no evidence that they work either (Brown *et al.*, 2000).

TAURINE

WHAT IS IT?

Taurine is a non-essential amino acid produced naturally in the body. It is also found in meat, fish, eggs and milk. It is the second most abundant amino acid in muscle tissue. Taurine is sold as a single supplement, but more commonly as an ingredient in certain protein drinks, creatine-based products and sports drinks. It is marketed to athletes for increasing muscle mass and reducing muscle tissue breakdown during intense exercise.

WHAT DOES IT DO?

Taurine has multiple roles in the body, including brain and nervous system function, blood pressure regulation, fat digestion, absorption of fat-soluble vitamins and control of blood cholesterol levels. It is used as a supplement because it is thought to decrease muscle breakdown during exercise. The theory behind taurine is that it may act in a similar way to insulin, transporting amino acids and sugar from the bloodstream into muscle cells. This would cause an increase in cell volume, triggering protein synthesis and decreasing protein breakdown.

WHAT IS THE EVIDENCE?

Intense exercise depletes taurine levels in the body, but there is no sound research to support the claims for taurine supplements.

DO I NEED IT?

As you can obtain taurine from food (animal protein sources), there appears to be no convincing reason to recommend taking the supplements for athletic performance or muscle gain.

ARE THERE ANY SIDE EFFECTS?

Taurine is harmless in the amounts found in protein and creatine supplements. Very high doses of single supplements may cause toxicity.

ZMA
WHAT IS IT?

ZMA (zinc monomethionine aspartate and magnesium aspartate) is a supplement that combines zinc, magnesium, vitamin B6 and aspartate in a specific formula. It is marketed to bodybuilders and strength athletes as a testosterone booster.

WHAT DOES IT DO?

Manufacturers claim that ZMA can boost testosterone production by up to 30%, strength by up to 11%, and improve muscle mass and recovery after exercise. The basis for these claims is that the supplement corrects underlying zinc and/or magnesium deficiencies, thus 'normalising' various body processes and improving testosterone levels (Brilla & Conte, 2000). Zinc is needed for growth, cell reproduction and testosterone production. In theory, a deficiency may reduce the body's anabolic hormone levels and adversely affect muscle mass and strength. Magnesium helps reduce levels of the stress hormone cortisol (high levels are produced during periods of intense training), which would otherwise promote muscle breakdown. A magnesium deficiency may increase catabolism. ZMA supplements may therefore help increase anabolic hormone levels and keep high levels of cortisol at bay by correcting a zinc and magnesium deficiency.

DO I NEED IT?

Strength and power athletes during periods of intense training may benefit from ZMA, but only if dietary levels of zinc and magnesium are low. Don't expect dramatic strength gains, though. You can obtain zinc from wholegrains, including wholemeal bread, nuts, beans and lentils. Magnesium is found in wholegrains, vegetables, fruit and milk.

ARE THERE ANY SIDE EFFECTS?

Do not exceed the safe upper limit of 25 mg daily for zinc; 400 mg daily for magnesium. High levels of zinc – more than 50 mg – can interfere with the absorption of iron and other minerals, leading to iron-deficiency. Check the zinc content of any other supplement you may be taking.

SUMMARY OF KEY POINTS

- Despite the widespread availability of sports supplements, there is no specific national or EU legislation governing their effectiveness, purity and safety. To reduce the risk of a positive doping test, the IAAF and British Olympic Association advise athletes against the use of supplements generally.
- Some supplements offer the potential of improved performance. These include beetroot juice, creatine, caffeine, sports drinks, gels and bars.
- Antioxidant supplementation provides many health benefits, but short-term benefits to performance are not clear.
- Caffeine increases alertness, concentration, and endurance and, taken in pharmacological doses, could benefit performance in endurance activities.
- Creatine supplementation may improve performance in single or multiple sprints, speed recovery between sets and increase lean and total body mass. However, it does not work for everyone and the long-term risks are not clear.
- There is no evidence that pre-hormones such as androstenedione enhance muscle mass or strength and their use may result in a positive doping test.
- Ephedrine-containing supplements are popular fat-loss aids and performance-enhancers, but they are associated with a number of side effects and many athletic bodies prohibit their use.
- There is insufficient evidence for the use of glutamine, HMB, taurine, ZMA and nitric oxide supplements.

// HYDRATION

7

Exercise is thirsty work.

Whenever you exercise you lose fluid, not only through sweating but also as water vapour in the air that you breathe out. Your body's fluid losses can be very high and, if the fluid is not replaced quickly, dehydration will follow. This will have an adverse effect on your physical performance and health. Exercise will be much harder and you will suffer fatigue sooner.

This chapter explains why it is important to drink fluids to avoid dehydration, when is the best time to drink, and how much to drink. It deals with the timing of fluid intake: before, during and after exercise, and considers the science behind the formulation of sports drinks. Do they offer an advantage over plain water and can they improve performance? Finally, this chapter looks at the effects of alcohol on performance and health, and gives a practical, sensible guide to drinking.

WHY DO I SWEAT?

First, let us consider what happens to your body when you exercise. When your muscles start exercising, they produce extra heat. In fact, about 75% of the energy you put into exercise is converted into heat, and is then lost. This is why exercise makes you feel warmer. Extra heat has to be dissi-

pated to keep your inner body temperature within safe limits – around 37–38°C. If your temperature rises too high, normal body functions are upset and eventually heat stroke can result.

The main method of heat dispersal during exercise is sweating. Water from your body is carried to your skin via your blood capillaries and as it evaporates you lose heat. For every litre of sweat that evaporates, you will lose around 600 kcal of heat energy from your body. (You can lose some heat through convection and radiation, but it is not very much compared with sweating.)

HOW MUCH FLUID DO I LOSE?

The amount of sweat that you produce and, therefore, the amount of fluid that you lose, depends on:

- how hard you are exercising
- how long you are exercising for
- the temperature and humidity of your surroundings
- individual body chemistry.

The harder and longer you exercise, and the hotter and more humid the environment, the more fluid you will lose. During one hour's exercise an average person could expect to lose around 1 litre of fluid – and even more in hot conditions. During more strenuous exercise in warm or humid conditions (e.g. marathon running), you could be losing as much as 2 litres an hour.

Some people sweat more profusely than others, even when they are doing the same exercise in the same surroundings. This depends partly on body weight and size (a smaller body produces less sweat), your fitness level (the fitter and better acclimatised to warm conditions you are, the more readily you sweat due to better thermoregulation), and individual factors (some people simply sweat more than others!). In general, women tend to produce less sweat than men, due to their smaller body size and their greater economy in fluid loss. The more you sweat, the more care you should take to avoid dehydration.

You can estimate your sweat loss and, therefore, how much fluid you should drink by weighing yourself before and after exercise. Every 1 kg decrease in weight represents a loss of approximately 1 litre of fluid.

WHAT ARE THE DANGERS OF DEHYDRATION?

An excessive loss of fluid (dehydration) impairs performance and has an adverse effect on health (Below *et al.*, 1995; McConnell *et al.*, 1997). As blood volume decreases and body temperature rises, it places extra strain on the heart, lungs and circulatory system, which means the heart has to work harder to pump blood round your body. The strain on your body's systems means that exercise becomes much harder and your performance drops.

The scientific consensus is that a loss of just 2% in your weight will affect your performance, and your maximal aerobic capacity will fall by 10–20%

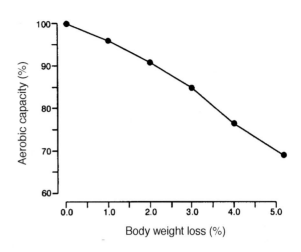

Figure 7.1 Fluid loss reduces exercise capacity

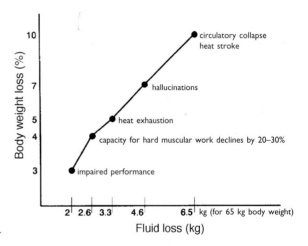

Figure 7.2 The dangers of dehydration

during endurance exercise lasting more than 90 minutes (Armstrong *et al.*, 1985). If you lose 4%, you may experience nausea, vomiting and diarrhoea. At 5% your aerobic capacity will decrease by 30%, while an 8% drop will cause dizziness, laboured breathing, weakness and confusion (see

Fig. 7.1). Greater drops have very serious consequences (Montain & Coyle, 1992; Noakes, 1993). Figure 7.2 shows the danger of dehydration with progressively greater fluid losses.

Ironically, the more dehydrated you become, the less able your body is to sweat. This is because dehydration results in a smaller blood volume (due to excessive loss of fluid), and so a compromise has to be made between maintaining the blood flow to muscles and maintaining the blood flow to the surface of the skin to carry away heat. Usually the blood flow to the skin is reduced, causing your body temperature to rise.

If you carry on exercising without replacing fluids you become more and more dehydrated.

A CONTROVERSY: DEHYDRATION AND PERFORMANCE

Not all scientists agree that dehydration impairs performance. Several studies have suggested that, contrary to popular dogma, dehydration up to 3 or 4% body weight loss can be well-tolerated and does not affect performance in elite athletes (Goulet 2011; Noakes, 2012). A study of elite Ethiopian distance runners found that they consumed comparatively little fluid (1.75l per day) and did not drink anything before or during training (Beis *et al.*, 2011). The researchers suggest that mild dehydration may actually be an advantage in elite runners as, theoretically, it will lower the energy cost of running.

Tim Noakes, a professor of sport and exercise science at the University of Cape Town, South Africa believes that few runners are in danger of dehydration or heat exhaustion during races such as a half-marathon or longer. Indeed, they are in greater danger of overhydration. He says that core temperature, hydration status and performance

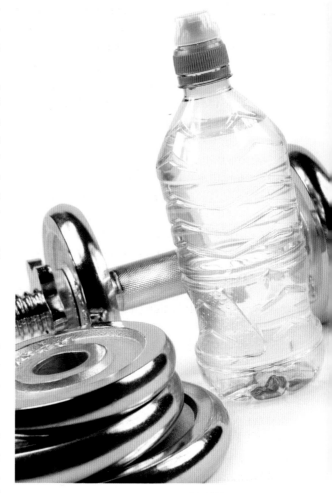

are unrelated. In other words, dehydration (or not drinking during exercise) does not result in a rise in core temperature, heat stroke or heat related illness. He also asserts that drinking during exercise will not reduce core temperature – this can only be achieved by reducing exercise intensity (e.g. walking instead of running) or exercising in cooler conditions. A 2006 study of Ironman triathletes in Australia found that quite large fluid losses of up to 3% of body mass had no adverse effect on performance (Laursen *et al*, 2006). There was little change in core temperature and other measures of dehydration stayed within normal ranges. Another study by researchers in France and South Africa found that dehydration equivalent to a 3% body weight loss had no adverse effect on performance during a marathon (Zouhal *et al*, 2011). In fact, those completing the marathon in the fastest times had the greatest body weight loss and there was a clear inverse relationship between body weight loss and performance time.

Professor Noakes believes that the body regulates its thermal response during prolonged exercise within a safe range, and warns against 'over-drinking' to maintain thermoregulation. Any rise in body temperature that occurs with dehydration is a biological adapatation that helps mammals conserve water (Noakes, 2012).

CAN I MINIMISE MY FLUID LOSS?

You cannot prevent your body from losing fluid. After all, this is a natural and desirable way to regulate body temperature. On the other hand, you can prevent your body from becoming dehydrated by offsetting fluid losses as far as possible. The best way to do this is to make sure you are well hydrated before you start exercising, and to drink adequate fluids (according to your thirst) during and after exercise (*see* 'When, what and how much should I drink?').

ARE YOU DEHYDRATED?

Many people, both athletes and non-athletes, suffer mild dehydration without realising it. Dehydration is cumulative, which means you can easily become dehydrated over successive days of training or competition if you fail to rehydrate fully between workouts or races. Symptoms of dehydration include sluggishness, a general sense of fatigue, headaches, loss of appetite, feeling excessively hot, lightheadedness and nausea.

From a practical point of view, you should be producing a dilute, pale-coloured urine. Concentrated, dark-coloured urine of a small volume indicates you are dehydrated and is a signal that you should drink more before you exercise. Indeed, many coaches and trainers advise their players or athletes to monitor their urine output and colour because this is a surprisingly accurate way of assessing hydration status. University of Connecticut researchers found that urine colour correlated very accurately with hydration status – as good as measurements of specific gravity and osmolality of the urine (Armstrong *et al.*, 1998). Urine described as 'very pale yellow' or 'pale yellow' indicates you are within 1% of optimal hydration.

HOW DO SWEATSUITS AFFECT FLUID LOSS?

Many athletes use sweatsuits, plastic, neoprene and other clothing to 'make' weight for competition. This is definitely not a good idea! By preventing sweat evaporation, the clothing prevents heat loss. This will cause the body temperature to rise more and more. In an attempt to expel this excess heat your body will continue to produce more sweat, thus losing increasing amounts of fluid. You will become dehydrated, with the undesirable consequences this entails.

As mentioned above, your ability to exercise will be impaired – you will suffer fatigue much sooner and will have to slow down or stop altogether. Obviously, this is not a good state in which to train or compete.

Losing weight through exercise in sweatsuits is not only potentially dangerous, but has no effect whatsoever on fat loss. Any weight loss will simply be fluid, which will be regained immediately when you next eat or drink. The exercise may seem harder because you will be sweating more, but this will not affect the body's rate of fat breakdown. If anything, you are likely to lose less fat, because you cannot exercise as hard or for as long when you wear a sweatsuit.

WHEN, WHAT AND HOW MUCH SHOULD I DRINK?
1. BEFORE EXERCISE

Your main priority is to ensure you are well-hydrated before exercise. It is clear that if you begin a training session or competition in a dehydrated state your performance will suffer and you will be at a competitive disadvantage. For example, in one study, runners performed a 5000 m run and a 10,000 m run in either a normally hydrated or slightly dehydrated condition (Armstrong *et al.*, 1985). When dehydrated by 2% of body weight their running speed dropped substantially (6–7%) in both events.

Obviously, prevention is better than cure. Make sure you are well hydrated before you begin exercising, especially in hot and humid weather. The easiest way to check your hydration status is by monitoring the colour and volume of your urine. It should be pale yellow, not completely clear. The American College of Sports Medicine (ACSM) recommends drinking 5–7 ml of fluid /kg BW slowly at least 4 hours before exercise to promote hydration and allow enough time for excretion of excess water (Sawka *et al.*, 2007). That's equivalent to 300–420 ml for a 60 kg person, or 350–490 ml for a 70 kg person. If this does not result in urine production within 2 hours or if your urine

is dark coloured, you should continue drinking. But don't force yourself to drink so much that you gain weight. The 2003 International Olympic Committee (IOC) Consensus Conference on Nutrition and Sport and the 2007 consensus statement of the International Association of Athletic Federations (IAAF) both caution against over-drinking before and during exercise, because of the risk of water intoxication.

2. DURING EXERCISE

There are no hard and fast rules about how much to drink, and old advice to 'drink before you feel thirsty' is no longer valid. The ACSM makes no specific recommendations about how much to drink because sweat rates and sweat composition vary considerably from one person to the next.

A small net fluid loss, equivalent to less than 2% of your body weight, is unlikely to affect your performance. However, greater losses will result in a drop in performance for most (non-elite) athletes, so experts advise limiting dehydration to less than 2% of your body weight (Sawka, 2007; IOC, 2004; Coyle, 2007). For example, this would mean 1 kg for a 50 kg person, 1.5 kg for a 75 kg person and 2 kg for a 100 kg person. However, in cold environments, dehydration greater than 2% is likely to be better tolerated. Also, dehydration of up to 3% has little effect on strength, power and sprint exercise.

Studies have shown that you can maintain optimal performance if you replace at least 80% of your sweat loss during exercise (Montain & Coyle, 1992). The best strategy is to work out how much fluid you lose through sweating by weighing yourself before and after a typical workout, then aim to drink sufficient to ensure a weight loss of no more than about 2%.

Can you 'fluid load' before exercise?

'Loading up' or 'hyper-hydrating' with fluid before an event seems advantageous for those competing in ultra-endurance events, activities during which there is little opportunity to drink, or in hot humid conditions. Unfortunately, you cannot achieve hyperhydration by simply consuming large volumes of water or sports drinks before the event. The body simply excretes surplus fluid and you will end up paying frequent visits to the toilet or bushes. However, there is a method of hyperhydration that involves the consumption of glycerol along with fluid 2 hours before exercise. Glycerol is a hyperhydrating agent, which, through its strong osmotic activity, drags water into both the extra-cellular and intra-cellular fluid. This results in an increase in total body fluid. In theory, you will be able to maintain blood volume, increase sweating and reduce the rise in core body temperature that occurs during exercise. Studies at the Australian Institute of Sport found that by doing this, athletes retained an extra 600 ml of fluid and improved performance in a time trial by 2.4% (Hitchins et al., 1999). A study at the University of Glasgow found that hyperhydrating with a combination of creatine and glycerol resulted in increased total body water but did not improve performance in a 16 km time trial compared with normal hydration (Easton et al., 2007). The potential performance benefits should be weighed up against the possible side effects, which include gastrointestinal upsets and headaches.

'DRINK ACCORDING TO YOUR THIRST'

Previous advice from the American College of Sports Medicine (ACSM, 1996; ACSM, 2000) to drink 'as much as possible' during exercise or 'to replace the weight lost during exercise' or *ad libitum*' has been replaced with advice to drink according to thirst because of the risk of hyponatraemia (water intoxication, a potentially fatal condition), particularly during prolonged exercise (Noakes, 2007; Noakes, 2010; Noakes, 2012). A Canadian study found that cyclists who drank according to thirst performed better than when they drank 'below' or 'above thirst' (Goulet 2011). Drinking when you're not thirsty confers no advantage.

Firstly, being slightly dehydrated does not harm performance or health, as was once believed to be the case. Second, the recommendation to drink enough fluid to prevent weight loss is based on the false assumption that all your weight loss is sweat. In fact, a significant amount of weight loss is due to the loss of water stored with fat and carbohydrate, which is released when these stores are converted into energy. This contributes to sweat loss, but does not cause dehydration because it does not reduce blood volume. Third, drinking too much water during exercise dilutes the concentration of sodium in the blood and may lead to hyponatraemia.

The new advice for regular exercisers and athletes is: don't force yourself to drink. The IAAF advises drinking when you're thirsty or drinking only to the point at which you're maintaining your weight, not gaining weight. Drink less if you begin to have a queasy sloshy feeling in your stomach. If you plan to run a marathon or exercise for more than four hours in warm weather, drink no more than 800 ml per hour, be guided by thirst and sip a sports drink containing sugar and salt instead of plain water.

PRACTICAL CONSIDERATIONS

From a practical point of view, the ACSM recommend cool drinks (15–22°C). You will also be inclined to drink more if the drink is palatable and in a container that makes it easy to drink. Studies have shown that during exercise athletes voluntarily drink more of a flavoured sweetened drink than water, be it a sports drink, diluted fruit juice, or fruit squash (Passe *et al.*, 2004; Wilk & Bar-Or, 1996; Minehan, 2002). Drinks bottles with sports caps are probably the most popular containers. It is also important to make drinks readily accessible: for example, for swim training have drinks bottles at the poolside; for games played on a pitch or court (soccer, hockey, rugby, netball, tennis), have the bottles available adjacent to the pitch or court.

SPORTS DRINKS VS WATER

During low or moderate-intensity activities such as 'easy pace' swimming, cycling, or power walking carried out for less than an hour, fluid losses are likely to be relatively small and can be replaced fast enough with plain water. There is little benefit to be gained from drinking sports drinks compared with water during these types of activities.

During high-intensity exercise lasting less than an hour, drinking a sports drink containing up to 8 g sugar/100 ml rather than water may benefit your performance (Wagenmakers *et al.*, 1996; Ball *et al.*, 1995). Examples of these activities include a 10 km run, tennis, squash, cycling, sprint training, circuit training and weight training.

During high-intensity exercise lasting longer than an hour (e.g. half-marathon, football match), you require rapid fluid replacement, as well as fuel replacement. In other words, you need to avoid early glycogen depletion and low

Is it possible to drink too much water?

Water intoxication or hyponatraemia sometimes happens in long distance runners or triathletes who consume a lot of water and lose a lot of salt through sweat (Noakes, 2000; Speedy *et al.*, 1999; Barr *et al.*, 1989). During intense exercise urine output is reduced, which further limits the body's ability to correct the imbalance. As the water content of the blood increases, the salt content is diluted. Consequently, the amount of salt available to body tissues decreases, which can lead to problems with brain, heart and muscle function. Initial symptoms of over-hydration include dizziness, nausea, bloating, lapses in consciousness and seizures due to swelling of the brain. However, these symptoms are also associated with dehydration so it's important to be aware of how much you are drinking. An advisory statement on fluid replacement in marathons written for the International Marathon Medical Directors Association and USA Track & Field advises endurance runners not to drink as much as possible but to drink *ad libitum* no more than 400–800 ml per hour (Noakes, 2002).

If you are sweating heavily for long periods of time, drink dilute electrolyte/carbohydrate drinks rather than plain water. These will help avoid hyponatraemia, maintain better fluid levels in the body, spare muscle glycogen and delay fatigue.

Table 7.1 Summary of recommendations for carbohydrate intake during exercise

Exercise duration	Recommended amount of carbohydrate	Type of carbohydrate
< 45 minutes	None	None
45–75 minutes	v small amounts (mouth rinse)	Any
1–2 hours	Up to 30 g/h	Any
2–3 hours	Up to 60 g/h	Glucose, maltodextrins
3 hours	Up to 90 g/h	Multiple transportable carbohydrates (glucose + fructose or maltodextrin + fructose in 2:1 ratio)

Table 7.2 Choosing the right type of drink

Exercise conditions	Drink
Exercise lasting <30 minutes	Nothing; water
Low–moderate intensity exercise lasting less than 1 hour	Water
High-intensity exercise lasting less than 1 hour	Hypotonic or isotonic sports drink
High-intensity exercise lasting more than 1 hour	Hypotonic or isotonic sports drink or glucose polymer drink

blood sugar, as well as dehydration, as all three can result in fatigue.

During hot and humid conditions you may be losing more than 1 litre of sweat per hour. Therefore, you should increase your drink volume (although still be guided by your thirst), if possible, and use a more dilute drink (around 20–40 g/L).

For exercise longer than 1 hour, the consensus recommendation is an intake of between 30–60 g carbohydrate/hour (IOC, 2011; Burke *et al.*, 2011; ACSM/ADA/DC, 2009; Coggan and Coyle, 1991) to maintain blood sugar levels and delay fatigue. Most commercial sports drinks

contain this level, which corresponds to the maximum rate at which fluid can be emptied from the stomach. More concentrated fluids take longer to absorb (ACSM, 1996).

For exercise lasting more than 3 hours, consuming 90g carbohydrate/hour can increase performance. However, this can be achieved only by consuming a mixture of carbohydrates ('multiple transportable carbohydrates'): glucose + fructose, or maltodextrin + fructose in a 2:1 ratio (IOC, 2010; Jeukendrup, 2008). This carbohydrate mixture appears to increase carbohydrate oxidation in the muscles as well as increase fluid uptake. It is possible to make up these drinks yourself although commercial sports drinks and gels with this formulation are becoming available.

Sports drinks based on glucose polymers may be a good choice if your sweat rate is low (e.g. during cold conditions) yet you are exercising hard, because they can provide more fuel than fluid replacers as well as reasonable amounts of fluid. In practice, many athletes find that glucose polymer drinks cause stomach discomfort and that sports drinks containing 4–8 g carbohydrate/100 ml do an equally good job.

The key to choosing the right drink during exercise is to experiment with different drinks in training to find one that suits you best (see Table 7.2).

WHY DO I FEEL NAUSEOUS WHEN I DRINK DURING EXERCISE?

If you feel nauseous or experience other gastro-intestinal symptoms when you drink during exercise, this may either indicate that you are dehydrated or be related to the fact you are exercising at a very high intensity for a prolonged period. In the former case, you need to be aware that even a fairly small degree of dehydration (around 2% of body weight) slows down stomach emptying and upsets the normal rhythmical movement of your gut. This can result in bloating, nausea and vomiting. Avoid this by ensuring you are well hydrated before exercise and then continue drinking little and often according to thirst during your workout. In the latter case, it is the nature of the training (i.e. high intensity prolonged exercise) that affects gut motility, causing discomfort and nausea. If you are prone to such symptoms during training or competition, ensure that you are well hydrated before exercise

Why do some people get stomach cramps from sports drinks?

There are lots of anecdotal reports suggesting sports drinks can cause cramping, discomfort or heaviness during exercise. Indeed, a study at the Gatorade Sports Science Institute, Illinois found that athletes experienced greater stomach discomfort during circuit training after drinking an 8% sports drink compared with a 6% drink (Shi et al., 2004). It is known that more concentrated drinks empty more slowly from the stomach and are absorbed more slowly from the intestines, which would explain the increased gastro-intestinal discomfort. Many people find that diluting sports drinks helps alleviate these problems, but there's a balance to be struck between obtaining enough carbohydrate to fuel your exercise and avoiding GI discomfort. If the drink is too dilute you may not consume enough carbohydrate to achieve peak performance. A study at the Georgia Institute of Technology found that athletes performed equally after drinking a 6% or 8% drink (Millard-Stafford et al., 2005). And researchers at the University of Iowa in the US found that diluting a 6% drink down to 3% (i.e. 3 g carbohydrate per 100 ml) had no effect on stomach emptying rate and resulted in a similar rate of water absorption (Rogers et al., 2005). The bottom line is: work out from trial and error the concentration of sports drink that suits you best.

so the risk of dehydration and therefore the need to drink during exercise will be less.

3. AFTER EXERCISE

Both water and sodium need to be replaced to restore normal fluid balance after exercise. This can be achieved by water (or non-sports drinks) plus accompanying food if there is no urgency for recovery (Shirreffs and Sawka, 2011). Researchers recommend you should consume approximately 1.2–1.5 times the weight of fluid lost during exercise (IAAF, 2007; Shirreffs et al., 2004; Shirreffs et al., 1996). The simplest way to work out how much you need to drink is to weigh yourself before and after training. Working on the basis that 1 litre of sweat is roughly equivalent to a 1 kg body weight loss, you need to drink 1.2–1.5 l fluid for each kg of weight lost during exercise.

You should not drink the whole amount straightaway, as a rapid increase in blood volume promotes urination and increases the risk of hyponatraemia. Consume as much as you feel comfortable with, then drink the remainder in divided doses until you are fully hydrated.

Sports drinks may be better than water at speeding recovery after exercise, particularly when fluid losses are high (e.g. a loss of more than 5% body mass) or for those athletes who train or compete twice a day. The problem with drinking water is that it causes a drop in blood osmolality (i.e. it dilutes sodium in the blood), reducing your thirst and increasing urine output, and so you may stop drinking before you are rehydrated (Maughan et al., 1996; Gonzalez-Alonzo et al., 1992). Sodium plays an important role in driving the thirst mechanism. A low sodium concentration in the blood signals to the brain a low thirst sensation. Conversely, a high sodium concentration in the blood signals greater thirst and thus drives you to drink. Hence, the popular strategy of putting salted peanuts and crisps at the bar to encourage customers to buy more drink to quench their thirst! Sports drinks, on the other hand, increase the urge to drink and decrease urine production.

But research at Loughborough University suggests that skimmed milk may be an even better option for promoting post-exercise rehydration (Shirreffs et al., 2007). Volunteers who drank skimmed milk after exercise achieved net positive hydration throughout the recovery period, but returned to net negative fluid balance one hour after drinking either water or a sports drink.

A further US study also suggests that consuming a drink containing carbohydrate with a small amount of protein improves fluid retention after exercise (Seifert et al., 2007). Those athletes who consumed the carbohydrate-protein drink retained 15% more fluid than carbohydrate-only and 40% more than water alone.

HOW MUCH SHOULD I DRINK ON NON-EXERCISING DAYS?

While there's no doubt that maintaining your fluid levels is very important, the belief that we need 8 glasses of water a day to stay healthy is a myth. A 2008 review of studies from the University of Pennsylvania in the US concluded that there is no clear evidence of any benefits from drinking so much. Most people can rely on their sense of thirst as a good indicator of when they should drink. Though 1.5–2 litres of water is the oft quoted amount needed to keep you hydrated, you shouldn't be too concerned about sticking to it rigidly. From a hydration point of view, it does not matter where you get your liquid from – coffee, tea, fruit juice, soup, squash and milk all count towards the total.

THE SCIENCE OF SPORTS DRINKS
WHAT TYPES OF SPORTS DRINKS ARE AVAILABLE?

Sports drinks can be divided into two main categories: fluid replacement drinks and carbohydrate (energy) drinks.

- Fluid replacement drinks are dilute solutions of electrolytes and sugars (carbohydrate). The sugars most commonly added are glucose, sucrose, fructose and glucose polymers (maltodextrins). The main aim of these drinks is to replace fluid faster than plain water, although the extra sugars will also help maintain blood sugar levels and spare glycogen. These drinks may be either hypotonic or isotonic (see below).
- Carbohydrate (energy) drinks provide more carbohydrate per 100 ml than fluid replacement drinks. The carbohydrate is mainly in the form of glucose polymers (maltodextrins). The main aim is to provide larger amounts of carbohydrate but at an equal or lower osmolality than the same concentration of glucose. They will, of course, provide fluid as well. Ready-to-drink brands are generally isotonic. Powders that you make up into a drink may be made hypotonic or isotonic (see below).

WHAT IS THE DIFFERENCE BETWEEN HYPOTONIC, ISOTONIC AND HYPERTONIC DRINKS?

- A hypotonic drink – often marketed as 'lite' or as 'sports water' – has a relatively low osmolality, which means it contains fewer particles (carbohydrate and electrolytes) per 100 ml than the body's own fluids. As it is more dilute, it is absorbed faster than plain water. Typically, a hypotonic drink contains less than 4 g carbohydrate/100 ml.
- An isotonic drink – a typical 'sports drink' – has the same osmolality as the body's fluids, which means it contains about the same number of particles (carbohydrate and electrolytes) per 100 ml and is therefore absorbed as fast as or faster than plain water. Most commercial isotonic drinks contain between 4 and 8 g carbohydrate/100 ml. In theory, isotonic drinks provide the ideal compromise between rehydration and refuelling.
- A hypertonic drink – such as cola and other ready-to-drink soft drinks – has a higher osmolality than body fluids, as it contains more particles (carbohydrate and electrolytes) per 100 ml than the body's fluids, i.e. it is more concentrated. This means it is absorbed more slowly than plain water. A hypertonic drink usually contains more than 8 g carbohydrate/100 ml.

WHEN SHOULD I OPT FOR A SPORTS DRINK INSTEAD OF WATER?

Opting for a sports drink would benefit your performance during any moderate or high intensity event lasting longer than about one hour. Numerous studies have shown that sports drinks containing about 40–80 g carbohydrate/litre promote both hydration and normal blood sugar levels, and enhance performance during intense and/or prolonged exercise (Coggan & Coyle, 1991; Coyle, 2004; Jeukendrup, 2004). If you are exercising longer than 2 hours or sweating very heavily, you should opt for a sports drink that also contains sodium (Coyle, 2007).

Researchers at the Medical School at the University of Aberdeen found that sports drinks containing glucose and sodium can delay fatigue (Galloway & Maughan, 2000). Cyclists given a dilute sports drink (2% carbohydrate) were able to keep going considerably longer (118 mins) than those drinking plain water (71 mins) or even a higher strength (15% carbohydrate) sports drink (84 mins). The success of the more dilute drink may be due to the larger volume drunk.

For example, in a study carried out by researchers at Loughborough University, seven endurance runners drank similar volumes of either water, a 5.5% sports drink (5.5 g carbohydrate/100 ml) or 6.9% (6.9 g carbohydrate/100 ml) sports drink before and during a 42 km treadmill run (Tsintzas *et al.*, 1995). Those who took the 5.5% sports drink produced running times on average 3.9 minutes faster compared with water, and 2.4 minutes faster compared with the 6.9% drink.

At Texas University, 8 cyclists performed a time trial lasting approximately 10 minutes after completing 50 minutes of high-intensity cycling at 85% VO_2max. Those who drank a sports drink (6 g carbohydrate/100 ml) during the 50 minute cycle reduced the time taken to cycle the final trial by 6% compared with those who drank water (Below *et al.*, 1995).

In a study at the University of South Carolina, cyclists who consumed a sports drink containing 6 g carbohydrate/100 ml knocked 3 minutes off their time during a time trial, compared with those who drank plain water (Davis *et al.*, 1988).

WHAT ARE ELECTROLYTES?

Electrolytes are mineral salts dissolved in the body's fluid. They include sodium, chloride, potassium and magnesium, and help to regulate the fluid balance between different body compartments (for example, the amount of fluid inside and outside a muscle cell), and the volume of fluid in the bloodstream. The water movement is controlled by the concentration of electrolytes on either side of the cell membrane. For example, an increase in the concentration of sodium outside a cell will cause water to move to it from inside the cell. Similarly, a drop in sodium concentration will cause water to move from the outside to the inside of the cell. Potassium draws water across a membrane, so a high potassium concentration inside cells increases the cell's water content.

Sports drinks and tooth enamel
Research at Birmingham University has found that sports drinks can dissolve tooth enamel and the hard dentine underneath, resulting in tooth erosion (Venables *et al.*, 2005). Their high acidity levels means that they can erode up to 30 times more tooth enamel than water. A 2007 study comparing the 'buffering capacity' of various drinks found that popular sports drinks and energy drinks have a greater potential to cause tooth erosion than cola (Owens 2007). Drinking them during exercise makes the effects worse because exercise reduces saliva needed to combat the drink's acidity. Similar erosive problems can occur when drinking soft drinks and fruit juice. Best advice is to drink quickly to minimise contact with the teeth, use chilled drinks (they are less erosive) and rinse your mouth with water after drinking them. Researchers are hoping to produce a sports drink that is less harmful to the teeth.

WHY DO SPORTS DRINKS CONTAIN ELECTROLYTES?

Electrolytes in sports drinks do not have a direct effect on performance. Sodium is the only electrolyte that has a potential benefit but only after, not during exercise: it increases the urge to drink, improves palatability and promotes fluid retention. The increase in sodium concentration and decrease in blood volume that accompany exercise increase your natural thirst sensation, making you want to drink. If you drink plain water it effectively dilutes the sodium, thus reducing your urge to drink before you are fully hydrated. Therefore, including a small amount of sodium (0.23–0.69 g/l) in a sports drink will encourage you to drink more fluid (Sawka *et al.*, 2007; ACSM, 1996; 2000).

It was originally thought that sodium also speeds water absorption in the intestines. However, research at the University of Iowa has since shown that adding sodium to a sports drink does not enhance fluid absorption (Gisolphi *et al.*, 1995). Researchers discovered that after you have consumed any kind of drink, sodium passes from the blood plasma into the intestine, where it then stimulates water absorption. In other words, the body sorts out the sodium concentration of the liquid in your intestines all by itself, so the addition of sodium to sports drinks is unnecessary.

Glucose is more important than sodium for promoting fluid absorption. That said, sodium remains a key ingredient in sports drinks – a marketing ploy by manufacturers! (Noakes, 2012). Other electrolytes, such as magnesium, potassium and calcium may be included in sports drinks, but there is no proven benefit to performance.

What does osmolality mean?

Osmolality is a measure of the number of dissolved particles in a fluid. A drink with a high osmolality means that it contains more particles per 100 ml than one with a low osmolality. These particles may include sugars, glucose polymers, sodium or other electrolytes. The osmolality of the drink determines which way the fluid will move across a membrane (e.g. the gut wall). For example, if a drink with a relatively high osmolality is consumed, then water moves from the bloodstream and gut cells into the gut. This is called net secretion. If a drink with a relatively low osmolality is consumed, then water is absorbed from the gut (i.e. the drink) to the gut cells and bloodstream. Thus there is net water absorption.

WHY DO SPORTS DRINKS CONTAIN CARBOHYDRATES (SUGARS)?

Carbohydrate in sports drinks serves two purposes: speeding up water absorption (Gisolphi *et al.*, 1992) and providing an additional source of energy (Coggan & Coyle, 1987).

Relatively dilute solutions of sugar (hypotonic or isotonic) stimulate water absorption from the small intestine into the bloodstream. A sugar concentration usually in the range 5 to 8 g/100 ml is used in isotonic sports drinks to accelerate water absorption. More concentrated drinks (hypertonic), above 8%, tend to slow down the stomach emptying and therefore reduce the speed of fluid replacement (Murray *et al.*, 1999).

Studies have shown that consuming extra carbohydrate during exercise can improve performance because it helps maintain blood glucose levels (Febbraio *et al.*, 2000; Bosch *et al.*, 1994).

WHAT ARE GLUCOSE POLYMERS?

Between a sugar (1–2 units) and a starch (several 100,000 units), although closer to the former, are glucose polymers (maltodextrins). These are chains of between 4 and 20 glucose molecules produced from boiling cornstarch under controlled commercial conditions.

The advantage of using glucose polymers instead of glucose or sucrose in a drink is that a higher concentration of carbohydrate can be achieved (usually between 10 and 20 g/100 ml) at a lower osmolality. That's because each molecule contains several glucose units yet still exerts the same osmotic pressure as just one molecule of glucose. So an isotonic or hypotonic drink can be produced with a carbohydrate content greater than 8 g/100 ml.

Also, glucose polymers are less sweet than simple sugars, so you can achieve a fairly concentrated drink that does not taste too sickly. In fact, most glucose polymer drinks are fairly tasteless unless they have added artificial flavours or sweeteners.

WHAT ARE 'MULTIPLE TRANSPORTABLE CARBOHYDRATES'?

This term refers to a mixture of carbohydrates (e.g. glucose and fructose; maltodextrin and fructose) in sports drinks. These carbohydrates are absorbed from the intestine by different transporters, and using a mixture rather than a single type of carbohydrate in a sports drink overcomes the usual limitation of gut uptake of carbohydrate. Studies show that such mixtures increase muscle carbohydrate uptake and oxidation during exercise compared with glucose-only drinks (Jeukendrup, 2010; IOC, 2010; Jeukendrup, 2008).

It means that more concentrated drinks can be consumed, providing the body with 90 g carbohydrate/hour instead of 30–60 g/hour. These drinks

How does weather affect performance?

Air temperature and wind speed can both affect performance. The hotter and more humid the weather, and the less wind there is, the more fluid your body will lose and the greater the chance of dehydration occurring.

In one study, 6 athletes cycled on a stationary bike at a set resistance. When the surrounding temperature was 2°C they could cycle for 73 minutes before experiencing exhaustion. When the surrounding temperature increased to 33°C, they could only cycle for 35 minutes. When the athletes were given a carbohydrate drink it was found that they could keep going for longer in the cold temperature. However, the drink made no difference in the hot temperature.

In hot conditions the body's priority is to replace water rather than carbohydrate. So drink water or a dilute carbohydrate electrolyte drink rather than a more concentrated carbohydrate drink. If you exercise in cold weather and sweat only a little, you may find a more concentrated carbohydrate drink beneficial.

would be appropriate only if you are exercising at a high intensity for three hours or longer.

SHOULD I CHOOSE STILL OR CARBONATED SPORTS DRINKS?

Experiments at East Carolina University and Ball State University found that carbonated and still sports drinks produced equal hydration in the body (Hickey *et al.*, 1994). However, the carbon-

Table 7.3 DIY sports drinks

Hypotonic	Isotonic
• 20–40 g sucrose I L warm water 1–1.5 g (¼ tsp) salt (optional) Sugar-free/low-calorie squash for flavouring (optional)	• 40–80 g sucrose I L warm water 1–1.5 g (¼ tsp) salt (optional) Sugar-free/low-calorie squash for flavouring (optional)
• 100 ml fruit squash 900 ml water 1–1.5 g (¼ tsp) salt (optional)	• 200 ml fruit squash 800 ml water 1–1.5 g (¼ tsp) salt (optional)
• 250 ml fruit juice 750 ml water 1–1.5 g (¼ tsp) salt (optional)	• 500 ml fruit juice 500 ml water 1–1.5 g (¼ tsp) salt (optional)

ated drinks tended to produce a higher incidence of mild heartburn and stomach discomfort. In practice, many athletes find that carbonated drinks make them feel full and 'gassy', which may well limit the amount they drink.

Should I take salt tablets in hot weather?

No, salt tablets are not a good idea, even if you are sweating heavily in hot weather. They produce a very concentrated sodium solution in your stomach (strongly hypertonic), which delays stomach emptying and rehydration as extra fluid must first be absorbed from your body into your stomach to dilute the sodium. The best way to replace fluid and electrolyte losses is by drinking a dilute sodium/carbohydrate drink (either hypotonic or isotonic) with a sodium concentration of 40–110 mg/100 ml.

CAN I MAKE MY OWN SPORTS DRINKS?

Definitely! Commercial sports drinks work out to be very expensive if you are drinking at least 1 litre per day to replace fluid losses during exercise. (If you need to drink less than 1 litre, you probably don't need a sports drink anyway.)

Table 7.3 includes some recipes for making your own sports drink.

OTHER NON-ALCOHOLIC DRINKS
CAN ORDINARY SOFT DRINKS AND FRUIT JUICE IMPROVE PERFORMANCE?

Ordinary soft drinks (typically between 9 and 20 g carbohydrate/100 ml) and fruit juices (typically between 11 and 13 g carbohydrate/100 ml) are hypertonic; in other words, they are more concentrated than body fluids, so are not ideal as fluid replacers during exercise. They empty more slowly from the stomach than plain water because they must first be diluted with water from the body, thus causing a temporary net reduction in body fluid.

If you dilute one part fruit juice with one part water, you will get an isotonic drink, ideal for rehydrating and refuelling during or after exercise (see Table 7.3).

CAN 'LITE', 'FITNESS' OR 'SPORTS WATERS' IMPROVE PERFORMANCE?

These types of drinks are hypotonic, containing around 2% sugar along with artificial sweeteners, flavourings, sodium and various vitamins and minerals. Their high sodium content means they may promote fluid retention and stimulate thirst more than plain water, and the flavours make the drinks palatable – but they don't deliver much carbohydrate energy (around 10 calories per 100 ml). They would therefore not be advantageous for intense workouts lasting longer than 1 hour and, even for shorter workouts, offer few advantages over plain water, apart from improving palatability and encouraging you to drink more.

ARE 'DIET' DRINKS SUITABLE DURING EXERCISE?

'Diet' or low-calorie drinks contain artificial sweeteners in place of sugars and have a very low sodium concentration. They are, therefore, useless as fuel replacers during exercise, although they will help replace fluid at approximately the same speed as plain water. Artificial sweeteners have no known advantage or disadvantage on performance. Choose these types of drink only if you dislike the taste of water, and under the same circumstances that you would normally choose

water, i.e. for low- to moderate-intensity exercise lasting less than 1 hour.

CAN CAFFEINE-CONTAINING ENERGY DRINKS IMPROVE MY PERFORMANCE?

A number of energy drinks containing caffeine claim to improve some aspect of performance, such as alertness, endurance or concentration during exercise. The exact mechanism is not clear, but it is thought that caffeine at doses of 1–3 mg/kg reduces the perception of fatigue and allows you to continue exercising at a higher intensity for a longer period (Graham & Spriet, 1995). For a 70kg person, this would be 210 mg, equivalent to about 2 cups of coffee or 2 cans of caffeinated energy drink. Performance benefits occur soon after consumption so caffeine may be consumed just before exercise, spread throughout exercise, or late in exercise as fatigue is beginning to occur. As individual responses vary, you should experiment during training to find the dose and protocol that suits you.

A study at the University of Saskatchewan tested the effects of Red Bull energy drink on weight training performance (Forbes et al., 2007). They found that consuming Red Bull (in amounts equivalent to 2 mg caffeine per kg body weight; each can contains 80 mg caffeine) one hour before exercise significantly increased bench press muscle endurance.

SHOULD I AVOID REHYDRATING WITH CAFFEINATED DRINKS?

It is a myth that you should completely avoid rehydrating with caffeinated drinks such as tea, coffee or cola. Researchers at the University of Maastricht found that cyclists were able to

Table 7.4	Caffeine content of various drinks and foods
Drink	**mg caffeine/cup**
Ground coffee	80–90
Instant coffee	60
Decaffeinated coffee	3
Tea	40
Energy/sports drinks	Up to 100 (per can)
Can of cola	40
Energy gel (1 sachet)	40
Chocolate (54 g bar)	40

rehydrate after a long cycle equally well with water or a caffeine-containing cola drink (Brouns, 1998). Urine output was the same after both drinks. However, large doses of caffeine – over 600 mg, enough to cause a marked ergogenic effect – may result in a larger fluid loss. A study at the University of Connecticut, US, found that both caffeine-containing cola and caffeine-free cola maintained hydration in athletes (during the non-exercise periods) over three successive days of training (Fiala *et al.*, 2004). The athletes drank water during training sessions but rehydrated with either caffeinated or caffeine-free drinks. A further study by the same researchers confirmed that moderate caffeine intakes (up to 452 mg caffeine/ kg body weight/ day) did not increase urine output compared with a placebo and concluded that caffeine does not cause a fluid electrolyte balance in the body (Armstrong *et al.*, 2005).

ALCOHOL
HOW DOES ALCOHOL AFFECT PERFORMANCE?

Drinking alcohol before exercise may appear to make you more alert and confident but, even in small amounts, it will certainly have the following negative effects:

* reduce coordination, reaction time, balance and judgement
* reduce strength, power, speed and endurance
* reduce your ability to regulate body temperature
* reduce blood sugar levels and increase the risk of hypoglycaemia
* increase water excretion (urination) and the risk of dehydration
* increase the risk of accident or injury.

CAN I DRINK ALCOHOL ON NON-TRAINING DAYS?

There is no reason why you cannot enjoy alcohol in moderation on non-training days. The Department of Health recommends up to 4 units a day for men and 3 units a day for women as a safe upper limit (see Table 7.5 for 1 unit equivalent measures). The daily limits are intended to discourage binge-drinking, which is dangerous to health. In fact, research has shown that alcohol drunk in moderation reduces the risk of heart disease. Moderate drinkers have a lower risk of death from heart disease than teetotallers or heavy drinkers. The exact mechanism is not certain, but it may work by increasing HDL cholesterol levels, the protective type of cholesterol in the blood. HDL transports cholesterol back to the liver for excretion, thereby reducing the chance of it sticking to artery walls. It may also reduce the stickiness of blood platelets, thus reducing the risk

Table 7.5	Alcoholic and calorie contents of drinks	
Drink equivalent to 1 unit	**% alcohol by volume**	**Calories**
½ pint ordinary beer/lager	3.0–3.5	90
1 measure spirits	38	50
1 measure vermouth/aperitif	18	60–80
125 ml glass of wine	11	75–100
1 measure sherry	16	55–70
1 measure liqueur	40	75–100

of blood clots (thrombosis). Red wine, in particular, may be especially good for the heart. Studies have shown that drinking up to two glasses a day can lower heart disease risk by 30–70%. It contains flavanoids from the grape skin, which have an antioxidant effect and thus protect the LDL cholesterol from free radical damage.

IS ALCOHOL FATTENING?

Any food or drink can be 'fattening' if you consume more calories than you need. Alcohol itself provides 7 kcal/g, and many alcoholic drinks also have quite a high sugar/carbohydrate content, boosting the total calorie content further (see Table 7.5). Excess calories from alcoholic drinks can, therefore, lead to fat gain.

WHAT EXACTLY HAPPENS TO ALCOHOL IN THE BODY?

When you drink alcohol, about 20% is absorbed into the bloodstream through the stomach and the remainder through the small intestine. Most of this alcohol is then broken down in the liver (it cannot be stored, as it is toxic) into a substance called acetyl CoA and then, ultimately, into ATP (adenosine triphosphate or energy). Obviously, whilst this is occurring, less glycogen and fat are used to produce ATP in other parts of the body.

However, the liver can carry out this job only at a fixed rate of approximately 1 unit alcohol/hour. If you drink more alcohol than this, it is dealt with by a different enzyme system in the liver (the microsomal ethanol oxidising system, MEO) to make it less toxic to the body. The more alcohol you drink on a regular basis, the more MEO enzymes are produced, which is why you can develop an increased tolerance to alcohol – you need to drink more to experience the same physiological effects.

Initially, alcohol reduces inhibitions, increases self-confidence and makes you feel more at ease. However, it is actually a depressant rather than a stimulant, reducing your psychomotor (coordination) skills. It is potentially toxic to all of the cells and organs in your body and, if it builds up to high concentrations, it can cause damage to the liver, stomach and brain.

Too much alcohol causes hangovers – headache, thirst, nausea, vomiting and heartburn. These symptoms are due partly to dehydration and a swelling of the blood vessels in the head. Congeners, substances found mainly in darker alcoholic drinks such as rum and red wine, are also responsible for many of the hangover symptoms. Prevention is better than cure, so make sure you follow the guidelines on page 120. The best way to deal with a hangover is to drink plenty of water or, better still, a sports drink. Avoid coffee or tea because these will make dehydration worse. Do not attempt to train or compete with a hangover!

SUMMARY OF KEY POINTS

- Dehydration causes cardiovascular stress, increases core body temperature and impairs performance.
- Fluid losses during exercise depend on exercise duration and intensity; temperature and humidity; body size; fitness level and the individual. They can be as high as 1–2 litres/hour.
- Always start exercise well hydrated.
- During exercise, drink only to the point at which you are maintaining not gaining weight. Drink according to thirst to avoid the risk of hyponatraemia.
- Aim to replace at least 80% of sweat loss during exercise.
- After exercise, replace by 150% any body weight deficit.

- Water is a suitable fluid replacement drink for low- or moderate-intensity exercise lasting less than 1 hour.
- For intense exercise, lasting up to 1 hour, a sports drink containing up to 8% carbohydrate (8 g carbohydrate/100 ml) can speed up water absorption, provide additional fuel, delay fatigue and improve performance.
- Consuming 20–60 g carbohydrate/hour can maintain blood sugar levels, and improve performance in intense exercise lasting more than 1 hour.
- Hypotonic (<4%) and isotonic (4–8%) sports drinks are most suitable when rapid fluid replacement is the main priority.
- Carbohydrate drinks based on glucose polymers also replace fluids, but provide greater amounts of carbohydrate (10–20%) at a lower osmolality. They are most suitable for prolonged intense exercise (>90 minutes), when fuel replacement is a major priority or fluid losses are small.
- The main purpose of sodium in a sports drink is to increase the urge to drink and increase palatability.
- Alcohol before exercise has a negative effect on strength, endurance, co-ordination, power and speed, and increases injury risk.
- Moderate amounts of alcohol (<4 units/day for men; <3 units/day for women) in the overall diet – particularly red wine, which is rich in antioxidants – may protect against heart disease.

BODY FAT AND DIETARY FAT

8

As athletes in almost every sport strive to get leaner and competitive standards get higher, the relationship between body fat, health and performance becomes increasingly important. However, the optimal body composition for fitness or sports performance is not necessarily a desirable one from a health point of view. This chapter deals with different methods for measuring body fat percentage and body fat distribution, and considers their relevance to performance. It highlights the dangers of attaining very low body fat levels, as well as the risks associated with a very low-fat diet. It gives realistic guidance on recommended body fat ranges and fat intakes, and explains the difference between the various types of fats found in the diet.

DOES BODY FAT AFFECT PERFORMANCE?

Carrying around excess body weight in the form of fat is a distinct disadvantage in almost every sport. It can adversely affect strength, speed and endurance. Surplus fat is basically surplus baggage. Carrying around this extra weight is not only unnecessary, but also costly in terms of energy expenditure.

For example, in endurance sports (e.g. long distance running) surplus fat can reduce speed and increase fatigue. It is like carrying a couple of shopping bags with you as you run; they make it harder for you to get up speed, slow you down and cause you to tire quickly. It is best to leave your shopping bags at home, or at least to lighten the load.

In explosive sports (e.g. sprinting/jumping), where you must transfer or lift the weight of your whole body very quickly, extra fat again is non-functional weight, slowing you down, reducing your power and decreasing your mechanical efficiency. Muscle is useful weight, whereas excess fat is not.

In weight-matched sports (e.g. boxing, karate, judo, lightweight rowing), greater emphasis is put on body weight, particularly during the competitive season. The person with the greatest percentage of muscle and the smallest percentage of fat has the advantage.

In virtually every sport, it is the leanest body that wins. Reducing your body fat while maintaining lean mass and health will result in improved performance.

IS BODY FAT AN ADVANTAGE IN CERTAIN SPORTS?

Until recently it was believed that extra weight – even in the form of fat – was an advantage for certain sports in which momentum is important (e.g. discus, hammer throwing, judo, wrestling).

A heavy body can generate more momentum to throw an object or knock over an opponent, but there is no reason why this weight should be fat. It would be better if it were in the form of muscle. Muscle is stronger and more powerful than fat – although, admittedly, it is harder to acquire! If two athletes both weighed 100 kg, but one comprised 90 kg lean (10 kg fat) mass, and the other 70 kg lean (30 kg fat) mass, the leaner one would obviously have the advantage. Perhaps the only sport where fat could be considered a necessary advantage is sumo wrestling – it would be almost impossible to acquire a very large body mass without fat gain.

HOW CAN I TELL IF I AM TOO FAT?

Looking in the mirror is the quickest and simplest way to see if you are too fat by everyday standards, but this will not give the accurate information that you need for your sport. Many women also tend to perceive themselves as fatter than they really are. It is useful, therefore, to employ some sort of measurement system so that you can work towards a definite goal.

Standing on a set of scales, reading your weight and comparing it to standard weight and height charts is easy. However, it has several drawbacks. Weights and heights given in charts are based on average weights of a sample population. They are only *average* weights for *average* people, not ideal weights, and give no indication of health risk.

To get a general picture of your health risk, you can calculate your Body Mass Index (BMI) from your weight and height measurements.

HOW MUCH BODY FAT DO I REALLY NEED?

A fat-free body would not survive. It is important to realise that a certain amount of body fat is absolutely vital. In fact, there are two components of body fat: essential fat and storage fat. *Essential fat* includes the fat that forms part of your cell membranes, brain tissue, nerve sheaths, bone marrow and the fat surrounding your organs (e.g. heart, liver, kidneys). Here it provides insulation, protection and cushioning against physical damage. In a healthy person, this accounts for about 3% of body weight.

Women have an additional essential fat requirement called sex-specific fat, which is stored mostly in the breasts and around the hips. This fat accounts for a further 5–9% of a woman's body weight and is involved in oestrogen production as well as the conversion of inactive oestrogen into its

Table 8.1	BMI classification	
<20	Underweight	increasing health risk
20–24.9	'Normal' weight (Grade 0)	lowest health risk
25–29.9	Overweight/'plump' (Grade I)	
30–40	Moderately obese (Grade II)	increasing health risk
40+	Severely obese (Grade III)	

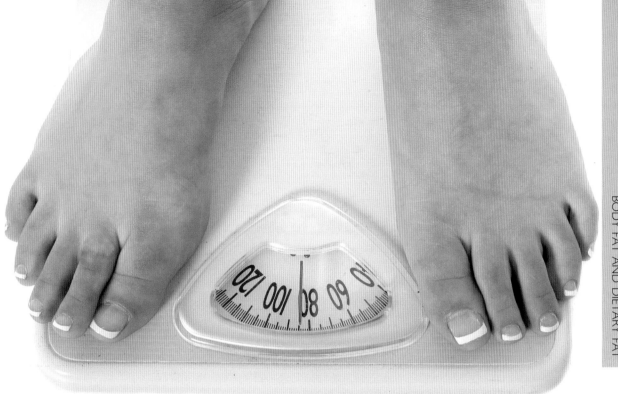

active form. So, this fat ensures normal hormonal balance and menstrual function. If stores fall too low, hormonal imbalance and menstrual irregularities result, although these can be reversed once body fat increases. There is some recent evidence that a certain amount of body fat in men is necessary for normal hormone production too.

The second component of body fat, *storage fat*, is an important energy reserve that takes the form of fat (adipose) cells under the skin (subcutaneous fat) and around the organs (intra-abdominal fat). Fat is used virtually all the time during any aerobic activity: while sleeping, sitting, standing and walking, as well as in most types of exercise. It is impossible to spot reduce fat selectively from adipose tissue sites by specific exercises or diets. The body generally uses fat from all sites, although the exact pattern of fat utilisation (and storage) is determined by your genetic make-up

and hormonal balance. An average person has enough fat for three days and three nights of continuous running – although, in practice, you would experience fatigue long before your fat reserves ran out. So, your fat stores are certainly not a redundant depot of unwanted energy!

WHAT IS THE BODY MASS INDEX?

Doctors and researchers often use a measurement called the Body Mass Index (BMI) to classify different grades of body weight and to assess health risk. It is sometimes referred to as the Quetelet Index after the Belgian statistician, Adolphe Quetelet, who observed that for normal weight people there is more or less a constant ratio between weight and the square of height. The BMI assumes that there is no single ideal weight for a person of a certain height, and that there is a healthy weight range for any given height.

The BMI is calculated by dividing a person's weight (in kg) by the square of his or her height (in m). For example, if your weight is 60 kg and height 1.7 m, your BMI is 21.

$$\frac{60}{1.7 \times 1.7} = 21$$

For a quick on-line BMI calculator and detailed BMI charts in imperial and metric measurements, log on to www.whathealth.com.

HOW USEFUL IS THE BMI?

Researchers and doctors use BMI measurements to assess a person's risk of acquiring certain health-related conditions, such as heart disease. Studies have shown that people with a BMI of between 18.5 and 25 have the lowest risk of developing diseases that are linked to obesity, e.g. cardiovascular disease, gall bladder disease, hypertension (high blood pressure) and diabetes. People with a BMI of between 25 and 30 are at moderate risk, while those with a BMI above 30 are at a greater risk.

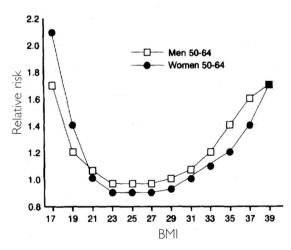

Figure 8.1 Relative risk of death according to BMI

It is not true that the lower a person's BMI the better, though (*see* Table 8.1). A very low BMI is also not desirable; people with a BMI below 20 have a higher risk of other health problems, such as respiratory disease, certain cancers and metabolic complications.

Both those with a BMI below 18.5 and those above 30 have an increased risk of premature death (*see* Fig. 8.1).

WHAT ARE THE LIMITATIONS OF THE BMI?

BMI does not give information about body composition, i.e. how much weight is fat and how much lean tissue. It simply gives the desirable weight of *average* people – not *sportspeople*!

When you stand on the scales you weigh everything – bone, muscle and water, as well as fat. Therefore you do not know how fat you actually are.

Overestimate

Individuals who are athletic and/or have a muscular build may be categorised as overweight. Body builders would be categorised as overweight or obese, as muscle weighs more than fat.

Underestimate

Body fat can be underestimated in individuals who have little muscle or who have lost muscle mass. This often occurs with older people.

IS THE DISTRIBUTION OF BODY FAT IMPORTANT?

Yes. Scientists believe that the distribution of your body fat is more important than the total amount of fat. This gives a more accurate assessment of your risk of metabolic disorders, such as heart disease, type 2 diabetes, high blood pressure and gall bladder disease. Fat stored mostly around the abdomen (visceral fat) gives rise to an 'apple' or 'barrel' shape, and this carries a much bigger health risk than fat stored mostly around the hips and thighs (peripheral or gynecoid obesity) in a pear shape. For most people, visceral fat is the largest store and is one of the first places where excess fat is laid down. When the store gets too large, it begins to pump out inflammatory and clot-producing compounds. This means that a man with a 'beer belly' but slim limbs may be at greater risk of heart disease and diabetes than a pear-shaped person with the same BMI but less visceral fat.

The way we distribute fat on our body is determined partly by our genetic make-up and partly by our natural hormonal balance. Men, for example, have higher levels of testosterone, which favours fat deposition around the abdomen, between the shoulder blades and close to the internal organs. Women have higher levels of oestrogen, which favours fat deposition around the hips, thighs, breasts and triceps. After the menopause, however, when oestrogen levels fall, fat tends to transfer from the hips and thighs to the abdomen, giving women more of an apple shape and pushing up their chances of heart disease.

HOW CAN I MEASURE MY BODY FAT DISTRIBUTION?

You can assess your body fat distribution by two methods:

1. The *waist/hip ratio*, which is your waist measurement (in inches or centimetres) divided by your hip measurement. For women (because of their proportionately larger pelvic hip bones), it should be 0.8 or less. For men, this ratio

Table 8.2	BMI categories
Category	**BMI**
Underweight	< 18.5
Ideal	18.5–24.9
Overweight	25–29.9
Obese	30–39.9
Very obese	40+

should be 0.95 or less. For example, a woman with a waist measurement of 66 cm and hips of 91.5 cm has a W/H ratio of 0.72 (66 ÷ 91.5).

2. *Waist circumference*: Scientists at the Royal Infirmary, Glasgow, have found that a simple waist circumference measurement correlates well with intra-abdominal fat and total body fat percentage (Lean *et al.*, 1995) and is more accurate than body weight or BMI in predicting type 2 diabetes (Wang *et al.*, 2005). A waist circumference of 94 cm or more in men, or 80 cm or more in women indicates excess abdominal fat.

Excess fat in the abdomen is a health risk. For example, a man with a W/H ratio of 1.1 has double the chance of having a heart attack as if it was below 0.95. The most likely explanation is to do with the close proximity of the intra-abdominal fat to the liver. Fatty acids from the adipose tissue are delivered into the portal vein that goes directly to the liver. The liver thus receives a continuous supply of fat-rich blood and this stimulates increased cholesterol synthesis. High blood cholesterol levels are a major risk factor for heart disease.

WHAT DOES BODY COMPOSITION MEAN?

The body is composed of two elements: lean body tissue (i.e. muscles, organs, bones and blood) and body fat (or adipose tissue). The proportion of these two components in the body is called body composition. This is more important than total weight.

For example, two people may weigh the same, but have a different body composition. Athletes usually have a smaller percentage of body fat and a higher percentage of lean weight than less physically active people. Lean body tissue is functional (or useful) weight, whereas fat is non-functional in terms of sports performance.

HOW CAN I MEASURE BODY COMPOSITION?

Clearly, height and weight measurements are not very accurate for assessing your body composition. To give you a more accurate idea of how much fat and how much muscle you have, there are a number of techniques for measuring body composition. These will tell you how much of your weight is muscle or fat as a percentage of your total weight.

The only method that is 100% accurate is cadaver analysis. Clearly this is impractical, so indirect methods must be used.

Underwater weighing

For a long time, this method was judged to be the most accurate. Its accuracy rate averages 97–98%. However, there are other methods, such as dual energy x-ray absorptiometry and magnetic resonance imaging, which produce similar, if not more accurate, results.

Underwater weighing works on the Archimedes' principle, which states that when an object is submerged under water it creates a buoyant coun-

ter force that is equal to the weight of water that it has displaced. Since bone and muscle are more dense than water, a person with a higher percentage of lean mass will weigh more in water, indicating a lower percentage of fat. Since fat is less dense than water, a person with a high fat percentage will weigh less in water than on land.

In this test, the person sits on a swing-seat and is then submerged into a water tank. After expelling as much air as possible from the lungs, the person's weight is recorded. This figure is then compared with the person's weight on dry land, using standard equations on a computer, and the fat percentage calculated.

The disadvantage of this method is that the specialised equipment is expensive and bulky and found only at research institutions or laboratories, i.e. it is not readily available to the public. The person also needs to be water-confident.

A newer method is the BOD POD, which is similar to the principle behind underwater weighing, but uses air displacement rather than weight under water. But, like underwater weighing, it is available only through university exercise science departments and is relatively expensive.

Skinfold callipers

The skinfold measurement method is widely available and used by many sports teams and in many health clubs. The callipers measure in millimetres the layer of fat just underneath the skin at various places on the body. This is done on three to seven specific places (such as the triceps, biceps, hip bone area, lower-back, abdomen, thigh and below the shoulder blade). Using these measurements, scientists have developed mathematical equations that account for age, sex, known body densities and estimated hidden fat that the callipers cannot measure. These equations produce a body density value, which another equation then changes into a body fat percentage.

The accuracy of this method depends almost entirely on the skill of the person taking the measurements. Also, it assumes that everyone has a predictable pattern of fat distribution as they age. Therefore, it becomes less accurate with elite athletes, as they tend to have a different pattern of fat distribution compared with sedentary people, and for very lean and obese people. There are different sets of equations to use, which take account of these factors. For the general population (over 15% body fat) the Durnin and Womersley (1974) equations are more suitable. The Jackson–Pollock (1984) equations apply best to lean and athletic people.

Kinanthropometry is the term for the recording of skinfold thickness measurements and body girth measurements (e.g. arms, chest, legs etc.) in order to monitor changes in body composition over time. The sites of girth measurements are shown in Figure 9.2 (Chapter 9, page 149).

An alternative is to present the body fat measurement as a 'sum of skinfolds'. This is the sum of the individual skinfold thicknesses from the seven specific sites.

Bioelectrical Impedance Analysis

Most body fat monitors and scales work using bioelectrical impedance analysis (BIA). These are widely used in gyms or available to buy from shops or mail-order companies. Here, a mild electrical current is sent through the body between electrodes attached to two specific points of the body (either between the hand and opposite foot, or from one foot to the other). The principle is that lean tissue (such as muscle and blood) contains high levels of water and electrolytes and is therefore a good conductor of electricity, whereas fat creates a resistance. Increasing levels of fat mass result in a higher impedance value and correspond to higher levels of body fat.

The advantages are the machine is portable, simple to operate and testing takes less than one minute. The disadvantage is the poor degree of accuracy compared with other methods. For example, changes in body fluid levels and skin temperature will affect the passage of the current and therefore the body fat reading. It tends to overestimate the body fat percentage of lean muscular people by 2–5% and underestimate the body fat percentage of overweight people by the same amount (Sun et al., 2005). It is important that you are well-hydrated when having a BIA measurement; if you are dehydrated, the current will not be conducted through your lean mass so well, giving you a higher body fat percentage reading.

Dual Energy X-ray Absorptiometry

Dual Energy X-ray Absorptiometry (DEXA) measures not only your total body fat but produces an accurate body fat map, showing exactly where your fat is distributed around the body. In this method, two types of x-rays are scanned over the whole body to measure fat, bone and muscle. The procedure takes about 5–20 minutes depending on the type of machine.

It is the most accurate method for assessing body fat. The disadvantages are the cost and size of the machine and lack of accessibility. DEXA machines are found in hospitals and research institutions. It may be possible to request a body fat analysis at your nearest site, but be prepared to pay considerably more than you would for the other methods.

Near-infrared interactance

In near-infrared interactance, an infra-red beam is shone perpendicularly through the upper arm. The amount of light reflected back to the analyser from the bone depends on the amount of fat located there, which is correlated to the body fat percentage. Age, weight, height, sex and activity level are all taken into account in the calculations.

The obvious disadvantage of this method is the assumption that fat in the arm is proportional to total body fat. However, it is a very fast, easy and cheap method. The equipment is portable, and anyone can operate it.

HOW ACCURATE ARE THESE METHODS?

Table 8.3 summarises studies that have assessed the accuracy of the various methods. DEXA and underwater weighing are regarded as the most accurate methods. Skinfold and BIA measurements – provided they are carefully carried out – can estimate body fat percentages with a 3–4% error (Houtkooper, 2000; Lohman, 1992). For example, if the actual body fat percentage is 15%, then predicted values could range from 12 to 18% (assuming a 3% error). But if poor measurement techniques or incorrectly calibrated instruments are used, then the margin of error could be greater. Since a relatively high degree of error is associated with these indirect body fat assessment methods, it is not recommended to set a specific body fat goal for athletes (ACSM, 2000). Instead, a range of target body fat values would be more realistic.

WHAT IS A DESIRABLE BODY FAT PERCENTAGE FOR ATHLETES?

Body fat percentages for athletes vary depending on the particular sport. According to scientists at the University of Arizona, the ideal body fat percentage, in terms of performance, for most male athletes lies between 6 and 15%, and for female athletes, 12 and 18% (Wilmore, J. H., 1983) In general, for men, middle- and long-distance runners and bodybuilders have the lowest body fat levels (less than 6%) while cyclists, gymnasts, sprinters, triathletes and basketball players average between 6 and 15% body fat (Sinning, 1998). In female athletes, the lowest body fat levels (6–15%) are observed in bodybuilders, cyclists, gymnasts, runners and triathletes (Sinning, 1998).

Physiologists recommend a minimum of 5% fat for men and 12% fat for women to cover the most basic functions associated with good health (Lohman, 1992). However, optimal body fat levels may be much higher than these minimums. The percentage (%) of fat associated with lowest health risk is 13–18% for men and 18–25% for women. Figure 8.2 gives the body fat percentages for standard (non-athletic) adults.

Clearly, there is no ideal body fat percentage for any particular sport. Each individual athlete has an optimal fat range at which their performance improves yet their health does not suffer.

Table 8.3	Accuracy of body fat measurement methods
Method	**Degree of inaccuracy**
DEXA	<2%
Skinfold measurement	3–4%
Underwater weighing	2–5%
Bioelectrical impedence	3–4%
Near-infrared interactance	5–10%

Table 8.4	Average body fat percentages in various sports	
Sport	**Men %**	**Women %**
Basketball	7–12	18–27
Bodybuilding (competitive)	6–7	8–10
Cycling	8–9	15–16
Football	8–18	(not available)
Gymnastics	3–6	8–18
Running	4–12	8–18
Swimming	4–10	12–23
Throwing	12–20	22–30
Tennis	12–16	22–26
Weight lifting	6–16	17–20

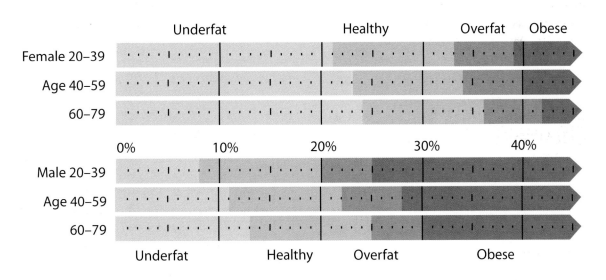

Figure 8.2 Healthy body ranges for adults

Based on NIH/WHO BMI Guidelines.
(Gallagher *et al* at NY Obesity Research Centre.)

HOW LOW CAN YOU GO?

Women and men who try to attain very low body fat levels, or a level that is unnatural for their genetic make-up, encounter problems. These problems can be serious, particularly for women, who may suffer long-term effects. Collectively known as the 'Female Athlete Triad', these problems are discussed in greater detail in Chapter 11.

WHAT ARE THE DANGERS FOR WOMEN WITH VERY LOW BODY FAT LEVELS?

One of the biggest problems for women with very low body fat levels is the resulting hormonal imbalance and amenorrhoea (absence of periods).

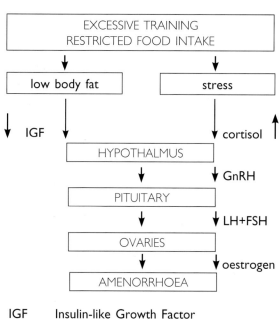

IGF	Insulin-like Growth Factor
GnRH	gonadotrophin-releasing hormone
LH	luteinising hormone
FSH	follicle-stimulating hormone

Figure 8.3 The development of amenorrhoea

As explained in more detail in Chapter 11, this tends to be triggered once body fat levels fall below 15–20% – the threshold level varies from one person to another. This fall in body fat, together with other factors such as low calorie intake and heavy training, is sensed by the hypothalamus of the brain, which then decreases its production of the hormone (gonadotrophin-releasing hormone) that acts on the pituitary gland. This, in turn, reduces the production of important hormones that act on the ovaries (luteinising hormone and follicle-stimulating hormone), causing them to produce less oestrogen and progesterone. The end result is a deficiency of oestrogen and progesterone and a cessation of menstrual periods (*see* Fig. 8.3).

Low body fat levels also upset the metabolism of the sex hormones, reducing their potency and thus fertility. Therefore, a very low body fat level drastically reduces a woman's chances of getting pregnant. However, the good news is that once your body fat level increases over your threshold and your training volume is reduced, your hormonal balance, periods and fertility generally return to normal.

WHAT ARE THE DANGERS FOR MEN WITH VERY LOW BODY FAT LEVELS?

Studies on competitive male wrestlers 'making weight' for contests found that once body fat levels fell below 5%, testosterone levels decreased, causing a drastic fall in sperm count, libido and sexual activity! Studies on male runners found similar changes. Thankfully, though, testosterone levels and libido return to normal once body fat increases. Team doctors in the US recommend a minimum of 7% fat before allowing wrestlers to compete.

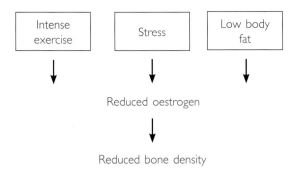

Intense exercise →

Stress → Reduced oestrogen

Low body fat →

Reduced oestrogen → Reduced bone density

Figure 8.4 Low body fat and bone density

CAN A LOW BODY FAT HARM YOUR BONES?

Amenorrhoea can lead to more serious problems such as bone loss. That's because low oestrogen levels result in loss of bone minerals and, therefore, bone density (*see* Fig. 8.4). In younger (premenopausal) women, this is called osteopoenia (i.e. lower bone density than normal for age), which is similar to the osteoporosis that affects post-menopausal women, where bones become thinner, lighter and more fragile. Amenorrhoeic athletes, therefore, run a greater risk of stress fractures. The British Olympic Medical Centre has reported cases of athletes in their twenties and thirties with osteoporotic-type fractures.

WHAT ARE THE PROBLEMS WITH LOW-FAT DIETS?

Very low fat intakes can leave you deficient in a variety of nutrients and lead to several health problems. You will certainly be missing out on the essential fatty acids (linoleic acid and linolenic acid) found in vegetable oils, seeds, nuts and oily fish (*see* pages 135–136), and will therefore be susceptible to dull flaky skin and other dermatological problems; cold extremities; prostaglandin (hormone) imbalance; poor control of inflammation, blood pressure, vasoconstriction and blood clotting.

Low-fat diets will be low in fat-soluble vitamins A, D and E. More importantly, fat is needed to enable your body to absorb and transport them, and to convert beta-carotene into vitamin A in the body. Although you can get vitamin D from UV light and vitamin A from beta-carotene in brightly coloured fruit and vegetables, getting enough vitamin E can be much more of a problem. It is found in significant quantities only in vegetable oils, seeds, nuts and egg yolk. Vitamin E is an important antioxidant that protects our cells from harmful free radical attack (*see* Chapter 5, page 74). It is thought to help prevent heart disease, certain cancers and even retard aging. It may also help reduce muscle soreness after hard exercise. So, cutting out oils, nuts and seeds means you are increasing your risk of free radical damage.

Chronically low-fat diets often result in a low-calorie and low-nutrient intake overall. Low-calorie diets quickly lead to depleted glycogen (carbohydrate) stores, resulting in poor energy levels, reduced capacity for exercise, fatigue, poor recovery between workouts and eventual burn-out. They can also increase protein breakdown – causing loss of muscle mass and strength or a lack of muscular development. This is just the opposite of what you should be achieving in your fitness programme.

FAT IN YOUR DIET
HOW MUCH FAT SHOULD I EAT?

The IOC and IAAF currently make no specific recommendation for fat intake. The focus should be on meeting carbohydrate and protein goals with fat making up the calorie balance. The American College of Sports Medicine (ACSM) and American Dietetic Association recommend fat provides 20–35% of calorie intake for athletes, which is consistent with the UK government recommendation of less than 35% for the general population (ACSM/ADA/DC, 2009). The emphasis should be on obtaining adequate energy, essential fatty acids and fat-soluble vitamins.

The International Conference on Foods, Nutrition and Sports Performance (1991) recommended a fat intake of between 15 and 30% of total calorie intake for sportspeople. Both recommendations are broadly in line with the maximum recommended by the World Health Organization (30% of calories) and the UK government (35% of calories). Using the lower limit of the ACSM recommendation and the upper limit of the UK recommendation, you should aim to achieve a fat intake between 20 and 35% of calories.

For example, an athlete consuming 3000 kcal a day would need:

- $(3000 \times 20\%) \div 9 = 66$ g
- $(3000 \times 35\%) \div 9 = 117$g

i.e. between 66 and 117g fat a day.

Although athletes need to focus on obtaining adequate carbohydrate, this does not mean reducing fat intake or eating a low fat diet. There is evidence that restricting fat may reduce your performance, and increasing fat intake does not appear to have any adverse effect on heart disease risk factors in athletes. In one study, runners who consumed a 42% fat diet had higher levels of HDL ('good') cholesterol and lower cardiovascular risk factors than those consuming a 16% fat diet (Leddy *et al.*, 2007). Another study by New Zealand researchers found that during periods of hard endurance training when energy requirements are high, increasing the percentage of fat in the diet to 50% of energy did not have an adverse effect on blood fats or cardiovascular risk (Brown & Cox, 1998).

In fact, recommendations to consume a low fat diet are no longer valid even for the general public. A large scale US trial involving nearly 49,000 women found that eating a low fat diet for 8 years had no effect on heart disease or stroke risk (Howard *et al.*, 2006).

The advice to limit saturated fat is misleading because many people replace saturated fat with carbohydrate, which raises blood triglyceride (fat) levels and actually increases cardiovascular risk. The Nurses Health study found that replacing saturated fat with unsaturated fat produced a more favourable change in blood fats and reduced cardiovascular risk. (Oh *et al.*, 2005). There was an inverse relationship between unsaturated fat intake and cardiovascular risk. In other words, the advice to 'limit saturated fat' should be replaced with 'replace saturated fat with unsaturated fat'.

Aim to eat a 'moderate fat' not a 'low fat' diet. Most of your fat intake should come from unsaturated fats, found in vegetable oils (e.g. olive, rapeseed, sunflower), nuts (all kinds), seeds (e.g. sunflower, sesame, pumpkin), oily fish (e.g. sardines, mackerel, salmon), peanut butter and avocado.

WHAT ARE FATS?

Fats and oils found in food consist mainly of *triglycerides*. These are made up of a unit of glycerol and three fatty acids. Each fatty acid is a chain of carbon and hydrogen atoms with a carboxyl group (–COOH) at one end and a methyl group at the other end (–CH3) – chain lengths between 14 and 22 carbon atoms are most common. These fatty acids are classified in three different groups, according to their chemical structure: saturated, monounsaturated and polyunsaturated. In food, the proportions of each group determine whether the fat is hard or liquid, how it is handled by the body and how it affects your health.

WHAT ARE SATURATED FATS?

Saturated fatty acids are fully saturated with the maximum amount of hydrogen; in other words, all of their carbon atoms are linked with a single bond to hydrogen atoms. Fats containing a high proportion of saturates are hard at room temperature and mostly come from animal products such as butter, lard, cheese and meat fat. Processed foods made from these fats include biscuits, cakes and pastry. Alternatives to animal fats are palm oil and coconut oil. Also highly saturated, these are often used in margarine, as well as in biscuits and bakery products.

Saturated fatty acids are considered the culprit fat in heart disease because they can increase total cholesterol and the more harmful low-density lipoprotein (LDL) cholesterol in the blood. The Department of Health (DoH) recommends a saturated fatty acid intake of no more than 10% of total calorie intake.

To achieve peak sports performance and health, you should minimise saturated fats: and eat instead unsaturated fats. Do not aim for a 'low fat diet'; eat a 'moderate fat' diet that includes mono and polyunsaturated fats.

WHAT ARE MONOUNSATURATED FATS?

Monounsaturated fatty acids have slightly less hydrogen because their carbon chains contain one double or unsaturated bond (hence 'mono'). Oils rich in monounsaturates are usually liquid at room temperature, but may solidify at cold temperatures. The richest sources include olive, rapeseed, groundnut, hazelnut and almond oil, avocados, olives, nuts and seeds.

Monounsaturated fatty acids are thought to have the greatest health benefits. They can reduce total cholesterol, in particular LDL cholesterol, without affecting the beneficial high-density lipoprotein (HDL) cholesterol. The DoH recommends a monounsaturated fatty acid intake of up to 12% of total calorie intake.

WHAT ARE POLYUNSATURATED FATS?

Polyunsaturated fatty acids have the least hydrogen – the carbon chains contain two or more double bonds (hence 'poly'). Oils rich in polyunsaturates are liquid at both room and cold temperatures. Rich sources include most vegetable oils and oily fish (and their oils).

Polyunsaturates can reduce LDL blood cholesterol levels – however, they can also lower the good HDL cholesterol slightly. It is a good idea to replace some with monounsaturates, if you eat a lot of them. For this reason, the DoH recommends a maximum intake of 10% of total calorie intake.

WHAT ARE THE ESSENTIAL FATTY ACIDS?

A sub-category of polyunsaturated fats, called essential fatty acids, cannot be made in your body, so they have to come from the food you eat. They are grouped into two series:

1. the omega-3 series, derived from alpha-linolenic acid (ALA)
2. the omega-6 series, derived from linoleic acid.

The series are called omega-3 and omega-6 because the last double bond is 3 and 6 carbon atoms from the last carbon in the chain respectively.

The omega-3 fatty acids can be further divided into two groups: long chain and short chain. The long-chain omega-3 fatty acids are eicosapentanoic acid (EPA) and docosahexanoic acid (DHA). They are found in oily fish and can also be formed in the body from ALA – the short-chain omega-3 fatty acid. EPA and DHA are then converted into hormone-like substances called prostaglandins, thromboxanes and leukotrienes. These control many key functions, such as blood clotting (making the blood less likely to form unwanted clots), inflammation (improving the ability to respond to injury or bacterial attack), the tone of blood vessel walls (widening and constriction of blood vessels) and your immune system.

Studies show that people with the highest intake of omega-3 fatty acids have a lower risk of heart attacks. This is because the prostaglandins reduce the ability of red blood cells to clot and reduce blood pressure.

The omega-6 fatty acids include linoleic acid, gamma-linolenic acid (GLA) and docosapentanoic acid (DPA) (see Fig. 8.5) and are important for healthy functioning of cell membranes. They are especially important for healthy skin. People on very low-fat diets, who are deficient in linoleic acid, often develop extremely dry, flaky

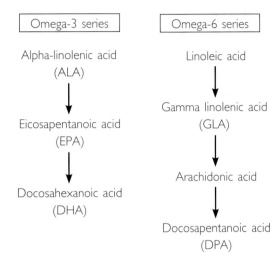

Figure 8.5 How the body uses and converts the omega-3 and omega-6 fatty acids

skin. Omega-6 fatty acids reduce LDL cholesterol, but a very high intake may also reduce HDL cholesterol. A high intake may also encourage increased free radical damage and, therefore, cancer risk. A moderate intake is recommended. Figure 8.5 shows how the body converts the two series of fatty acids.

WHAT ARE THE BEST FOOD SOURCES OF ESSENTIAL FATTY ACIDS?

Oily fish such as mackerel, fresh tuna (not tinned), salmon and sardines are undoubtedly the richest sources of DHA and EPA, but don't worry if you are a vegetarian or do not eat fish, because you can also get reasonably good amounts of ALA from certain plant sources. The richest plant sources include linseeds (flax seeds), linseed (flax) oil, pumpkin seeds, walnuts, rapeseed oil and soybeans. The dark green leaves of leafy vegetables (e.g. spinach, curly kale) also contain small amounts. There is an increasing range of omega-3 enriched foods, including omega-3 eggs (achieved by feeding hens on omega-3 enriched feed), bread and margarine. It is easier to meet your requirement for omega-6 fatty acids because they are found in more commonly eaten foods: vegetable oils, polyunsaturated margarine and many dishes and processed foods made from these oils and fats (e.g. fried foods, cakes, stir-fry, sandwiches spread with margarine, biscuits, crisps, cakes).

HOW MUCH DO I NEED?

We need both omega-3s and omega-6s to be healthy, but our diets are more often deficient in omega-3s. Most people have a far greater intake of omega-6 compared with omega-3; we tend to get most of our unsaturated fats from margarines and oils, processed foods containing vegetable oils, and oily fish. Experts recommend shifting this balance in favour of omega-3s.

The right balance between omega-3 and omega-6 fatty acids is the most important factor if you are to get enough EPA and DHA. That's because both ALA (omega-3) and linoleic acid (omega-6) compete for the same enzymes to metabolise them. You should also aim to achieve an LA to ALA ratio of around 5:1 or even lower, i.e. at least 1 g omega-3s for every 5 g of omega-6s (Simopoulos and Robinson, 1998). A high intake of LA interferes with the conversion process of ~~LA~~ LNA to EPA and DHA. The best way to correct

this is to eat more oily fish or other ALA-rich foods (*see* above) or take supplements.

There is no RDA in the UK for omega-3 and omega-6 fatty acids but the DoH recommends a minimum of 0.2% total energy as linolenic acid and advises people eat a minimum of 2 portions of fish a week, one of which should be oily fish. This will supply about 2–3 g omega-3 fatty acids per week. In 1999 at the XXIst Congress of the European Society of Cardiology in Barcelona, scientists concluded that 0.9 g omega-3 fatty acids/day will lower blood fats and heart disease risk. To get 0.9 g a day you can eat one of the following:

- 32 g mackerel
- 45 g (half a small tin) tuna in oil (0.45 g) plus 1 small (120 g) chicken leg portion (0.45 g)
- 2 tbsp (30 g) linseeds
- 4 tbsp (40 g) pumpkin seeds
- 12–15 g walnuts
- 1 level tbsp linseed oil
- 1 omega-3 fortified egg*
- (0.7 g) plus 2 tbsp (0.2 g) spinach

* from hens fed a omega-3 rich diet

Most fish oil-based supplements supply 0.1 g omega-3 fatty acids. Taking 9 supplements a day may be unrealistic, so get as close as possible to the recommended intake from food and then top

Table 8.5	Omega-3 fatty acid content of some fish
Weight	**Source**
0.5 g or less	Cod, haddock, mullet, halibut, skipjack tuna, clams, scallops, crab, prawns
0.6–1 g	Red snapper, yellow fin tuna, turbot, swordfish, mussels, oysters
1 g or more	Rainbow trout, mackerel, herring, sardines, salmon, blue fin tuna

up with a supplement if you need to (*see* Table 8.5 for fish sources of omega-3).

In addition, the DoH advises a minimum of 1% energy as linoleic acid. This can be met by consuming:

- 1 tbsp (15 g) sunflower seeds
- 1 tbsp (15 g) sesame seeds
- 0.5 tbsp (7.5 ml) sunflower, corn, safflower or sesame oil
- 1 tbsp (15 g) polyunsaturated margarine

HOW CAN OMEGA-3 FATTY ACIDS HELP ATHLETIC PERFORMANCE?

Studies have shown that omega-3 fatty acids can lead to improvements in strength and endurance by enhancing aerobic metabolism (Brilla and Landerholm, 1990; Bucci, 1993) – a critical energy system for all types of activities. Omega-3 fats have been shown to minimise post exercise soreness (Jouris *et al*, 2011). The benefits of omega-3 fatty acids can be summarised as follows:

- improved delivery of oxygen and nutrients to cells because of reduced blood viscosity
- more flexible red blood cell membranes and improved oxygen delivery
- enhanced aerobic metabolism
- increased energy levels and stamina
- increased exercise duration and intensity
- improved release of growth hormone in response to sleep and exercise, improving recovery and promoting anabolic (or anti-catabolic) environment
- anti-inflammatory, preventing joint, tendon, ligament strains
- reduction of inflammation caused by over-training, assisting injury healing.

WHAT ARE TRANS FATTY ACIDS?

Small amounts of trans fatty acids are found naturally in meat and dairy products, but most come from processed fats. These are produced by hydrogenation, a process that changes liquid oils into solid or spreadable fats. During this highly pressurised heat treatment, the geometrical arrangement of the atoms changes. Technically speaking, one or more of the unsaturated double bonds in the fatty acid is altered from the usual cis form to the unusual *trans* form. Hydrogenated fats and oils are used in many foods, including cakes, biscuits, margarine, low-fat spreads and pastries – check the ingredients.

The exact effect of trans fatty acids on the body is not certain, but it is thought that they may be worse than saturates: they could lower HDL and raise LDL levels. They may also increase levels of a substance that promotes blood clot formation and stops your body using essential fatty acids properly. A US study in 1993 of 85,000 nurses by researchers at Harvard Medical School linked high intakes of trans fatty acids (from processed fats, not natural fats) with a 50% increase in the risk of heart disease. In 2002, the US Institute of Medicine advised that zero is the only safe level of intake. The UK's Food Standards Agency states that 'trans fats have no known nutritional benefits… evidence suggests the effects of trans fats are worse than saturated fats'.

In the UK, the average intake is estimated to be around 4–6 g. The DoH recommends that trans fatty acids make up no more than 2% of total calorie intake – roughly 5 g per day – and the FSA recommends keeping your intake to 'a minimum'.

As there is no law requiring trans fats to be listed on food labels, the best advice is to avoid any foods that list hydrogenated or partially

Table 8.6	Sources of omega-3 fatty acids		
	g/100 g	Portion	g/portion
Salmon	2.5 g	100 g	2.5 g
Mackerel	2.8 g	160 g	4.5 g
Sardines (tinned)	2.0 g	100 g	2.0 g
Trout	1.3 g	230 g	2.9 g
Tuna (canned in oil, drained)	1.1 g	100 g	1.1 g
Cod liver oil	24 g	1 teaspoon (5 ml)	1.2 g
Flaxseed oil	57 g	1 tablespoon (14 g)	8.0 g
Flaxseeds (ground)	16 g	1 tablespoon (24 g)	3.8 g
Rape seed oil	9.6 g	1 tablespoon (14 g)	1.3 g
Walnuts	7.5 g	1 tablespoon (28 g)	2.6 g
Walnut oil	11.5 g	1 tablespoon (14 g)	1.6 g
Peanuts	0.4 g	Handful (50 g)	0.2 g
Broccoli	0.1 g	3 tablespoons (125 g)	1.3 g
Pumpkin seeds	8.5 g	2 tablespoons (25 g)	2.1 g
Omega-3 eggs	0.2 g	One egg	0.1 g
Typical omega-3 supplement		8 capsules	0.5 g

Source: MAFF/ RSC (1991); British Nutrition Foundation (1999)

hydrogenated oils on the label. Cut down on the following:

1. Spreads made with hydrogenated oils. Expect around 2.8 g per tablespoon in hard margarine and 0.6 g per tablespoon in soft (spreadable) margarine.
2. Fast food. Most are fried in partially hydrogenated oil – expect up to 14 g in a medium portion of takeaway chips.
3. Cakes and biscuits. More hydrogenated fat and shortening (high in trans fats) is used in shop-bought cakes and biscuits than any other food – a doughnut contains around 5 g trans fat, a sandwich biscuit as much as 1.9 g.
4. Crisps and snacks. Those fried in hydrogenated fat can contain up to 3.2 g per packet.
5. Chocolate bars. The innocent sounding vegetable fat on the label means hydrogenated fat.

WHAT IS CHOLESTEROL?

Cholesterol is an essential part of our bodies; it makes up part of all cell membranes and helps produce several hormones. Some cholesterol comes from our diet, but most is made in the liver from saturated fats. In fact, the cholesterol we eat has only a small effect on our LDL cholesterol; if we eat more cholesterol (from meat, offal, eggs, dairy products, seafood) the liver compensates by making less, and vice versa. This keeps a steady level of cholesterol in the bloodstream.

Several factors can push up blood cholesterol levels. The major ones are obesity (especially android or central obesity), lack of exercise and the amount of saturated fatty acids we eat. Studies have shown that replacing saturated fatty acids with carbohydrates or unsaturated fatty acids can lower total and LDL cholesterol levels.

SO, WHICH ARE THE BEST TYPES OF FATS TO EAT?

Fats should make up 20–35% of your total calorie intake. Use all spreading fats sparingly; opt for a spread with a high content of olive oil and avoid those containing hydrogenated vegetable oil or partially hydrogenated oil. Avoid hard margarines and vegetable fats because they have the highest content of hydrogenated fats and trans fatty acids.

For cooking and salad dressings, choose oils that are high in omega-3 fatty acids or monounsaturated fatty acids – olive, rapeseed, flax and nut oils are good choices for health as well as taste. These are healthier than oils rich in omega-6 fats, such as sunflower and corn oil, which disrupt the formation of EPA and DHA. Include nuts and seeds in your daily diet; they provide many valuable nutrients apart from omega-3 fatty acids and monounsaturates. If you eat fish, include one to two portions of oily fish (e.g. mackerel, herring, salmon) per week. Vegetarians should make sure they include plant sources of omega-3 fatty acids in their daily diet.

SUMMARY OF KEY POINTS

- Excess body fat is a disadvantage in almost all sports and fitness programmes, reducing power, speed and performance.
- Very low body fat does not guarantee improved performance either. There appears to be an optimal fat range for each individual, which cannot be predicted by a standard linear relationship.
- There are three main components of body-fat: essential fat (for tissue structure); sex-specific fat (for hormonal function); and storage fat (for energy).
- The minimum percentage of fat recommended for men is 5% and for women, 10%. However, for normal health, the recommended ranges are 13–18% and 18–25% respectively. In practice, many athletes fall below these recommended ranges.
- Very low body fat levels are associated with hormonal imbalance in both sexes, and amenorrhoea, infertility, reduced bone density and increased risk of osteoporosis in women.
- Very low-fat diets can lead to deficient intakes of essential fatty acids and fat-soluble vitamins.
- A fat intake of 20–35% of energy is recommended for athletes and active people.
- Unsaturated fatty acids should make up the majority of your fat intake, with saturated fatty acids and trans fatty acids kept to a minimum.
- Greater emphasis should be placed on omega-3 fatty acids to improve the omega-3:omega-6 ratio. Include oily fish 1–2 times a week or consume 1–3 tbsp of linseed oil, pumpkin seeds, walnuts and rapeseed oil a day.
- Omega-3 fatty acids can enhance oxygen delivery to cells and therefore improve athletic performance.

WEIGHT LOSS

9

Many athletes and fitness participants wish to lose weight, either for health or performance reasons, or in order to make a competitive weight category. However, rapid weight loss can have serious health consequences, leading to a marked reduction in performance. A knowledge of safe weight loss methods is, therefore, essential. Since 95% of dieters fail to maintain their weight loss within a five-year period, lifestyle management is the key to long-term weight management.

This chapter examines the effects of weight loss on performance and health, and highlights the dangers of rapid weight loss methods. It presents a simple step-by-step guide to calculating your calorie, carbohydrate, protein and fat intake on a fat-loss programme. Both nutritional and exercise strategies are given, including a detailed fat-loss exercise plan designed to minimise muscle loss and maximise fat burning. It examines the reasons why many people find it hard to lose and maintain weight, and the barriers to long-term success. Up-to-date research on appetite control and metabolism is presented, along with the dangers of 'yo-yo' dieting (repeated dieting and weight gain, also known as 'weight cycling'). It explodes many of the myths and fallacies about metabolic rates and, finally, gives safe and simple step-by-step strategies for successful weight loss.

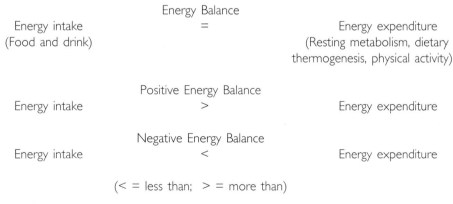

Energy Balance

| Energy intake (Food and drink) | = | Energy expenditure (Resting metabolism, dietary thermogenesis, physical activity) |

Positive Energy Balance

Energy intake > Energy expenditure

Negative Energy Balance

Energy intake < Energy expenditure

(< = less than; > = more than)

Figure 9.1 Energy balance equations

To lose body fat, you have to expend more energy (calories) than you consume. In other words, you have to achieve a negative energy balance (see Fig. 9.1).

Research has shown that a combination of diet and activity is more likely to result in long-term success than diet or exercise alone. Unfortunately, there are no miracle solutions or short cuts. The objectives of a healthy diet and exercise programme are to:

- achieve a modest negative energy (calorie) balance
- maintain (or even increase) lean tissue
- gradually reduce body fat percentage
- avoid a significant reduction in your resting metabolic rate (see definition below)
- achieve an optimal intake of vitamins and minerals.

WILL DIETING AFFECT MY HEALTH OR PERFORMANCE?

Reducing body fat levels can be advantageous to performance in many sports (see 'Does body fat affect performance?' on page 123). However, it is important to achieve this through scientifically proven methods.

Unfortunately, many athletes use rapid weight loss methods that have an adverse effect on their performance and their health. The two most common are crash dieting and dehydration. Clearly, an athlete may achieve a desirable appearance, but to the detriment of his or her performance.

Rapid weight loss results in a diminished aerobic capacity (Fogelholm, 1994). A drop of up to 5% has been measured in athletes who had lost just 2–3% of body weight through dehydration. A loss of 10% can occur in those who lose

Rapid weight loss

To make weight for a competition (e.g. boxing, bodybuilding, judo), athletes may resort to rapid weight loss methods, such as fasting, dehydration, exercising in sweatsuits, saunas, diet pills, laxatives, diuretics or self-induced vomiting. Weight losses of 4.5 kg in 3 days are not uncommon. In a study of 180 female athletes (Rosen et al., 1986), 32% admitted they used more than one of these methods. In another (Drummer et al., 1987), 15% of young female swimmers said they had tried one of these methods.

weight through strict dieting. Anaerobic performance, strength and muscular endurance are also decreased, although researchers have found that strength (expressed against body weight) can actually improve after gradual weight loss (Tiptan, 1987).

Prolonged dieting can have more serious health consequences. In female athletes, low body weight and body fat have been linked with menstrual irregularities, amenorrhoea and stress fractures; in male athletes, with reduced testosterone production. It has also been suggested that the combination of intense training, food restriction and the psychological pressure for extreme leanness may precipitate disordered eating and clinical eating disorders in some athletes. Scientists say that those who attempt to lose body fat for appearance are more likely to develop an eating disorder than those who control it only for performance purposes.

There is a fine line between dieting and obsessive eating behaviour, and many female athletes, in particular, are under pressure to be thin and improve their performance. The warning signs and health consequences of eating disorders are discussed in Chapter 11.

WHAT HAPPENS TO THE BODY DURING RAPID WEIGHT LOSS BY DEHYDRATION?

Dehydration results in a reduced cardiac output and stroke volume, reduced plasma volume, slower nutrient exchange and slower waste removal, all of which have an impact on health and performance (Fogelholm, 1994; Fleck and Reimers, 1994). In moderate-intensity exercise lasting more than 30 seconds, even dehydration of less than 5% body weight will diminish strength or performance, although it does not appear to affect exercise lasting less than 30 seconds. So, for athletes relying on pure strength (e.g. weightlifting), rapid weight loss may not be as detrimental.

IS REPEATED WEIGHT LOSS HARMFUL?

Repeated weight fluctuations, or yo-yo dieting, have been linked with an increased risk of heart disease, secondary diabetes, gall bladder disease and premature death. However, researchers are divided as to the exact reason. One explanation is that fat tends to be re-deposited intra-abdominally, closer to the liver, rather than in the peripheral regions of the body, such as the hips, thighs and arms, and thus poses a greater heart disease risk. Another explanation is that repeated severe dieting can lead to a loss of lean tissue (including organ tissue) and nutritional deficiencies that can damage heart muscle. Contrary to popular belief, there is no evidence that yo-yo dieting permanently slows your metabolism (it returns to its original levels once normal eating

is resumed). But yo-yo dieting can be bad for your psychological health. Each time you regain weight, you experience a sense of failure, which can lower your confidence and self-esteem.

WILL I STILL BE ABLE TO TRAIN HARD WHILST LOSING WEIGHT?

The problem with most weight-loss diets is they do not provide enough calories or carbohydrate to support intense training. They can leave you with depleted muscle glycogen stores, which results in lethargy, fatigue and poor performance. However, you can continue training hard provided you reduce your calorie intake by approximately 10–20% (ACSM/ADA/DC, 2000). This modest change should produce weight loss in the region of 0.5 kg per week without you feeling deprived, tired or overly hungry. One consistent finding from studies is that an adequate carbohydrate intake (50–60% of energy) is critical for preserving muscular strength, endurance, and both aerobic and anaerobic capacity. A lower intake can result in glycogen depletion and increased protein oxidation (muscle loss). Retaining lean mass is also vital for losing fat. The less muscle you have the lower your resting metabolic rate and the harder it is to lose fat (*see* page 156).

CAN CARBOHYDRATE MAKE ME FAT?

Studies have shown that eating carbohydrates increases your metabolic rate: about 10–15% of the carbohydrate calories are expended as heat (*see* page 153, 'What is thermogenesis?'). That gives you a little leeway in your carbohydrate intake by allowing you to overconsume by around 10–15% (relative to your requirements).

So what happens to the excess carbohydrate? Well, it is converted preferentially into glycogen

– provided there is spare storage capacity and provided there is only a modest rise in blood glucose. A rapid rise in blood glucose produced by high GI carbohydrates (*see* Appendix One) can lead to fat storage. This is because it provokes a rapid release of insulin. The more insulin that is present in the bloodstream in response to high GI carbohydrates, the more likely that this insulin will turn excess carbohydrates into fat and deposit it in your fat cells.

The key to keeping insulin levels low is to eat low GI meals. In practice that means you need to eat balanced amounts of carbohydrate, protein and healthy (unsaturated) fats at each meal.

CAN PROTEIN MAKE ME FAT?

When protein is overeaten, the amino part of the molecule is excreted and the remainder of the molecule provides an energy substrate. This can

Fat makes you fat

The hypothesis that fat is more fattening, calorie for calorie, than carbohydrate, is supported by a number of studies (Flatt, 1993; Danforth, 1985). In one study, men were fed 150% of their calorie requirements for two 14-day periods. In one period, the excess calories came from fat; in the other, from carbohydrate (Horton et al., 1995). Overfeeding fat caused much greater deposition of body fat than overfeeding carbohydrate. Other researchers believe that it is unimportant whether the excess calories come from carbohydrate or fat. The best way to avoid obesity is to limit your total calories, not just the fat calories (Willett & Stampfer, 2002).

either be used directly for energy production or else stored – preferably as glycogen rather than fat. Furthermore, protein ingestion stimulates thermogenesis (*see* page 153), so a significant proportion of protein calories are given off as heat.

Researchers believe that protein is the most effective nutrient for switching off hunger signals, so it helps you to stop overeating. The most likely explanation is that we have no capacity to store excess protein, so the brain readily detects when you have eaten enough and switches off hunger signals.

By including adequate amounts of protein in your meals on a fat-loss programme, you can help control hunger.

CAN FAT MAKE ME FAT?

Dietary fat is far more likely to make you fat than any other nutrient, as it is stored as adipose tissue if it is not required straight away. In contrast to carbohydrate and protein, overeating fat does not increase fat oxidation; this occurs only when total energy demands exceed total energy intake or during aerobic exercise.

Fat is very calorie-dense; it contains more than double the calories per gram (9 kcal/g) of carbohydrate and protein (both 4 kcal/g), but it is much easier to overconsume, as it is less satiating for two reasons. Firstly, carbohydrate and protein produce a rise in blood glucose, which reduces the appetite. Fat, on the other hand, is digested and absorbed less rapidly, and often actually depresses blood glucose, thereby failing to satisfy the appetite as efficiently. Secondly, fatty foods usually have a high calorie density and low bulk, again making them less satisfying, even in the short term, and easier to overeat.

The fats you do eat should comprise unsaturated fatty acids, particularly the mono-unsaturated fats omega-3 and omega-6 fatty acids (*see* pages 136–138).

CAN ALCOHOL MAKE ME FAT?

Indirectly, alcohol can encourage fat storage. Since alcohol cannot be stored in the body, it must be oxidised and converted into energy (*see* page 16. Whilst this is happening, the oxidation of fat and carbohydrate is suppressed, and these are channelled into storage instead.

Alcohol provides 7 kcal/g, which can significantly increase your total calorie intake if you consume large quantities. Also, many alcoholic drinks contain sugars and other carbohydrates, which increase the calorie content further.

HOW MUCH CARBOHYDRATE, PROTEIN AND FAT SHOULD I CONSUME FOR WEIGHT LOSS?

The key to successful body fat loss is to cut your dietary fat to 20–25% of total calories (Walberg-Rankin, 2000) and to reduce carbohydrates by 15%, proportional to your drop in calories. Ideally, you should aim to consume 4–7 g/kg body weight daily if you want to maintain your usual training volume and intensity. If you consume too little carbohydrate (less than 4 g/kg BW/day), your glycogen stores become depleted, and not only does fat oxidation increase but protein oxidation also increases. Clearly, this is not a desirable state for athletes, as it results in a loss of lean tissue. This will, of course, affect your performance and cause a reduction in your metabolic rate (*see* box: 'What exactly is metabolism?'). The less lean tissue you have, the lower your metabolic rate, and the fewer calories you burn just to maintain your weight.

A higher protein intake can offset some of the lean tissue loss. Most researchers recommend around 1.6 g/kg body weight/day on a fat-loss programme, which is consistent with the range recommended generally for athletes (1.2–1.7 g). For example, a 75 kg athlete would need to consume 120 g protein/day. In other words, you should maintain or slightly increase your protein intake and cut calories from carbohydrate and fat.

HOW TO CALCULATE YOUR CALORIE, CARBOHYDRATE, PROTEIN AND FAT REQUIREMENTS ON A WEIGHT-LOSS PROGRAMME

Aim to reduce your usual calorie intake by 10–20%. This relatively modest reduction in calories will avoid the metabolic slowdown that is associated with more severe calorie reductions. The body will recognise and react to a smaller deficit by oxidising more fat. If you cut calories more drastically, it will not make you shed fat faster. Instead it will cause your body to lower its metabolic rate in an attempt to conserve energy stores. It will also increase protein oxidation and glycogen depletion. The end result is likely to be loss of lean muscle tissue, low energy levels, and extreme hunger.

In theory, 0.5 kg (500 g) of fat can be shed when a deficit of 4500 kcal is created since 1 g fat yields 9 kcal (9 × 500 = 4500 kcal). However, in practice, it may not work exactly like this because it depends on your initial calorie intake. For example, athlete A (male) normally eats 3000 kcal/day and athlete B (female) normally eats 2000 kcal/day. If both athletes reduced their calorie intake by 643 kcal/day (equivalent to 4500 kcal/week), athlete A now eats 2357 kcal/day and athlete B now eats 1357 kcal/day. The two athletes will, in practice, get very different results in terms of their body composition. Athlete A will almost certainly lose around 0.5 kg fat/week because his deficit is a 15% (modest) reduction. Athlete B will probably lose 0.5 kg fat/week for the first week or two, but after that she will lose muscle tissue. That's because she has cut her calories by 32%, which is too severe. In general, calorie reductions of greater than 15% will lead to a metabolic slowdown and muscle loss, making fat loss slower. Athlete B may well lose 0.5 kg of fat/week, but some will come from muscle and a loss of muscle will slow her metabolism.

So, for fat loss, aim for a reduction of calories as a percentage of your maintenance calorie intake. Reducing calorie intake by approximately 15% (or 10–20%) will lead to fat loss without slowing the metabolism. It may not allow you to lose 0.5 kg of fat/week – it may be 0.5 kg/10 days – but at least it will be fat, not muscle. Athlete B should eat 1700 kcal a day. This will produce a loss of 0.5 kg fat every 11 or 12 days.

To help guide you through, calculations are shown for a 65 kg male cyclist, aged 30, who leads a mostly sedentary lifestyle and trains 10 hours on his bike (16 km/h) per week.

Step 1: Estimate your RMR (see Table 9.1)
Example:
- RMR = $(65 \times 15.3) + 679 = 1673$ kcal

Step 2: Calculate your daily energy expenditure
Multiply your RMR by the appropriate number below:

a) If you are mostly sedentary (mostly seated or standing activities during the day):
   RMR × 1.4
b) If you are moderately active (regular brisk walking or equivalent during the day):
   RMR × 1.7
c) If you are very active (generally physically active during the day):
   RMR × 2.0

Example:
- Daily energy expenditure = $1673 \times 1.4 = 2342$ kcal

Step 3: Estimate the number of calories expended during exercise (see Table 9.2)
It's best to estimate your exercise calorie expenditure over a week (7 days) then divide by 7 to get a daily average.

Example:
- Exercise calories/week = $10 \times 385 = 3850$ kcal
- Exercise calories/day = $3850 \div 7 = 550$ kcal

Table 9.1	Resting metabolic rate (RMR) in athletes	
Age	**Male**	**Female**
10–18 years	(body weight in kg × 17.5) + 651	(body weight in kg × 12.2) + 746
18–30 years	(body weight in kg × 15.3) + 679	(body weight in kg × 14.7) + 496
31–60 years	(body weight in kg × 11.6) + 879	(body weight in kg × 8.7) + 829

(Reference: Goran and Astrup, 2002)

Table 9.2	Calories expended during exercise
Sport	**kcal/hour***
Aerobics (high intensity)	520
Aerobics (low intensity)	400
Badminton	370
Boxing (sparring)	865
Cycling (16 km/hour)	385
Cycling (9 km/hour)	250
Judo	760
Rowing machine	445
Running (3.8 min/km)	1000
Running (5.6 min/km)	750
Squash	615
Swimming (fast)	630
Tennis (singles)	415
Weight training	270–450

* Figures are based on the calorie expenditure of an athlete weighing 65 kg. Values will be greater for heavier body weights; lower for smaller body weights.

Step 4: Add figures from steps 2 and 3

This is the number of calories you need to maintain your body weight. Regard this figure as your maintenance intake. If your current calorie intake is higher or lower than your maintenance intake, gradually adjust your intake until it almost matches. This may take a few weeks.

Example:
- Maintenance calorie intake = 2342 + 550 = 2892 kcal

Step 5: Reduce your calorie intake by 15%

To do this, multiply your maintenance calories, as calculated in step 4, by 0.85 (85%) to give you your new total daily calorie intake.

Example:
- New total daily calorie intake = 2892 × 85% = 2458 kcal

Step 6: Calculate your carbohydrate needs

In a 24-hour period during low or moderate intensity training days you should get 5–7 g/kg of body weight. During moderate to heavy endurance training 7–10 g/kg is recommended. However, as your calorie needs decrease by 15%, so should your usual carbohydrate intake. In practice, aim to eat about 50–100 g less carbohydrate.

Step 7: Calculate your protein needs

This is based on the recommended requirement of 1.6 g/kg body weight/day (*see above, p. 145*). Multiply your weight in kg × 1.6 to give you your daily protein intake in grams.

For example, if you weigh 65 kg:
Protein intake = 65 × 1.6 = 104 g

Step 8: Calculate your fat needs

Your fat intake as a percentage of total calories is the balance left once you have calculated the carbohydrate and protein percentages.

HOW CAN I SPEED UP MY FAT LOSS?

Increasing exercise calorie expenditure will help speed up fat loss. This can have a dual effect. Firstly, any additional aerobic exercise you perform on top of your regular training will increase fat oxidation during exercise as well as increase your metabolic rate for a while afterwards (*see* pages 156–160 for more information on exercise and fat loss). Secondly, adding or increasing weight training exercises will offset any loss of lean tissue and maintain muscle mass.

WEIGHT LOSS STRATEGY

Step 1: Set realistic goals

Before embarking on a weight loss plan, write down your goals clearly, as research has proven that by writing down your intentions, you are far more likely to turn them into actions.

These goals should be specific, positive and realistic ('I will lose 5 kg of body fat') rather than hopeful ('I would like to lose some weight'). Try to allow a suitable time frame (*see* Step 3): to lose 15 kg one month before a summer holiday is, obviously, unrealistic! Make sure, also, that you are clear about your reasons for wanting to lose weight: many normal-weight women wrongly believe that losing weight will solve their emotional or body image problems.

Step 2: Monitor body composition changes

The best way to ensure you are losing fat not muscle is to measure your body composition

The psychology of dieting

Researchers believe that a psychological difference exists between dieters (or restrained eaters) and non-dieters. In dieters and restrained eaters, the normal regulation of food intake becomes undermined as normal appetite and hunger cues are ignored. This leads to periods of restraint and semi-starvation, followed by overindulgence and guilt, followed by restraint, and so on.

Psychologists have shown that habitual dieters tend to have a more emotional personality than those who are not preoccupied with weight. They also tend to be more obsessive and less able to concentrate. Dieters usually live by a set of rules centred around 'allowed' foods and 'banned'/'naughty' foods.

At the University of Toronto, dieters and non-dieters were given a high-calorie milkshake, followed by free access to ice cream (Herman & Polivy, 1991). The dieters actually went on to eat more ice cream than the non-dieters. This is due to a phenomenon known as 'counter regulation'; having lost the inbuilt regulation system of non-dieters, they were unable to detect and thus compensate for the calorie pre-load.

Dr Barbara Rolls and colleagues at Penn State University (Rolls & Shide, 1992) demonstrated that weight worriers appear to lack the internal 'calorie counter' possessed by people who don't worry about their weight. When given a yoghurt half an hour before lunch, those who worried about their weight ate more for lunch than those who were not weight concerned. It appears that such dieters have poor appetite control and are unable to compensate for previous food intake.

once a month. The simplest method is to use a combination of simple girth or circumference measurements (e.g. chest, waist, hips, arms, legs), as shown in Figure 9.2, and skinfold thickness measurements, obtained by callipers (*see* Chapter 8, page 128). Exercise physiologists recommend keeping a record of the skinfold thickness measurements themselves rather than converting them into body fat percentages. This is because the conversion charts are based on equations for the average, sedentary person and may not be appropriate for sportspeople or very lean or fat individuals. Monitoring changes in measurements at specific sites of the body allows you to see how your shape is changing and where most fat is being lost. This is a far better motivator than weighing scales! Alternatively, you can use one of the other methods of body composition measurement described in Chapter 8.

Step 3: Aim to lose no more than 0.5 kg/week

Weekly or fortnightly weighing can be useful for checking the speed of weight/fat loss, but do not rely exclusively on this method because it does not reflect changes in body composition! Avoid more frequent weighing because this can lead to an obsession with weight. Bear in mind that weight loss in the first week may be as much as 2 kg, but this is mostly glycogen and its accompanying fluid (0.5 kg glycogen is stored with up to 1.5–2 kg water). Afterwards, aim to lose no more than 0.5 kg fat/week. Faster weight loss usually suggests a loss of lean tissue.

Step 4: Keep a food diary

A food diary is a written record of your daily food and drink intake. It is a very good way to evaluate

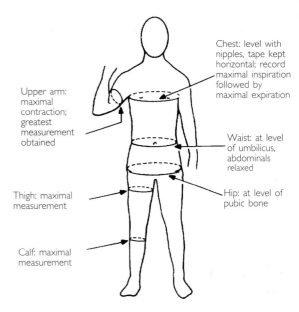

Upper arm: maximal contraction; greatest measurement obtained

Chest: level with nipples, tape kept horizontal; record maximal inspiration followed by maximal expiration

Waist: at level of umbilicus, abdominals relaxed

Thigh: maximal measurement

Hip: at level of pubic bone

Calf: maximal measurement

All measurements are recorded before a workout with the muscles still cold. The tape should be horizontal and taut, but not compressing the skin.

Figure 9.2 Girth measurements

your present eating habits and to find out exactly what, why and when you are eating. It will allow you to check whether your diet is well balanced or lacking in any important nutrients, and to take a more careful look at your usual meal patterns and lifestyle.

Weigh and write down everything you eat and drink for at least three consecutive days – ideally seven. This period should include at least one weekend day. It is important not to change your usual diet at this time and to be completely honest! Every spoonful of sugar in tea, every scrape of butter on bread should be recorded.

Use your food diary to find out about:

- the main sources of saturated fat in your diet which you need to eliminate

- the GI of your meals and snacks. Aim to consume low-GI food during the day and before exercise
- your fibre intake. Check that most meals are based on fibre-rich foods (*see* page 152)
- the timing of your meals and snacks. Aim to eat approximately six times a day.

Step 5: Never consume fewer calories than your RMR

Calorie intake should never be less than your RMR, otherwise you risk losing excessive lean tissue, severely depleting your glycogen stores and having an inadequate nutrient intake. It is erroneous and potentially dangerous to prescribe

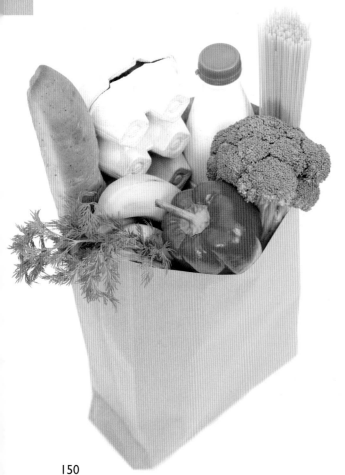

low-calorie diets of 1000 kcal or less. Keep to the 15% rule.

Step 6: Trim saturated and hydrogenated fat

Look carefully at your food diary and identify the foods containing saturated and hydrogenated fats that you are currently eating. Fat puts on more body fat than any other nutrient. When protein or carbohydrate is eaten in excess, the body makes metabolic adjustments to promote glycogen storage and increase the use of protein or carbohydrate for fuel. You have to overeat fairly large amounts of these foods before they are converted into body fat. In contrast, excess saturated fats cause virtually no change in metabolism and are readily converted into body fat. Focus on cutting saturated rather than unsaturated fats. Table 9.3 provides practical tips for weight loss.

Step 7: Include healthy fats

Don't cut fat out of your diet completely. You need a certain amount each day to provide essential fatty acids, stimulate hormone production, keep your skin healthy, and absorb and transport fat-soluble vitamins. Dr Udo Erasmus (1996) believes that the essential fatty acids in foods such as nuts, seeds and oily fish help burn fat by assisting the transport of oxygen to the body's tissues. So, if you want to lose weight, cut down on saturated and trans fatty acids; the remainder should come from unsaturated fats. Aim for 15–20% of your total calories.

Step 8: Go for the (slow) burn

Make all of your meals low GI. This helps improve appetite regulation, increases feelings of fullness and delays hunger between meals.

Table 9.3 Eating for weight loss – top tips

Making small changes to the way you eat through the day can yield big results. You don't have to cut out all the foods you love – cut out only what doesn't benefit your body.

Trim the fat
Cut down on foods high in saturated and hydrogenated fats – butter, hard margarine, fried food, fatty meats, burgers, pastry dishes, cakes, biscuits, puddings and chocolate. Choose leaner meats, skinless poultry and fish instead of fatty meat, and use less oil in cooking.

Start the day with breakfast
Don't even think about skipping breakfast. People who do so are more likely to overeat later in the day and pile on unwanted pounds. When you start your day off with a healthy, filling breakfast, you dramatically increase your chances of eating healthily throughout the day. You also fuel your body, so you feel happy and energised for the rest of the day. Studies show that when you eat a filling high-fibre breakfast you'll eat 100–150 fewer calories for breakfast and lunch.

Pack lunch
Bring your own lunch from home – you'll have more control over how many calories you eat. A study found that people who eat in restaurants daily consume 300 more calories a day than those who prepare their own food.

Start with salad, fruit or soup
Eating a low-fat salad or a dish of fruit as a starter can cut the number of calories you eat in your main meal by 12%, according to a study published in the Journal of the American Dietetic Association (Rolls et al., 2004). All that fibre and water takes the edge off your appetite so you eat less of the higher calorie foods. Starting your meal with a bowl of chunky soup can cut your calories by 20%.

Plan ahead
Plan your meals for the whole week. Making a shopping list before you go shopping means that you're more likely to stick to it, and planning ahead means you won't get home from work tired and hungry, only to discover there's nothing healthy in your fridge.

Be size-wise at mealtimes
Stuff yourself with carbohydrate before bedtime and you definitely won't burn all the calories you've taken in. Go easy on the pasta and potatoes and increase the vegetables, fresh fruit and lean protein. Replace half of your usual portion of pasta with veg and you won't eat any less food, just fewer calories. As a guide, a healthy serving of pasta or rice should be around 60 g/2 oz (dry weight) and a serving of potato around 150 g (5 oz), or the size of two eggs.

Veg out
Aim for 3–5 portions of veggies a day. Vegetables help you feel full without boosting your daily calorie intake. Three generous sprigs of broccoli contain just 45 calories, about the same as a nibble (one square) of chocolate.

Table 9.3 Eating for weight loss – top tips cont.

Slow down

You'll eat 15% fewer calories if you sit down and slow down your meal rather than eating on the hoof. Studies show that people eat up to 15% more calories when they rush at mealtimes. Scoffing your meal means that your hypothalamus – the part of the brain that senses when you are full – doesn't receive the right signals and explains why you may feel hungrier sooner.

Get fruity

Eating more fruit is one of the best things you can do for your health. Aim for 2–4 daily portions. Place at least two portions of fruit – apples, grapes, cherries, whatever fruit you like – on your desk. Promise to eat them before you leave work.

Drink wisely

Unsurprisingly, alcohol is the diet downfall of many people. A bottle of wine totals about 500 calories, so you can undo a whole day's good behaviour in just one boozy night. Alcohol can encourage fat storage. It's high in calories and puts undue stress on the liver. Alcohol calories can't be stored and have to be used as they are consumed – and this means that calories excess to requirements from other foods get stored as fat instead.

Remember that adding protein, fat or soluble fibre to carbohydrate always reduces the speed of absorption and produces a lower blood sugar rise. In practice, this is easy to achieve if you plan to eat a carbohydrate source (e.g. potatoes) with a high-protein source (e.g. fish) and add vegetables. Better still, choose low-GI carbohydrates, such as lentils and beans.

Step 9: Bulk up

The most filling foods are those with a high volume per calorie. Water and fibre add bulk to foods, so load up on foods naturally high in these components. Fruit, vegetables, pulses and wholegrain foods give maximum fill for minimum calories. If you can eat a plate of food that is low in calories relative to its volume, you're likely to feel just as satisfied as eating smaller amounts of high-calorie food.

Step 10: Eat more fibre

Apart from reducing your risk of various cancers and heart disease, fibre slows down the emptying of food from your stomach and helps to keep you feeling full. Fibre also gives food more texture so you need to chew your food more. This slows down your eating speed, reducing the chances of overeating and gives better meal satisfaction.

Fibre also slows the digestion and absorption of carbohydrates and fats, resulting in a slow steady energy uptake and stable insulin levels (Albrink, 1978). Non-fluctuating glucose and insulin levels will encourage the use of food for energy rather than for storage as body fat; it also reduces hunger and satisfies the appetite.

Step 11: Indulge yourself

Don't cut out your favourite comfort foods. Many people find that a 'day off' from healthy eating or dieting once a week satisfies their cravings and keeps them well-motivated to eat well week after week. This means you can allow yourself to have chocolate, or your favourite ice cream or that extra large hamburger, without feeling guilty. If you know you can eat a little of your favourite food every week you'll stop thinking of it as a forbid-

Healthy weight loss checklist

- Keep a food diary for a week, writing down the weight of everything you normally eat and drink. This helps you become aware of your true eating pattern.
- Do not skip meals or starve yourself during the day.
- Plan regular meals and snacks throughout the day, thereby eliminating excessive hunger, satisfying appetite, facilitating efficient glycogen refuelling, and improving energy levels and health.
- Set yourself a realistic weight goal that is right for your body type.
- Avoid weekday dieting and weekend splurging. Aim to eat about the same amount of food each day and don't worry if you occasionally overdo it.
- Remember, there are no banned foods; all foods are allowed.
- Do not set yourself rigid eating and exercising rules. Be flexible and never feel guilty if you overindulge or miss an exercise session.
- Examine your feelings and emotions when you eat. Food should not be used as a shield for emotional problems. Solve these with the help of a trained counsellor or eating disorder specialist.

What is thermogenesis?

Thermogenesis means heat production. Every time you consume food your metabolic rate (MR) increases and your body temperature rises a little. If you can get your body to produce more heat by eating the right ratio of fuels, then more of the calories you consume will be burned off as heat. Some nutrients have a higher thermic effect than others. Protein exerts the strongest thermic effect, carbohydrates exert a milder effect, but fat exerts only a tiny thermic effect. When you eat 100 kcal fat only 3 kcal will be burned off as heat. When you eat 100 kcal carbohydrate, 12–15 kcal are 'wasted' as heat. When you eat protein, approximately 20 kcal are wasted (Swaminathan et al., 1985). So eating protein and carbohydrate increases the MR, whereas fat causes very little increase in MR and most of the calories will be converted into body fat. That's a good reason to keep your fat intake low.

den food and won't want to overeat on it. Studies have shown that not banning 'naughty' foods and enjoying the occasional high-fat indulgence without feeling guilty is a successful strategy for maintaining weight loss.

Step 12: Eat regularly and frequently

Plan to eat 4–6 times a day, at regular intervals. This does not mean increasing the amount eaten, but eating moderate-sized meals or snacks more frequently. Studies have shown that eating regularly is associated with a lower total energy intake and an elevated metabolic rate after eating

Table 9.4 Healthy snacks

If you feel hungry between meals, here are some suggestions on what to eat. The snacks are designed to provide balanced amounts of carbohydrate, protein and healthy fat and a low–moderate GI.

- Wholemeal sandwiches, rolls, toast, bagels with healthy fillings (e.g. cottage cheese, tuna, chicken, peanut butter)
- Wholemeal English muffins, fruit buns, scones with olive oil spread
- Smoothies (home-made or ready-made) made with crushed fruit and yoghurt
- Oat/Scotch/homemade pancakes
- Oatcakes and rice cakes with healthy toppings (e.g. peanut butter, avocado)
- Baked beans on wholemeal toast
- Fresh fruit
- Dried fruit and nuts
- Meal replacement shake or bar
- Home-made shakes made with low-fat milk, fruit and yoghurt
- Low-fat yoghurt and fromage frais

(Farschi *et al.*, 2005). After eating, the metabolic rate increases by approximately 10% for a short while afterwards. This phenomenon is the *thermic effect of food*, or dietary-induced *thermogenesis* (see box: 'What is thermogenesis? on page 153). Researchers at the University of Nottingham, UK have also found that eating meals at regular intervals keeps blood sugar and insulin levels more stable, as well as helping to control blood cholesterol levels. For regular exercisers, eating six times a day is especially beneficial for efficient glycogen replenishment between workouts, and for minimising fat deposition. A regular food intake also ensures a constant flux of nutrients for repairing body tissues.

Some suggestions for healthy snacks are given in Table 9.4.

Step 13: Make gradual lifestyle changes

Long-term weight management can be achieved with healthy eating and regular exercise. However, one of the biggest barriers to this is an unwillingness to commit to a few necessary changes in lifestyle. Table 9.5 lists some of the common reasons why many people fail to manage their weight in the long term, together with some suggestions as to how to overcome them.

METABOLIC RATE
DEFINITIONS

Metabolism is the term given to all processes by which your body converts food into energy. The *metabolic rate* is the rate at which your body burns

Table 9.5	Lifestyle changes
Lifestyle	**Suggestion**
Not enough time to prepare healthy meals	Plan meals in advance so all ingredients are at hand. Make meals in bulk and refrigerate/freeze portions. Cook baked potatoes, pasta and rice in larger quantities and save
Work shifts	Plan regular snack breaks and take own food with you
Work involves lots of travelling	Take portable snacks (e.g. rolls, fruit, nuts, energy bars, muffins, dried fruit, diluted fruit juice)
Need to cook for rest of family	Adapt favourite family meals (e.g. spaghetti bolognese) to contain less fat, more carbohydrate and fibre (e.g. leaner mince, more vegetables, wholemeal pasta). Make meals that everyone enjoys
Overeat when stressed	Consider stress counselling or relaxation courses to learn to handle stressful situations; take up new sport/hobby/leisure interests
Eat out frequently	Choose lower fat meals in restaurants (e.g. pasta with vegetable sauces, chicken tikka with chappati, stir fried vegetables with rice)

calories. Your *basal metabolic rate (BMR)* is the rate at which you burn calories on essential body functions, such as breathing and blood circulation during sleep. In practice, the *resting metabolic rate (RMR)* is used, and is measured while you are awake and in a non-fasting state. It accounts for 60–75% of the calories you burn daily.

Several equations have been developed to estimate RMR from body weight. The classic equations of Harris and Benedict, developed in the early 1900s, have been frequently used, but have been superseded by new equations, developed in larger groups of subjects, which have been shown to be more accurate (Goran and Astrup, 2005). These are shown in Table 9.1.

As a rule of thumb, BMR uses 11 calories for every half-kilo (1 lb) of a woman's body weight and 12 calories per half kilo (1 lb) of a man's body weight.

- Women: BMR = weight in kilos x 2 x 11 (alternatively weight in pounds x 11)
- Men: BMR = weight in kilos x 2 x 12 (alternatively weight in pounds x 12)

WHAT MAKES YOUR RMR HIGH OR LOW?

The most important factor that determines your RMR is the amount of fat-free mass you have (muscle, bone and vital organs). This is calorie-burning tissue, so the more fat-free mass you have, the higher your RMR will be.

Your total body weight also affects your RMR. The more you weigh, the higher your RMR, because the larger your body the more calories it needs for basic maintenance.

It is a myth that overweight people have a lower RMR (except in clinical conditions such as hypothyroidism or Cushing's syndrome). Numerous studies have shown a linear relationship between total weight and metabolic rate, i.e. the RMR increases with increasing body weight. Genetics undoubtedly play a role – some people are simply born with a more 'revved-up' metabolism than others.

DOES YOUR METABOLISM SLOW DOWN AS YOU GET OLDER?

Unless you exercise regularly, you'll lose around 0.25 kg (½ lb) of muscle every year after your late twenties. And as you lose muscle, your BMR drops about 2% every decade, so your body burns fewer calories. You can combat age-related muscle loss with twice-weekly weight training.

CAN DIETING SLOW DOWN MY RMR?

Strict dieting will sabotage long-term efforts at weight control because it sends the body into 'famine' mode. When you restrict your calories, your RMR slows down as your body becomes more energy efficient. You need fewer calories just to maintain your weight. The more severe the calorie drop, the greater the decrease in your RMR. Generally the decrease is between 10–30%. However, the effect is not permanent because the RMR returns to its original level once normal eating is resumed.

Avoid a big drop in your RMR by cutting your calories as modestly as possible (15% is recommended) and always consume more calories than your RMR. For example, if your maintenance calorie intake is 2500 kcal, you should reduce this to 2125 kcal.

HOW CAN I INCREASE MY METABOLIC RATE?

Exercise

During the hour or two after vigorous exercise, you continue burning calories faster than normal as your body pays off the oxygen debt, replenishes its energy reserves (PC and ATP) and repairs muscle tissue. The longer and more intense the workout, the greater this 'after-burn' will be. This post-exercise increase in RMR is called the excess post-exercise oxygen consumption or 'after-burn' and comes chiefly from the body's fat stores.

Add muscle

To increase your metabolic rate in the long term, you have to add muscle. Studies have shown that regular weight training will raise your RMR in as little as three months (Thompson et al., 1996).

The American College of Sports Medicine recommends two weight training sessions a week. Adding two pounds (1 kg) of muscle burns an extra 65 calories a day; that's 2015 calories per month, equivalent to losing ½ lb (0.25 kg) of fat.

Eat small meals often through the day

Small regular meals increase the metabolic rate for a short while after eating (see 'Eat regularly and frequently' above). Plan three meals and two or three snacks a day, spacing them at 2–3-hour intervals. Your metabolism is boosted by about ten per cent for two to three hours after you eat. Avoid skipping meals or leaving more than five hours between meals.

Get enough protein

While eating anything raises your metabolic rate, protein boosts it the most. Up to 20% of such a meal's calories may be burned off as heat. Protein is also the most satisfying nutrient, so helps stop you overeating.

Eat a good breakfast

Breakfast kick-starts your metabolism and allows you the whole day to burn up those calories. A combination of carbohydrate and protein (say, porridge made with milk) will give you sustained energy.

Go for a walk after a meal

Moderate exercise, such as walking, after eating may turn more of the calories you have just eaten into heat and make your body burn more calories. Similarly, eating in the hour after vigorous exercise encourages it to be turned into energy rather than being stored as fat, as the metabolic rate is speeded up during this time.

Check portion sizes

Use smaller plates and opt for smaller packages. US researchers have found that the bigger the portion or serving size, the more calories are consumed (Wansink, 2005; Wansink et al., 2005). People who were given large containers of popcorn or soup consumed 45% and 73% more calories respectively than those given smaller containers.

EXERCISE AND WEIGHT LOSS
WHAT IS THE BEST TYPE OF EXERCISE FOR FAT LOSS?

Anyone on a calorie-reduced programme will lose both muscle and fat. On a severe calorie-reduced programme, muscle loss can account for up to 50% of weight loss. However, muscle loss can be minimised by the right choice of exercise.

When weight training exercise is added to a weight-loss programme, more muscle is preserved and a greater proportion of weight loss is fat loss. Intense resistance exercise should be included in your fat-loss programme for two reasons. Firstly, your RMR will be elevated for up to 15 hours post-exercise, due to the oxidation of body fat (Melby et al., 1993). Secondly, weight training acts as the stimulus to muscle retention. The more muscle you have, the faster your metabolism.

Muscle accounts for at least 60% of EPOC (excess post-exercise oxygen consumption). So, the more muscle tissue you have, the greater the EPOC (Bosselaers et al., 1994).

CAN AEROBIC EXERCISE SPEED UP FAT LOSS?

Adding aerobic exercise to your fat-loss programme will burn more calories and offset some of the muscle wastage, but don't rely on aerobic exercise exclusively. You could still lose substantial amounts of muscle tissue with aerobic exercise – some studies have estimated as much as 40% (Aceto, 1997). This is because aerobic exercise does not act as sufficient stimulus to ensure muscle retention while you are on a calorie-reduced programme. Muscle loss will subsequentially result in a lowering of your metabolic rate.

IS HIGH-INTENSITY AEROBICS BETTER THAN LOW-INTENSITY?

Despite what many people believe, low-intensity, long-duration aerobic exercise is not the best method for shedding fat. Research indicates that not only does high-intensity aerobic exercise burn fat more effectively but it also speeds up your metabolism and keeps it revved-up for a while after your workout. What actually counts is the number of calories burned per unit of time. The more calories you expend, the more fat you break down. For example, walking (i.e. low-intensity aerobic exercise) for 60 minutes burns 270 kcal, of which 160 kcal (60% calories) comes from fat. Running (i.e. high-intensity aerobic exercise) for the same amount of time burns 680 kcal, of which 270 kcal (40% calories) comes from fat. Therefore, high-intensity aerobic exercise results in greater fat loss over the same time period. This principle applies to everyone no matter what your level of fitness – exercise intensity is always relative to the individual. Walking at 6 km/h may represent high-intensity exercise for an unconditioned individual; running at 10 km/h may represent low-intensity exercise for a well-conditioned athlete.

HOW SHOULD I CONSTRUCT MY FAT BURNING EXERCISE PROGRAMME?

You have two parts to your fat burning exercise programme:

1. weight training
2. high-intensity aerobic exercise.

Ideally, they should be performed on alternate days so you will have adequate time for recuperation between workouts and maximum energy for each workout. Here is a plan to achieve effective

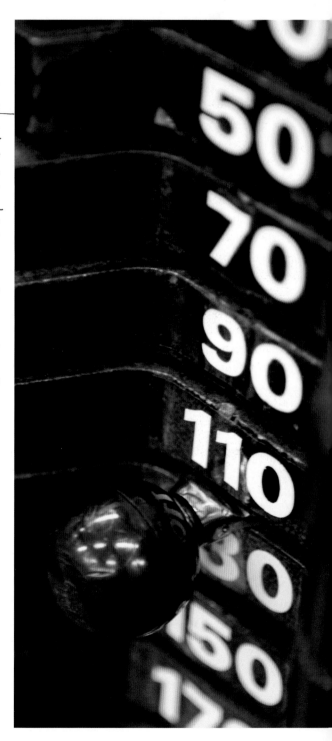

fat loss, and preservation (or building) of muscle mass and the metabolic rate:

- Perform your weight training workout 3 times a week on alternate days (e.g. Monday, Wednesday, Friday). Training sessions should be intense, causing you to reach muscular failure (maximum rating of intensity or perceived exertion on the last set of each exercise).
- Each weight training session should last 40–45 minutes.
- Alternate training the muscles of the upper and lower body (i.e. a two-way split). For example, train upper body on Monday, lower body on Wednesday, upper body on Friday, etc.
- Perform a total of 6 sets for each muscle group, choosing one or two different exercises that target that muscle group. (*See* Table 9.6.)
- Maintain super-strict form and focus on each repetition, keeping the weight fully in control. The importance of technique cannot be stressed enough.

- Lift and lower for a count of two on each part of the movement, and aim to hold the fully contracted position for a count of one.
- Perform your aerobic training sessions three times a week on alternate days (e.g. Tuesday, Thursday, Saturday). Each session should take approximately 20–25 minutes.
- Suitable activities include running, cycling (stationary bike or outdoor cycling), stepping, swimming, rowing or any cardiovascular apparatus. The important factor is that the activity is continuous and you are able to vary your intensity.
- Start with a 3–5 minute warm-up phase. Increase the intensity gradually over the next 4 minutes until you have reached a high-intensity effort. Maintain for 1 minute then reduce the intensity back to a moderate level for 1 minute. Repeat that pattern 4 times. Finish with a gradual reduction in intensity over 2–3 minutes.

Table 9.6	Sample fat-burning exercise plan					
Monday	**Tuesday**	**Wednesday**	**Thursday**	**Friday**	**Saturday**	**Sunday**
Week 1						
UBWT: Chest, back, shoulders, arms	AT: 20–25 minutes on stationary bike	LBWT: Legs, calves, abdominals	AT: 20–25 minute run	UBWT: Chest, back, shoulders, arms	AT: 20–25 minute swim	No training
Week 2						
LBWT: Legs, calves, abdominals	AT: 20–25 minutes on stationary bike	UBWT: Chest, back shoulders, arms	AT: 20–25 minute run	LBWT: Legs, calves, abdominals	AT: 20–25 minute swim	No training
Key:	UBWT = Upper body weight training					
	LBWT = Lower body weight training					
	AT = Aerobic training					

Table 9.7	Sample weight training plan (upper body workout)	
Muscle group	**Exercise**	**Reps**
Chest	Bench press (warm-up)	1 × 12–15
	Bench press	3 × 8–10
	Dumb-bell flyes	3 × 8–10
Back	Lat pulldown (warm-up)	1 × 12–15
	Lat pulldown	3 × 8–10
	Seated row	3 × 8–10
Shoulders	Dumb-bell shoulder press (warm-up)	1 × 12–15
	Dumb-bell shoulder press	3 × 8–10
	Lateral raise	3 × 8–10
Arms	Barbell curl (warm-up)	1 × 12–15
	Barbell curl	3 × 8–10
	Lying tricep extension (warm-up)	1 × 12–15
	Lying tricep extension	3 × 8–10

Table 9.8	Sample weight training plan (lower body workout)	
Muscle group	**Exercise**	**Reps**
Legs	Squat (warm-up)	1 × 12–15
	Squat	3 × 8–10
	Lunges	3 × 8–10
	Calf raise (warm-up)	1 × 12–15
	Calf raise	3 × 8–10
Abdominals	Crunches	2 × 10–15
	Oblique crunches	2 × 10–15
	Reverse curl-ups	2 × 10–15

Note: For a full description of the exercises in Tables 9.7 and 9.8 see *The Complete Guide to Strength Training* (4th edition) by Anita Bean (A & C Black, 2008).

COMMERCIAL WEIGHT LOSS DIETS

HOW EFFECTIVE ARE LOW-CARBOHYDRATE DIETS?

Proponents of low-carbohydrate diets (e.g. Atkins, the South Beach Diet) claim that people lose weight more effectively when insulin levels are kept as low as possible. According to the low-carb theory carbohydrate causes frequent insulin surges, which in turn, encourages the body to store fat. Over time, this may result in a metabolic disorder called insulin resistance, which means that the body becomes unresponsive to the actions of insulin and, as a result, produces more of it, further pushing the body into fat-storage mode. The solution, according to low-carb authors is to cut carbohydrate intake dramatically and force the body to go into ketosis, i.e. fat is broken down in a different way to release ketones.

Low-carb diets have been criticised by eminent researchers who state that it is not the insulin that makes people put on weight; the opposite is more likely to be true. In most cases, it's being fat that makes people insulin resistant. When you lose weight, resistance returns to normal.

Low-carbohydrate diets may work in the short term, but only because you eat fewer calories. If you cut out virtually all sugar and starch, you automatically restrict the foods you can eat. It's difficult to overeat meat and eggs and with so few choices most people end up consuming fewer calories. It's a simple negative energy balance explanation. In a year-long study at the University of Pennsylvania, obese people on the Atkins diet lost 10 lbs more after 6 months than volunteers on a conventional diet (Samaha, 2003). But by the end of the year, the differences between the two groups were not significant, suggesting the Atkins diet is no better at helping overweight people shed weight than traditional diets. The novelty of such a 'different' eating system appeals to certain people and that in itself is motivating. However, these diets are highly unsuitable for athletes as they provide too little carbohydrates to support athletic performance. They would empty your glycogen reserves, produce fatigue and limit your endurance.

Worse still is the threat of ketosis and muscle-wasting brought on by eating a low-carb diet. Low glycogen and blood sugar levels cause the body to break down protein for energy.

Other risks of low-carb dieting include headaches, constipation and halitosis (bad breath). Ketosis can upset electrolyte balance in the body and, potentially, cause cardiac arrhythmias. One of the biggest concerns with low-carb diets is that they are nutritionally unbalanced – they provide low amounts of fibre, vitamins C, E, and beta-carotene, calcium and lycopene. They also tend to be high in fat, particularly saturated fat, which can increase blood cholesterol levels and promote heart disease.

ARE POPULAR DIETS HEALTHY AND EFFECTIVE?

Most diets work in the short term, but not all are healthy and most are not sustainable in the long term. The more extreme the diet, the lower the chance of adhering to it. A year-long study at the Tufts-New England Medical Centre in the US compared four different diets (Atkins diet, Ornish low-fat diet, Weight Watchers and the Zone diet) and found that all produced a similar, albeit small, weight loss (three-quarters of them lost less than 5% of their body weight in

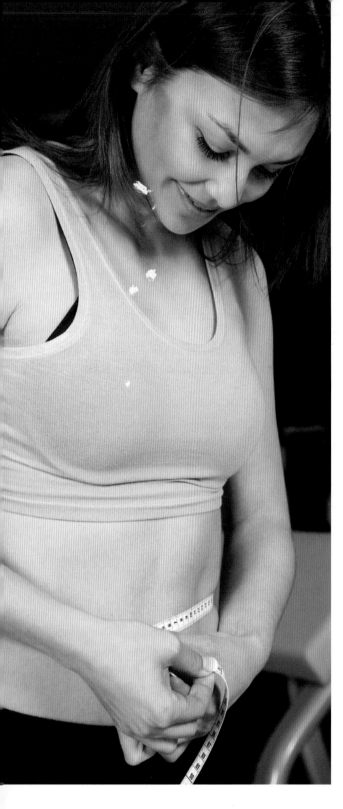

a year) but that few dieters could stick to them for long enough to make a permanent difference (Dansinger *et al.*, 2005). They found that most dieters reduced their calorie intake initially but levels crept back up again. Of the diets tested, the low-carb Atkins diet achieved the lowest weight loss over 12 months and had the lowest adherence.

A 2008 UK study compared the effectiveness and nutritional content of four commercial slimming programmes: Slim Fast, Atkins, WeightWatchers and Rosemary Conley's Eat Yourself Slim diet (Truby *et al.*, 2008). The researchers found that all the diets result in a reduced calorie intake, resulting in an average weight loss after eight weeks of between 3.7 kg and 5.2 kg. There was no significant difference in weight loss between the diets themselves. On the whole, the diets provided the RDAs for most nutrients, but dieters failed to increase significantly their consumption of fruit and vegetables as recommended.

The secret to losing weight is to eat more healthily, increase your activity and make easy changes to your lifestyle that you are comfortable with and will be able to adopt long term. Failing to keep to a diet can not only affect your health and metabolism but can cause psychological problems. A two-year study at the University of California found that overweight women who did not follow a set diet, but who simply ate more healthily and listened to hunger and satiety cues, improved their health (e.g. blood pressure and cholesterol levels) and had higher self esteem (Bacon *et al.*, 2005). In contrast, those who dieted for six months regained their weight and reported significant drops in confidence and self-esteem.

SUMMARY OF KEY POINTS

- Rapid weight loss can result in an excessive loss of lean tissue, dehydration, and a reduction in aerobic capacity (up to 10%), strength and endurance.
- Effective fat loss can be achieved by reducing calorie intake by no more than 15%; this will minimise both lean tissue loss and resting metabolic rate (RMR) reduction.
- The recommended rate of fat loss is no more than 0.5 kg/week.
- Carbohydrate should be reduced by only a modest amount, but still contribute 60% of calories.
- Protein intake should be approx 1.6 g/ kg body weight/ day to offset lean tissue loss.
- A reduction in saturated fat while maintaining essential fatty acids will result in an effective body-fat loss.
- Additional aerobic exercise performed for 20 minutes 3 times a week together with high intensity weight training performed on alternate days will maintain muscle mass and RMR while losing body fat.
- Your diet should be based on low GI meals, and foods with a high fibre and/or water content.
- Eating carbohydrate and protein, minimising fat and increasing meal frequency can optimise thermogenesis and, therefore, fat loss.
- The most effective way of increasing your RMR is to increase lean mass and follow a high intensity aerobic and weight training programme.
- Appetite regulation is enhanced by a high protein, high carbohydrate, low-fat eating programme.
- Yo-yo dieting can have an adverse effect on body composition, and overall physical and mental health.
- Failed attempts to lose body fat permanently may be due to inconsistent patterns of food intake, negative body image, poor motivation, unnecessary food restriction or avoidance, or a negative mental attitude.

10

// WEIGHT GAIN

There are two ways to gain weight: either by increasing your lean mass or by increasing your fat mass. Both will register as weight gain on the scales but result in a very different body composition and appearance!

Lean weight gain can be achieved by combining a consistent well-planned resistance training programme with a balanced diet. Resistance training provides the stimulus for muscle growth while your diet provides the right amount of energy (calories) and nutrients to enable your muscles to grow at the optimal rate. One without the other would result in only minimal lean weight gain.

WHAT TYPE OF TRAINING IS BEST FOR GAINING WEIGHT?

Resistance training (weight training) is the best way to stimulate muscle growth. Research shows that the fastest gains in size and strength are achieved using relatively heavy weights that can be lifted strictly for 6–10 repetitions per set. If you can do more than 10–12 repetitions at a particular weight, your size gains will be less, but you may still achieve improvements in muscular endurance, strength and power.

Concentrate on the 'compound' exercises, such as bench press, squat, shoulder press and lat pull-down, as these work the largest muscle groups of the body together with neighbouring muscles that act as 'assistors' or 'synergists'. These types of exercises stimulate the largest number of muscle fibres in one movement and are therefore the most effective and quickest way to gain muscle mass. Keep the smaller isolation exercises, such as biceps concentration curls or tricep kickbacks, to a minimum; these produce slower mass gains and should be added to your workout only occasionally for variety.

HOW MUCH WEIGHT CAN I EXPECT TO GAIN?

The amount of muscle weight you can expect to gain depends on several genetic factors, including your body type, muscle fibre mix, the arrangement of your motor units and your hormonal balance, as well as your training programme and diet.

Your genetic make up determines the proportion of different types of fibres in your muscles. The fast-twitch (type II) fibres generate power and increase in size more readily than the slow-twitch (type I or endurance) fibres. So, if you naturally have plenty of fast-twitch fibres in your muscles, you will probably respond faster to a strength training programme than someone who has a higher proportion of slow-twitch fibres. Unfortunately, you cannot convert slow-twitch into fast-twitch fibres – hence two people can follow exactly the same training programme, yet the one with lots of fast twitch muscle fibres will naturally gain weight faster than the other.

Your natural body type also affects how fast you gain lean weight. An ectomorph (naturally slim build with long lean limbs, narrow shoulders and hips) will find it harder to gain weight than a mesomorph (muscular, athletic build with wide shoulders and narrow hips) who tends to gain muscle readily. An endomorph (stocky, rounded build with wide shoulders and hips and an even distribution of fat) gains both fat and muscle readily.

People with a higher natural level of the male (anabolic) sex hormones, such as testosterone, will also gain muscle faster. That is why women cannot achieve the muscle mass or size of men unless they take anabolic steroids.

However, no matter what your genetics, natural build and hormonal balance, everyone can gain muscle and improve their shape with strength training. It is just that it takes some people longer than others.

HOW FAST CAN I EXPECT TO GAIN WEIGHT?

Mass gains of 20% of starting body weight are common after the first year of training. However, the rate of weight gain will gradually drop off over the years as you approach your genetic potential. Men can expect to gain 0.5–1 kg per month (GSSI, 1995). Women usually experience about 50–75% of the gains of men – i.e. 0.25–0.75 kg/month – partly due to their smaller initial body weight and smaller muscle mass, and partly due

Training for muscle gain

Certain compound exercises, such as dead lifts, clean and jerks, snatches and squats, not only stimulate the 'prime mover' muscles, but also have a powerful anabolic ('systemic') effect on the whole body and the central nervous system. These are the classic mass builders and should be included once a week in any serious muscle/strength training programme.

To stimulate the maximal number of muscle fibres in a muscle group, select one to three basic exercises and aim to do 4–12 total sets for that muscle group. Latest research suggests that doing fewer sets (4–8) but using heavier weights (80–90% of your one-rep maximum – i.e. the maximum weight which can be lifted through one complete repetition) results in faster size and strength gains. If you exercise that muscle group to exhaustion, you will need to allow up to 7 days for recuperation before repeating the same workout. So, aim to train each muscle group once a week (on average). In practice, divide your body parts (e.g. chest, legs, shoulders, back, arms) into three or four, and train one part per workout.

Always use strict training form and, ideally, have a partner to 'spot' for you so that you can use near-maximal weights safely. Always remember to warm up each muscle group beforehand with light aerobic training (e.g. exercise bike) and some relevant stretches. Ensure you also stretch the muscles after (and, ideally, in between each part of) the workout to help relieve soreness.

to lower levels of anabolic hormones. Monitor your body composition rather than simply your weight. If you gain weight much more than 1 kg per month on an established programme, then you are likely to be gaining fat!

HOW MUCH SHOULD I EAT?

To gain lean weight and muscle strength at the optimal rate, you need to be in a positive energy balance, i.e. consuming more calories than you need for maintenance. This cannot be stressed too much. These additional calories should come from a balanced ratio of carbohydrate, protein and fat.

1 CALORIES

Estimate your maintenance calorie intake using the formulae in Steps 1–4, Chapter 9, p. 146. To gain muscle, increase your calorie intake by 20%, i.e. multiply your maintenance calories by 1.2 (120%).

Example:

• If your maintenance calorie requirement is 2700 kcal, you will need to eat 2700 × 1.2 = 3240 kcal.

In practice, most athletes will need to add roughly an extra 500 kcal to their daily diet. Not all of these extra calories are converted into muscle –

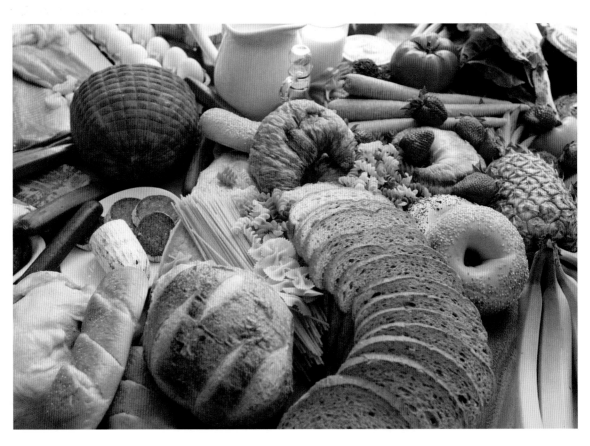

some will be used for digestion and absorption, given off as heat or used for physical activity. Increase your calorie intake gradually, say 200 a day for a while, then after a week or two, increase it by a further 200 kcal. Slow gainers may need to increase their calorie intake by as much as 1000 kcal a day.

2 CARBOHYDRATE

In order to gain muscle, you need to train very hard, and that requires a lot of fuel. The key fuel for this type of exercise is, of course, muscle glycogen. Therefore, you must consume enough carbohydrate to achieve high muscle glycogen levels. If you train with low levels of muscle glycogen, you risk excessive protein (muscle) breakdown, which is just the opposite of what you are aiming for.

In a 24-hour period during low or moderate intensity training days, you should get 5–7 g/kg of body weight. During moderate to heavy endurance training 7–10 g/kg is recommended. As your calorie needs increase by 20%, so should your usual carbohydrate intake. In practice, aim to eat an extra 50–100 g carbohydrate.

3 PROTEIN

The recommendation for strength training is 1.4–1.7 g/kg body weight/day (Tarnopolsky *et al.*, 1992; Lemon *et al.*, 1992). This level of protein intake should support muscle growth – studies show that increasing your intake above 2.0 g/kg body weight produces no further benefit.

For example, if you weigh 80 kg you would need between 112 g and 136 g protein a day.

4 FAT

Fat should comprise between 20 and 33% of total calories, or the balance of calories once you have met your needs for carbohydrate and protein. Most of your fat should come from unsaturated sources, such as olive oil and other vegetable oils, avocado, oily fish, nuts and seeds.

For example, if you consume 3000 kcal a day, your fat intake should be:

- $(3000 \times 20\%) \div 9 = 66$ g
- $(3000 \times 33\%) \div 9 = 110$ g

i.e. between 66 and 110 g fat a day.

WHAT IS THE IDEAL POST-WORKOUT MEAL?

Begin refuelling as soon as possible after training. You can optimise glycogen recovery after training by consuming 1 g carbohydrate/kg body weight during the 2-hour post exercise period (Ivy *et al.*, 1988). So, for example, if you weigh 80 kg you need to consume 80 g carbohydrate within 2 hours after exercise.

However, it's not only carbohydrate that aids recovery after training: several studies suggest that taking carbohydrate combined with protein after exercise, helps create the ideal hormonal environment for glycogen storage and muscle building (Zawadzki *et al.*, 1992; Bloomer *et al.*, 2000; Gibala, 2000; Krieder *et al.*, 1996). Both trigger the release of insulin and growth hormone in your body. These are powerful anabolic hormones. Insulin transports amino acids into cells, reassembles them into proteins, and prevents muscle breakdown. It also transports glucose into muscle cells and stimulates glycogen storage. Growth hormone increases protein manufacture and muscle building.

In the study, nine weight trainers were given water, a carbohydrate supplement, a protein supplement or a carbohydrate–protein supplement immediately after training and again 2 hours later. Blood levels of insulin and growth hormone were greatest during the 8 hours after exercise in those trainers who consumed the carbohydrate–protein supplement. Therefore, it seems that the combination of post-workout carbohydrate and protein promotes the best hormonal environment for muscle growth.

The optimal post-workout meal or drink should comprise protein and carbohydrate in a ratio of 1:4, e.g. 15–30 g protein and 60–120 g carbohydrate. Suitable snacks are suggested in the box 'Post-workout snacks'.

To optimise glycogen storage and muscle growth, you should ensure a relatively steady supply of nutrients into the bloodstream by dividing your food intake into five or six meals and snacks throughout the day. Avoid leav-ing gaps longer than 3–4 hours because this would encourage protein breakdown and slow down glycogen storage. Avoid consuming large infrequent meals or lots of high GI meals because they will produce large fluctuations in blood sugar and insulin and therefore reduce glycogen storage.

WILL WEIGHT GAIN SUPPLEMENTS HELP?

There are literally dozens of supplements on the market that claim to enhance muscle mass, although many of the claims are not supported by scientific research, lack safety data and some have even been found to contain illegal substances! For more information on supplements, *see* Chapter 6. Supplements that may be worth considering for weight gain include:

- Creatine may help increase performance, strength and muscle mass. Dozens of studies since the mid 1990s show significant increases in lean mass and total mass, typically between 1–3% lean body weight (approx. 0.8–3 kg) after a 5-day loading dose, compared with controls. See also Chapter 6, pp. 90–94.

  For example, in a study carried out at Pennsylvania State University, 13 weight trainers gained an average 1.3 kg body mass after taking creatine supplements for 7 days (Volek, 1997). The same team of researchers measured total weight gain of 1.7 kg and muscle mass gain of 1.5 kg after one week of creatine supplementation among 19 weight trainers (Volek, 1999). After 12 weeks, total weight gain averaged 4.8 kg and muscle gain averaged 4.3 kg.

Post-workout snacks

To be eaten within 2 hours after exercise:

- 1–2 portions of fresh fruit with a drink of milk
- 1 or 2 cartons of yoghurt
- A smoothie (crushed fresh fruit and yoghurt whizzed in a blender)
- A homemade milkshake (milk with fresh fruit and yoghurt)
- A yoghurt drink
- A sandwich/bagel/roll/wrap filled with lean protein – tuna, chicken, cottage cheese, peanut butter or egg
- A handful of dried fruit and nuts
- Jacket potato with tuna, baked beans or cottage cheese

The observed gains in weight are due partly to an increase in cell fluid volume and partly to muscle synthesis. However, not all studies have shown a positive effect on muscle mass; some have found gains in total body weight only.

- Meal replacement supplements provide a convenient alternative to solid food. They will not necessarily improve your performance but can be a helpful and convenient addition (rather than replacement) to your diet if you struggle to eat enough real food, you need to eat on the move or you need the extra nutrients they provide.
- Protein supplements may benefit you if you have particularly high protein requirements or cannot consume enough protein from food alone (e.g. a vegetarian or vegan diet).

WEIGHT GAIN TIPS

Put more total eating time into your daily routine. This may mean rescheduling other activities. Plan your meal and snack times in advance and never skip or rush them, no matter how busy you are.

- increase your meal frequency – eat at least three meals and three snacks daily.
- eat regularly – every 2–3 hours – and avoid gaps longer than three hours.
- plan nutritious high-calorie low-bulk snacks – e.g. shakes, smoothies, yoghurt, nuts, dried fruit, energy/protein bars.
- eat larger meals but avoid overfilling!
- if you are finding it hard to eat enough food, have more drinks such as meal replacement or protein supplements once or twice a day to help bring up your calorie, carbohydrate and protein intake.

How does creatine cause weight gain?

Weight gain is due partly to water retention in the muscle cells and partly to increased muscle growth. Researchers have found that urine volume is reduced markedly during the initial days of supplementation with creatine, which indicates the body is retaining extra water (Hultman, 1996).

Creatine draws water in to the muscle cells, thus increasing cell volume. In one study with cross-trained athletes, thigh muscle volume increased 6.6% and intra-cellular volume increased 2–3% after a creatine-loading dose (Ziegenfuss et al., 1997). It is thought that the greater cell volume caused by creatine supplementation acts as an anabolic signal for protein synthesis and therefore muscle growth (Haussinger et al., 1996). It also reduces protein breakdown during intense exercise.

The fact that studies show a substantially greater muscle mass even after long-term creatine supplementation indicates that creatine must have a direct effect on muscle growth. In studies at the University of Memphis, athletes taking creatine gained more body mass than those taking the placebo, yet both groups ended up with the same body water content (Kreider et al., 1996). If creatine allows you to train more intensely, it follows that you will gain more muscle mass. For more details on creatine supplement doses see Chapter 6, pp. 90–94.

- boost the calorie and nutritional content of your meals – e.g. add dried fruit, bananas, honey, chopped nuts or seeds to breakfast cereal or yoghurt. This is more nutritious than the common practice of adding sugar or jam ('empty calories').

SUMMARY OF KEY POINTS

- To build muscle, an intense weight-training programme must be combined with a balanced intake of calories, carbohydrate, protein and fat.
- Aim to gain 0.5–1 kg lean weight per month.
- The amount of lean weight you gain depends on your genetic make-up, body type and hormonal balance.
- To gain lean weight, increase your maintenance calorie intake by 20%, or about 500 kcal daily.
- A protein intake of 1.4–1.7 g/kg body weight will meet your protein needs; carbohydrates should supply about 60% of your total calories. As your calorie needs increase by 20%, so should your usual carbohydrate intake.
- Consume 1 g carbohydrate/kg body weight immediately after training, ideally combined with protein in a ratio of 4:1.

High calorie snacks for hard gainers

- Nuts
- Dried fruit – raisins, sultanas, dates, apricots, mango, blueberries, apples and peaches
- Milkshake
- Smoothie
- Yoghurt
- Yoghurt drink
- Sandwich, bagel, roll, pitta or muffin
- Cereal or breakfast bar
- Flapjack
- Meal replacement shake
- Sports or protein bar

- Increase your meal frequency – eat at least 3 meals and 3 snacks daily.
- Plan nutritious high-calorie low-bulk snacks – eg. shakes, smoothies, yoghurt, nuts, dried fruit, energy/protein bars.
- Creatine may help increase performance, strength and muscle mass.

THE FEMALE ATHLETE

11

This chapter covers the issues that relate specifically to female athletes. These centre around disordered eating, amenorrhoea and bone loss, which are closely linked and relatively common among female athletes. In 1992 this combination of disorders was given the formal name of the 'female athlete triad' during a consensus conference convened by the American College of Sports Medicine, and documented in a position stand published in 1997 (Otis *et al.*, 1997).

The emphasis placed on being lean or attaining a very low body weight in many sports is now greater than ever. To achieve this goal, many female athletes undertake an intense and excessive training programme and combine it with a restrictive diet. However, in some athletes, this can lead to an obsessive preoccupation with body weight and calorie intake, and eventually disordered eating. This chapter examines why female athletes are more prone to disordered eating and gives some of the warning signs to look out for. It considers the effects on health and how to help someone suspected of having an eating disorder.

This chapter aslo considers the causes and treatment of amenorrhoea and explains the effect it has on health and performance. One of the most serious effects is the reduction in bone density and increased risk of bone loss, osteoporosis and stress fractures.

Female athletes are more prone than non-athletes to iron-deficiency anaemia, due to increased losses associated with training or a low dietary intake. This chapter describes the symptoms of this condition and also explains the causes of related conditions, sports anaemia and latent iron deficiency. The appropriate use of iron supplements is also covered.

Finally, details of specific nutritional considerations for female athletes during pregnancy are given, and the effect a low body fat percentage may have on the chances of conception and successful pregnancy are discussed.

DISORDERED EATING OR EATING DISORDER?

Many athletes are very careful about what they eat and often experiment with different dietary programmes in order to improve their performance. However, there is a thin line between paying attention to detail and obsessive eating behaviour. The pressure to be thin or attain higher performance makes some athletes develop eating habits that not only put their performance at risk but also endanger their health.

Disordered eating is one of the risk factors for the development of amenorrhoea, a loss of normal menstrual periods. This condition is often the result of a chronic low calorie intake, low body fat and weight, high-intensity training and volume, and psychological stress.

Eating disorders represent the extremes in a continuum of eating behaviours. An eating disorder is defined as: a *distorted pattern of thinking and behaviour about food*. In all cases, preoccupation and obsession with food occurs and eating is out of control. It's as much about attitude and behaviour towards food as it is about consumption of food.

Clinical eating disorders such as anorexia, bulimia and compulsive eating are defined by official, specific criteria by the American Psychiatric Association (APA). *Anorexia nervosa* is the extreme of restrictive eating behaviour in which the individual continues to restrict food and feel fat in spite of being 15% or more below an ideal body weight. *Bulimia* refers to a cycle of food restriction followed by bingeing and purging. Compulsive eating is a psychological craving for food that results in uncontrollable eating.

However, many people who don't fall into these clinical categories may still have a sub-clinical eating disorder. This is often called *disordered eating*. Sufferers have an intense fear of gaining weight or becoming fat even though their weight is normal or below normal. They are preoccupied with food, their weight and body shape. Like anorexics, they have a distorted body image, imagining they are larger than they really are. They attempt to lose weight by restricting their food, usually consuming less than 1200 kcal a day, and may exercise excessively to burn more calories. The result is a chaotic eating pattern and lifestyle.

ARE FEMALE ATHLETES MORE LIKELY TO DEVELOP DISORDERED EATING?

Female athletes are more vulnerable to disordered eating than the general population – disordered eating may affect up to 60% of female athletes in certain sports (Sundgot-Borgon, 1994 (a) and (b); Petrie, 1993). Disordered eating appears to be more common in athletes in sports where a low body weight, body fat level or thin physique is perceived to be advantageous (see Table 11.1) (Beals & Manore, 2002; Sundgot-Borgon & Torstveit, 2004). In a US study 30% of elite female skaters considered themselves overweight, had a poor body image and indicated a preference for a thinner body shape (Jonnalagadda *et al.*, 2004). Another study suggests that females

Table 11.1	Eating disorders – high risk sports
Lean sports	Distance running and cycling, horse racing
Aesthetic sports	Gymnastics, figure skating, ballet, competitive aerobics, bodybuilding, synchronised swimming
Weight category sports	Lightweight rowing, judo, karate, weightlifting, bodybuilding

Source: Beal & Manore, 1994.

involved in sports that favour leanness, such as figure skating and gymnastics, are more likely to be at risk of developing disordered eating and be over-concerned about their body weight and dieting (Zucker *et al.*, 1999).

The causes differ depending on the sport. Distance runners are at greater risk of developing disordered eating because of the close link between low body weight and performance. Those participating in aesthetic sports such as dancing, bodybuilding and gymnastics are at risk because success depends on body shape as well as physical skill. Athletes competing in weight category sports such as judo and lightweight rowing are also more likely to develop eating disorders due to the pressures of meeting the weight criteria.

There is no single cause of disordered eating but, typically, it stems from a belief that a lower body weight enhances athletic success. The athlete begins to diet and, for reasons not completely understood, then adopts more restrictive and unhealthy eating behaviour.

The demands of certain sports or training programmes or the requests made by coaches to lose weight may trigger an eating disorder in susceptible individuals. It is possible that some people with a predisposition to eating disorders are attracted to certain sports. Studies have shown that athletes in sports demanding a high degree of leanness have a more distorted body image, and are more dissatisfied with their body weight and shape compared to the general population. Researchers have found that the personality characteristics of elite athletes are very similar to those with eating disorders: obsession, competitiveness, perfectionism, compulsiveness and self-motivation. Training then becomes a way to lose weight and the positive relationship between

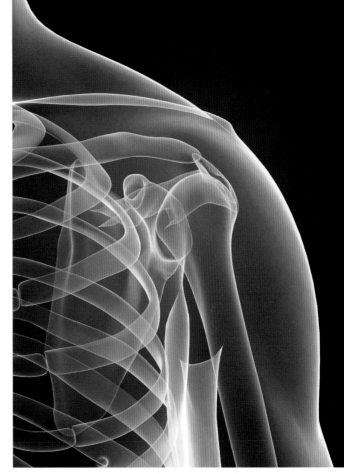

leanness and performance further legitimises the athlete's pursuit of thinness.

Evidence is also emerging that sufferers have a disturbed body chemistry as well as a psychological predisposition to disordered eating. For example, studies have found that more than half of those suffering from anorexia have a severe zinc deficiency and that recovery is more successful if zinc supplements are given (Bryce-Smith and Simpson, 1984). There may also be a genetic link. Around 10% of anorexics have siblings similarly affected, and it occurs more commonly than would be expected in identical twins. Researchers have identified certain genes that influence personality traits such as perfectionism and thus predispose an individual to eating disorders (Garfinkel

Table 11.2	Characteristics of anorexia nervosa	
Physical signs	**Psychological signs**	**Behavioural signs**
Severe weight loss	Obsessive about food, dieting and thinness	Eating very little
Well below average weight	Claiming to be fat when thin	Relentless exercise
Emaciated appearance	Obsessive fear of weight gain	Great interest in food and calories
Periods stop or become irregular	Low self-esteem	Anxiety and arguments about food
Growth or downy hair on face, arms and legs	Depression and anxiety	Refusing to eat in company
Feeling cold, bluish extremities	Perfectionism	Lying about eating meals
Restless, sleeping very little	High need for approval	Obsessive weighing
Dry/yellow skin	Social withdrawal	Rituals around eating

Table 11.3	Characteristics of bulimia nervosa	
Physical signs	**Psychological signs**	**Behavioural signs**
Tooth decay, enamel erosion	Low self-esteem and self-control	Out of control bingeing on large amounts of food (up to 5000 kcal)
Puffy face due to swollen salivary glands	Impulsive	Eating to numb feeling/provide comfort
Normal weight or extreme weight fluctuations	Depression, anxiety, anger	Guilt, shame, withdrawal and self-deprecation after bingeing
Abrasions on knuckles from self-induced vomiting	Body dissatisfaction and distortion	Purging – vomiting, laxative abuse
Menstrual irregularities	Preoccupied with food, body image, appearance and weight	Frequent weighing
Muscle cramps/weakness		Disappearing after meals to get rid of food
Frequently dehydrated		Secretive eating
		May steal food/laxatives

and Garner, 1982; Davis, 1993). Scientists have recently proposed that sufferers have a defective gene that results in abnormally high levels of the brain chemical, serotonin. This causes a reduction in appetite, lowered mood and anxiety. They suggest that anorexics use starvation as a means of escaping anxiety.

WHAT ARE THE WARNING SIGNS?

Athletes with disordered eating try to keep their disorder a secret. However, there are physical and behavioural signs you can look out for. These are detailed in Tables 11.2 and 11.3 (*see also* 'Have you got disordered eating?').

WHAT ARE THE HEALTH EFFECTS OF DISORDERED EATING?

The chaotic and restricted eating patterns of disordered eating often result in menstrual and fertility problems. Menstrual dysfunction (irregularities in the menstrual cycle − oligomenorrhoea − or a complete loss of menstrual periods − amenorrhoea) is common among anorexics. The combination of low body fat levels, restricted calorie intake, low calcium intake, intense training and stress can result in bone thinning, stress fractures and other injuries, and, ultimately premature osteoporosis. One study found that disordered eating was associated with low bone mineral density in runners who had regular menstrual cycles (Cobb *et al.*, 2003). Another found that 45 out of 53 female competitive track and field runners had suffered stress fractures, and this was correlated with high levels of weight and eating concerns (Bennell *et al.*, 1995). Researchers at the University of British Columbia, Vancouver, found that women runners with a recent stress fracture were more likely to have a high degree of

Have you got disordered eating?

This questionnaire is not intended as a diagnostic method for disordered eating or as a substitute for a full diagnosis by an eating disorders specialist. If you answer yes to six or more of the following questions you could be at risk of developing disordered eating and may benefit from further help.

- Do you count the calories of everything you eat?
- Do you think about food most of the time?
- Do you worry about gaining weight?
- Do you worry about or dislike your body shape?
- Do you diet excessively?
- Do you feel guilty during or after eating?
- Do you feel your weight is one aspect of your life you can control?
- Do your friends and family insist that you are slim while you feel fat?
- Do you exercise to compensate for eating extra calories?
- Does your weight fluctuate dramatically?
- Do you ever induce vomiting after eating?
- Have you become isolated from family and friends?
- Do you avoid certain foods even though you want to eat them?
- Do you feel stressed or guilty if your normal diet or exercise routine are interrupted?
- Do you often decline invitations to meals and social occasions involving food in case you might have to eat something fattening?

dietary restraint compared with runners without a history of stress fractures (Guest and Barr, 2005). Gastrointestinal problems, electrolyte imbalances, kidney and bowel disorders, and depression are also common. Anorexics may develop low blood pressure and chronic low core body temperature.

Improve your body image

This guide is not intended as a treatment for disordered eating. Treatment should always be sought from an eating disorders specialist.

- Learn to accept your body's shape – emphasise your good points.
- Realise that reducing your body fat will not solve deep-rooted problems or an emotional crisis.
- Don't set rigid eating rules for yourself and feel guilty when you break them.
- Don't ban any foods or feel guilty about eating anything.
- Don't count calories.
- Think of foods in terms of taste and health rather than a source of calories.
- Establish a sensible healthy eating pattern rather than a strict diet.
- Listen to your natural appetite cues – learn to eat when you are hungry.
- If you do overeat, don't try to 'pay for it' later by starving yourself or exercising to burn off calories.
- Enjoy your exercise or sport for its own sake; have fun instead of enduring torture to lose body fat.
- Set positive exercise goals not related to losing weight.

In bulimics, repeated vomiting and use of laxatives can lead to stomach and oesophagus pain, enamel erosion and tooth decay.

HOW CAN ATHLETES WITH DISORDERED EATING CONTINUE TRAINING?

It seems extraordinary that athletes with apparently very low calorie intake continue to exercise and compete, apparently unabated. Undoubtedly, a combination of psychological and physiological factors are involved.

On the psychological side, anorexics are able to motivate and push themselves to exercise, despite feelings of exhaustion. Sufferers are strong willed, highly driven and have a strong desire to succeed.

Some scientists believe that some athletes under-report their food intake and, in fact, eat more than they admit. For example, a study at Indiana University on nine highly trained cross-country runners found that they were eating, on average, 2100 kcal per day but their predicted energy expenditure was 3000 kcal (Edwards, 1993). After analysing the results of a Food Attitude Questionnaire, the researchers suggested that many had a poor body image and had inaccurately reported what they ate during the study.

On the physiological side, it is likely that the body adapts by becoming more energy efficient, reducing its metabolic rate (10–30% is possible). This would allow the athlete to train and maintain energy balance on fewer calories than would be expected. Some scientists, however, suggest that excessive exercise during dieting may augment the fall in metabolic rate.

To overcome physical and emotional fatigue, many anorexics and bulimics use caffeine-containing drinks such as strong coffee and 'diet' cola.

However, in the long term, performance ultimately falls. As glycogen and nutrient stores become chronically depleted, the athlete's health will suffer and optimal performance cannot be sustained indefinitely. Maximal oxygen consumption decreases, chronic fatigue sets in and the athlete becomes more susceptible to injury and infection.

HOW SHOULD I APPROACH SOMEONE SUSPECTED OF HAVING DISORDERED EATING?

Approaching someone you suspect has disordered eating requires great tact and sensitivity. Sufferers are likely to deny that that have a problem; they may feel embarrassed and their self-esteem threatened, so it is vital to avoid a direct confrontation about their eating behaviour or physical symptoms. Be tactful, tread very gently – do not suddenly present 'evidence' – and avoid accusations.

If the sufferer admits to having an eating problem (see box 'Have you got disordered eating'), suggest that it would be best to consult an eating disorders specialist. Various forms of specialist help are available, such as trained counsellors from a self-help organisation or private eating disorders clinic (see pp. 325–327 for a list of useful organisations), or with a GP's referral, treatment within a multidisciplinary team of psychologists and dietitians.

MENSTRUAL DYSFUNCTION AND BONE LOSS

ARE FEMALE ATHLETES AT GREATER RISK OF MENSTRUAL DYSFUNCTION?

Female athletes are more likely to develop menstrual dysfunction. Several studies have found that menstrual dysfunction is more prevalent among female athletes participating in endurance or aesthetic sports (Beals & Hill, 2006; Torstveit and Sundgot-Borgon, 2005; Sundgot-Borgon, 1994; Sundgot-Borgon and Larsen, 1993).

In a study at the University of Utah and the University of Indianapolis, significantly more lean-build athletes suffered menstrual irregularities than non lean-build athletes (Beals & Hill, 2006). This may be due to the greater volume of training associated with endurance sports. However, a study at San Diego State University indicates that approximately 20% of female high school athletes, regardless of sport, are at risk of disordered eating or menstrual dysfunction and that the two conditions are often inter-related (Nichols *et al.*, 2007). Nearly 27% of lean-build athletes had menstrual dysfunction, compared with 17% non lean-build athletes.

Menstrual dysfunction is unlikely to develop as a result of exercise alone, nor does there seem to be a specific body fat percentage below which regular periods stop. Studies have shown that female athletes who have a restricted calorie intake are at increased risk of menstrual dysfunction (Louks, 2003). A combination of factors, such as restricted calorie intake, disordered eating, intense training before menarche, high-intensity training and volume, low body-fat levels and physical and emotional stress are usually involved (*see* Fig. 11.1). The more of these risk factors that you have, the greater the chance of developing menstrual dysfunction.

Girls who begin intense training pre-puberty usually start their periods at a later age than the average. This may be due to a combination of high-volume exercise and low body-fat levels. Some female athletes, particularly runners, may

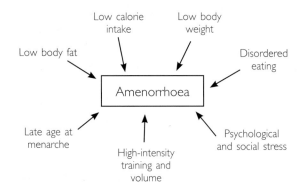

Figure 11.1 Risk factors for amenorrhoea among athletes

have shorter than average menstrual cycles due to anovulatory cycles, which are cycles during which an egg is not produced. This pattern is linked to low levels of female hormones: oestrogen and progesterone, follicle-stimulating hormone (FSH) and luteinising hormone (LH).

ARE DISORDERED EATING AND MENSTRUAL DYSFUNCTION LINKED?

Studies show that female athletes who consistently eat fewer calories than they would seem to need for their activity (i.e. they are in chronic negative energy balance) are more likely to have menstrual dysfunction. It has been suggested that this is an energy-conserving adaptation by the body to a very low calorie intake. In other words, the body tries to save energy by economising on the energy costs of menstruation i.e. 'shutting down' the normal menstrual function.

The body mechanism is as follows: the combination of mental or physiological stress and a chronic negative energy balance increases cortisol production by the adrenals, which disrupts the release of gonadotrophin-releasing hormone (GnRH) from the brain. This, in turn, reduces the production of the gonadotrophin-releasing hormone, luteinising hormone (LH) and follicle-stimulating hormone (FSH), oestrogen and progesterone (Loucks *et al.*, 1989; Edwards *et al.*, 1993).

HOW DOES MENSTRUAL DYSFUNCTION CAUSE BONE LOSS?

It's a myth that amenorrhoea is simply a consequence of hard training; it should be regarded as a clinical state of overtraining, because of the adverse effects it has on many systems in the body.

One of the most severe effects is the reduction in bone density and increased risk of early osteoporosis and stress fractures. This is partly due to low levels of oestrogen and progesterone, both of which act directly on bone cells to maintain bone turnover (Drinkwater *et al.*, 1984). When hormone levels drop, the natural breakdown of old bone exceeds the speed of formation of new bone. The result is loss of bone minerals and a loss of bone density. Training, then, no longer has a positive effect on bone density: it cannot compensate for the negative effects of low oestrogen and progesterone. But high levels of cortisol and poor nutritional status – both linked to menstrual dysfunction – are also thought to contribute to bone loss and low bone density (Carbon, 2002). Canadian researchers have found that disordered eating is correlated with menstrual irregularities and increased cortisol levels, all of which are risk factors for stress fractures (Guest and Barr, 2005).

Studies have found that the bone mineral density in the lumbar spine can be as much as 20–30% lower in amenorrhoeic distance runners compared with normally menstruating runners (Cann *et al.*, 1984; Nelson *et al.*, 1986). Whether bone mineral density 'catches up' once menstruation resumes is not known for certain. One long-term study found that bone mass increased initially, but in the long term, it remained lower compared to active and inactive women (Drinkwater, 1986).

DOES MENSTRUAL DYSFUNCTION AFFECT PERFORMANCE?

Menstrual dysfunction results in many performance-hindering effects, all of which are linked to very low oestrogen levels. These include an increased risk of soft tissue injuries, stress fractures, prolonged healing of injuries and reduced ability to recover from hard training sessions (Lloyd *et al.*, 1986). For example, low oestrogen levels result in a loss of suppleness in the ligaments, which then become more susceptible to injury. Low oestrogen levels slow down bone adaptation to exercise and micro-fractures occur more readily and heal more slowly.

The good news is that performance will most likely improve once menstruation resumes. Studies show that when amenorrhoeic athletes improve their diet and restructure their training programme to improve energy balance, normal menstruation resumes within about three months and performance improves consistently (Dueck *et al.*, 1996). This is perhaps the most persuasive reason to seek treatment if you have amenorrhoea.

HOW CAN MENSTRUAL DYSFUNCTION BE TREATED?

You should definitely seek advice if you have suffered amenorrhoea (absence of periods) for longer than six months. An initial consultation with your GP will rule out medical causes of amenorrhoea. You should then get a referral to a specialist, such as a gynaecologist, sports physician, endocrinologist or bone specialist. As part of your treatment you should consider advice from a sports nutritionist, exercise physiologist or sports psychologist. Treatment will centre on resuming 'normal' body weight and body fat, and reducing or changing your training programme. For example, you may have to reduce your training frequency, volume and intensity or change your current programme to include more cross-training. You may need to increase your food intake in order to bring your body weight and body fat within the normal range. If you have some degree of disordered eating, you will need help in overcoming this problem (*see* page 177).

If amenorrhoea persists after this type of treatment, hormone therapy may be prescribed to prevent further loss of bone mineral density. Doses of oestrogen and progesterone, similar to those used for treating postmenopausal women, are usually used. Supplements containing calcium, magnesium and other key minerals may be advised simultaneously.

IRON DEFICIENCY
ARE FEMALE ATHLETES MORE LIKELY TO BE IRON DEFICIENT?

It has been estimated that up to 80% of elite female endurance athletes are iron deficient. However, this is based on measurements of low blood ferritin or haemoglobin, which does not give a true indication of total body iron content. In fact, iron-deficiency anaemia occurs no more frequently among athletes than in non-athletes. It is easily confused with sports anaemia, which is more common among female athletes and is simply an adaptation to endurance training. Unlike iron-deficiency anaemia, sports anaemia does not benefit from iron supplements.

SO, WHAT'S THE DIFFERENCE BETWEEN IRON-DEFICIENCY ANAEMIA AND SPORTS ANAEMIA?

Iron-deficiency anaemia occurs when there is insufficient haemoglobin to meet the body's needs. It is characterised by a low concentration of haemoglobin in the blood (the normal range is 11.5–16.5 g/100 ml) and/or a low level of ferritin in the blood, the storage form of iron (the normal level is above 12 µg/L). Sports anaemia, although associated with a low haemoglobin concentration, is not really anaemia. It arises as a consequence of regular aerobic training, which causes an increase in blood plasma volume. As a result the red blood cells are more diluted, and measures of haemoglobin and ferritin appear lower since they have effectively been 'watered down'.

WHAT ARE THE CAUSES OF IRON-DEFICIENCY ANAEMIA IN FEMALE ATHLETES?

Iron-deficiency anaemia may be the result of increased blood losses associated with training or a deficient dietary intake.

Training effects

Blood losses in the urine, a condition called *haematuria*, may occur in female distance runners. This is due to bruising of the bladder lining caused by repeated pounding by the abdominal contents during running. Another condition, called *haemoglobinuria* (the presence of haemoglobin in the urine), can result from repetitive foot strikes associated with poor running gait or pounding on hard surfaces. This causes some destruction of red blood cells in the soles of the feet. In haematuria, the urine has a cloudy appearance, whereas in haemoglobinuria it is clear like rosé wine. Another route of blood loss in distance runners may be via the digestive tract and may be visible with diarrhoea. This is caused by the repeated minor trauma as the abdominal contents bounce up and down with each foot strike. However, iron losses via any of these routes are relatively small.

Diet

Studies reveal that many female athletes consume less than the RDA of iron. This may be due to a low food or calorie intake, which is common among weight-conscious athletes and those involved in sports requiring a low body fat level. It is very difficult to consume enough iron on a calorie intake of less than 1500 kcal a day. Many female athletes avoid red meat (a readily absorbed source of iron) or eat very little and perhaps do not compensate by eating other sources of iron.

WHAT ARE THE SYMPTOMS OF IRON-DEFICIENCY ANAEMIA?

The main symptoms of iron-deficiency anaemia are fatigue, headaches, light-headedness and above-normal breathlessness during exercise. Unfortunately, many of these symptoms are not specific to anaemia. Fatigue and tiredness are associated with stress and many other illnesses, making iron-deficiency anaemia difficult to diagnose without blood tests. Anaemia will affect aerobic performance, so if you notice an unexplained drop in your performance and you feel excessively tired despite plenty of rest and you have no other symptoms, you should consult your GP for a blood test.

WHAT IS LATENT IRON DEFICIENCY?

Many athletes have a lower concentration of ferritin in the blood than non-athletes. Values below 12 µg/L would normally indicate depleted iron stores, but in athletes this does not correlate with iron deficiency (Ashenden *et al.*, 1998). This combination of low ferritin yet normal haemoglobin is sometimes referred to as *latent iron deficiency*. There has been considerable research investigating the possible adverse effect of low serum ferritin on sports performance. The current consensus is that a low ferritin value in the absence of symptoms of iron-deficiency anaemia does not affect your performance. This is surprising, but repeated studies have found that physical training reduces serum ferritin concentration without producing any symptoms of iron-deficiency anaemia and that iron supplementation in cases of low

ferritin has no beneficial effect on performance (Cook, 1994).

CAN IRON SUPPLEMENTS IMPROVE PERFORMANCE?

When athletes with iron-deficiency anaemia are given iron supplements, their performance will improve. The usual recommended dose is 200 mg iron sulphate 3 times a day for 1 month. However, studies have shown that iron supplementation does not increase performance in athletes with sports anaemia or latent iron deficiency (see above). In other words, the discovery of sports anaemia or latent iron deficiency should not automatically be accompanied by supplementation (Ashenden

Food	Portion size	Mg iron
Calves liver	Average (100 g)	12.2
Bran flakes	1 bowlful (50 g)	10.0
Dried apricots (ready to eat)	5 (200 g)	7.0
Red lentils (boiled)	4 tbsp (160 g)	4.0
Prunes (ready to eat)	10 (110 g)	3.0
Baked beans	1 small tin (205 g)	2.9
Chick peas (boiled)	4 tbsp (140 g)	2.8
Lean beef fillet (grilled)	Average (105 g)	2.4
Wholemeal bread	2 large slices (80 g)	2.0
Wholemeal roll	1 (50 g)	1.8
Cashew nuts	30 (30 g)	1.8
Walnuts	12 halves (40 g)	1.2
Eggs	1 large (61 g)	1.2
Broccoli	2 spears (90 g)	1.0
Dark chicken meat	2 slices (100 g)	0.8

Table 11.4 The iron content of various foods

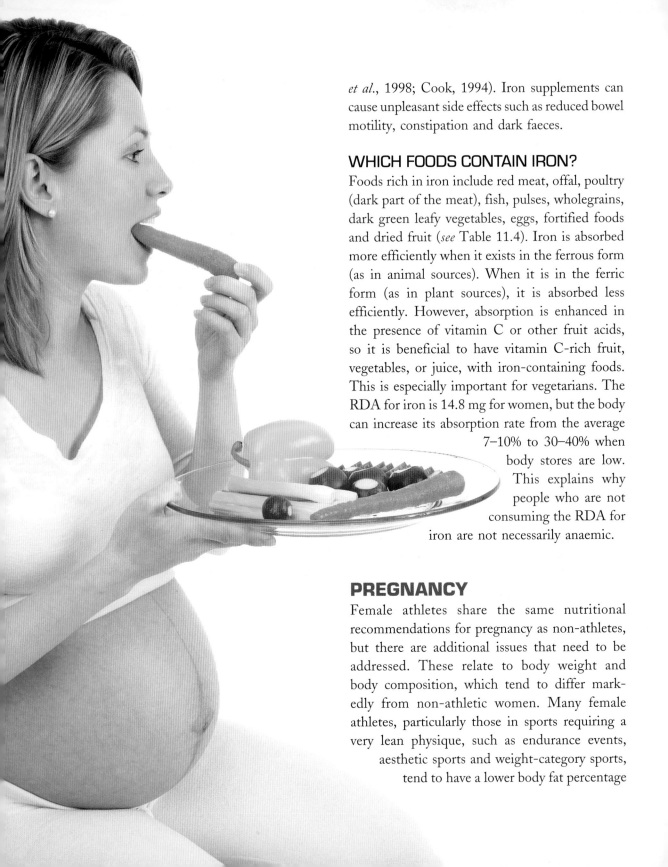

et al., 1998; Cook, 1994). Iron supplements can cause unpleasant side effects such as reduced bowel motility, constipation and dark faeces.

WHICH FOODS CONTAIN IRON?

Foods rich in iron include red meat, offal, poultry (dark part of the meat), fish, pulses, wholegrains, dark green leafy vegetables, eggs, fortified foods and dried fruit (*see* Table 11.4). Iron is absorbed more efficiently when it exists in the ferrous form (as in animal sources). When it is in the ferric form (as in plant sources), it is absorbed less efficiently. However, absorption is enhanced in the presence of vitamin C or other fruit acids, so it is beneficial to have vitamin C-rich fruit, vegetables, or juice, with iron-containing foods. This is especially important for vegetarians. The RDA for iron is 14.8 mg for women, but the body can increase its absorption rate from the average 7–10% to 30–40% when body stores are low. This explains why people who are not consuming the RDA for iron are not necessarily anaemic.

PREGNANCY

Female athletes share the same nutritional recommendations for pregnancy as non-athletes, but there are additional issues that need to be addressed. These relate to body weight and body composition, which tend to differ markedly from non-athletic women. Many female athletes, particularly those in sports requiring a very lean physique, such as endurance events, aesthetic sports and weight-category sports, tend to have a lower body fat percentage than non-athletic women. In addition the physical and psychological demands of regular exercise may affect your chances of conception and of a successful pregnancy. This section highlights the sports-specific issues associated with pregnancy.

DOES MY BODY FAT LEVEL AFFECT MY FERTILITY?

A lower than average body fat level is often associated with a drop in oestrogen production which, in turn, affects normal menstrual function and can result in oligomenorrhoea or amenorrhoea (*see* p. 177 'Are female athletes at greater risk of menstrual dysfunction?'). Research shows that body fat is important for oestrogen production and for converting the hormone from its inactive form into its active form. However, as explained on p. 177, loss of normal menstrual function is not simply a result of attaining a very low body fat percentage. It is often the result of a combination of factors, including a chronic low calorie intake, high training volume and intensity, and emotional and physical stress. Many female athletes are affected by one or more of these factors and, thus, fertility can be low and the chances of pregnancy small. Normal menstrual function and fertility can usually be restored within 6 months by adopting a more appropriate training programme, increasing your food intake so that energy intake matches energy output, and reducing stress.

WHAT ARE THE PROBLEMS WITH HAVING A VERY LOW BODY FAT PERCENTAGE DURING PREGNANCY?

A low body fat level is less likely to be a problem than a small pregnancy weight gain. Provided you are in good health and are gaining weight at the recommended rate (*see* Table 11.5), low body fat levels should not present a problem. However, a small weight gain suggesting prolonged food restriction, can have an adverse effect on the baby. The baby is more likely to be underweight when born, shorter in length and have a smaller head circumference than normal. Dieting or restricting your weight gain during pregnancy is not recommended.

Table 11.5	Guidelines for weight gain during pregnancy	
Body Mass Index* category	**Recommended total weight gain (kg)**	**Approx. rate of gain in 2nd and 3rd trimesters (kg/week)**
Underweight < 19.8	12.5–18	0.5
Normal 19.8–26	11.5–16	0.4
Overweight 26–29	7.0–11.5	0.3
Obese > 29	At least 6.0	No recommended value

Source: Institute of Medicine, 1990.
* (see p. 125 'What is the body mass index?')

Short-term dietary imbalances (e.g. during the first trimester due to sickness) do not affect the baby. Hormones are produced by the mother and placenta to ensure the baby continues to receive the necessary growth factors and nutrients during occasional times of adversity. During these periods, it is the mother's health that is more likely to suffer.

HOW MUCH WEIGHT SHOULD I GAIN DURING PREGNANCY?

The recommended average weight gain is 12.5 kg over 40 weeks although anywhere between 11.5 and 16 kg is considered healthy. The recommended weight gain guidelines are shown in Table 11.5. Distribution of weight gain (body component changes) is shown in Table 11.6. The increased level of progesterone favours body fat deposition, mainly subcutaneously (76%) in the thighs, hips and abdomen (Sohlstrom and Forsum, 1995). This extra fat deposit acts as a buffer of energy for late pregnancy when the developing baby's energy needs are highest. The hormone lactogen is produced during late pregnancy and post-pregnancy to mobilise these fat stores to provide energy for the developing baby and breast milk production should your calorie intake drop. In practice, this extra fat is not necessary because there is little danger of a drop in food supply (i.e. famine). Most women have already got enough body fat to buffer against a food shortage.

Gaining extra body fat, therefore, is certainly not advantageous for female athletes because it represents surplus baggage that can potentially reduce your performance once you resume training. Thus, the 3.35 kg fat allowance in the recommended 12.5 kg pregnancy weight gain may be regarded as optional for female athletes. Provided you consume a well-balanced diet during pregnancy, you can aim to gain 9–10 kg. However, do not try to stay below this level.

HOW MANY CALORIES SHOULD I EAT?

The Department of Health recommends no change in calorie intake during the first two trimesters of pregnancy for the general population. However, as an athlete, you may need to adjust your food intake if you reduce your training substantially during pregnancy. It is fine to continue exercising during pregnancy, but you will almost certainly need to reduce the intensity and/or frequency of your training particularly during the third trimester (due to your increased

Table 11.6	Body component changes during pregnancy
Body component	**Average increase in weight (kg)**
Baby	3.4
Placenta	0.65
Amniotic fluid	0.8
Uterus	0.97
Breasts	0.41
Blood	1.25
Extracellular fluid	1.68
Fat	3.35
Total	**12.5**

Source: Hytten and Leitch, 1971

weight and the physiological changes associated with pregnancy). Prolonged high-impact activities such as running, jumping, plyometrics and high-impact aerobics, and heavy weight training are not recommended during the second and third trimesters as they cause undue stress on the joints. During pregnancy, the ligaments, which support the joints, become softer and more lax owing to the effects of the hormone relaxin. Therefore, if you omit these activities from your routine your energy expenditure may be considerably lower than normal and you risk unnecessary fat gain unless you eat less or substitute an alternative exercise programme.

During the third trimester, there is a greater increase in your energy needs as the baby grows larger and additional pregnancy-related tissues are laid down. The DoH recommends an extra 200 kcal daily during this time. However, you may not need to eat more food because the discomfort of the growing bump may curtail your normal physical activity level. Your training may be further reduced or even stopped during the last few weeks of pregnancy, so there may be no change in your net calorie intake.

GENERAL NUTRITIONAL GUIDELINES FOR PREGNANCY

- Include foods rich in omega-3 and omega-6 fatty acids in your diet. These are needed for the normal development of brain tissue, and for brain, central nervous system and eye function. (*See* Chapter 8 p. 136 'What are the best food sources of essential fatty acids?').
- A daily multivitamin and mineral supplement may be useful to help meet your increased needs. *See* Chapter 5 pp. 65–76
- The DoH recommends taking a daily folic

acid supplement containing 400 µg (0.4 mg) prior to pregnancy and during the first 12 weeks to reduce the risk of neural tube defects. *See* Appendix Two, 'Glossary of Vitamins and Minerals', for food sources of folic acid.
- It is safest to avoid alcohol altogether, especially during the first trimester. After that, the Royal College of Physicians advises limiting alcohol to a maximum of two units a day (equivalent to 2 glasses of wine or 1 pint of beer).
- You should avoid vitamin A supplements (*see* Appendix Two, 'Glossary of Vitamins and Minerals'), fish liver oil supplements, liver and liver pate since very high doses (more than 10 times the RDA) may lead to birth defects.
- Avoid raw or lightly cooked eggs and products made with them to reduce the risks of salmonella poisoning.
- Avoid mould-ripened soft cheeses such as Camembert and Brie, and also blue-veined cheeses to reduce the risk of listeria poisoning.

SUMMARY OF KEY POINTS
- Three conditions – disordered eating, amenorrhoea and bone loss are increasingly common among female athletes.
- Intense and excessive training programmes combined with restrictive diets may lead to an obsessive preoccupation with body weight and calorie intake and eventually disordered eating.
- Eating disorders are much more common in athletes in sports where a low body weight, body fat level or thin physique is perceived to be advantageous.
- It is possible that some people with a predisposition to eating disorders are attracted to certain sports.

- It has been estimated that menstrual irregularities such as amenorrhoea affect up to 62% of endurance athletes.
- Amenorrhoea develops due to a combination of factors, such as restricted calorie intake, disordered eating, the commencement of intense training before menarche, high training intensity and volume, low body fat levels and physical and emotional stress.
- Amenorrhoea has an adverse effect on many systems in the body, including a reduction in bone density, putting you at risk of early osteoporosis and stress fractures; soft tissue injuries; prolonged healing of injuries and reduced ability to recover from hard training sessions.
- Iron-deficiency anaemia is characterised by a concentration of haemoglobin in the blood below 11.5 g/dl and/or a level of ferritin below 12 μg/L, but occurs no more frequently among athletes than in non-athletes.

- Iron-deficiency anaemia may be the result of increased blood losses associated with training or a deficient dietary intake.
- Sports anaemia, although associated with a low haemoglobin concentration, arises as a consequence of regular aerobic training, which causes an increase in blood plasma volume.
- The physical and psychological demands of regular exercise, together with a very low body fat, may reduce your chances of conception.
- A low body fat level is less likely to be a problem than a small pregnancy weight gain, which may result in reduced growth of the developing baby. Dieting or restricting your weight gain during pregnancy is not recommended.
- You may need to reduce your food intake if you reduce your training substantially during pregnancy.

THE YOUNG ATHLETE

12

Like adults, young athletes need to eat a balanced diet to maintain good health and achieve peak performance. While there has been relatively limited research performed with active children, it is possible to adapt nutritional guidelines for children and adolescents to the specific demands of exercise and sport as well as use some of the research on adult athletes. This chapter deals with energy, protein and fluid needs for young athletes as well as meal timing, travelling and competing. Weight is also an important issue for some young athletes. Being overweight not only affects their health but also reduces their athletic performance and their self-esteem. Similarly some young athletes struggle to keep up their weight or put on weight because of the high energy demands of their sport. This chapter details some key strategies to help parents and coaches manage these issues.

HOW MUCH ENERGY DO YOUNG ATHLETES REQUIRE?

There are no specific data on energy requirements for children who train regularly, but you can get a rough estimate using the values in Tables 12.1 and 12.2. Table 12.1 shows the estimated average requirements for children for standard ages published by the Department of Health. These figures do not take account of regular exercise or sport, so you will need to make an allowance for this.

More relevant to young athletes are the figures shown in Table 12.2, which shows energy requirements according to body weight and physical activity level (PAL). PAL is the ratio of overall daily energy expenditure to BMR based on the intensity and time spent being active. You can work out the PAL from Table 12.3. Sedentary children (and adults) would have a PAL of 1.4, while active children are likely to have a PAL between 1.6 and 2.0.

Table 12.4 lists the estimated calorie expenditure for various activities for a 10-year-old child weighing 33 kg. These values are based on measurements made on adults, scaled down to the body weight of a child, with an added margin of 25% (Astrand, 1952). (There are no published values relating to children.) This margin takes account of the relative 'wastefulness' of energy in children compared with adults performing the same activity, due mainly to their lack of coordination between agonist and antagonist muscle groups. This makes children metabolically less economical than adolescents and adults. Also they are biomechanically less efficient (e.g. they tend

Table 12.1	Estimated average requirements for energy of children*	
Age	Boys (kcal)	Girls (kcal)
4–6 years	1715	1545
7–10 years	1970	1740
11–14 years	2220	1845
15–18 years	2755	2110

* Dept. of Health Dietary reference values for food energy and nutrients for the United Kingdom (1991) London: HMSO

Table 12.2	Estimated average requirements of children and adolescents according to body weight and physical activity level					
Weight (kg)	BMR kcal/d	PAL 1.4	1.5	1.6	1.8	2.0
Boys						
30	1189	1675	1794	1914	2153	2368
35	1278	1794	1914	2057	2297	2559
40	1366	1914	2057	2177	2464	2727
45	1455	2033	2177	2320	2632	2919
50	1543	2153	2321	2464	2775	3086
55	1632	2297	2440	2608	2943	3253
60	1720	2416	2584	2751	3086	3445
Girls						
30	1095	1531	1651	1746	1962	2201
35	1163	1627	1715	1866	2081	2321
40	1229	1722	1842	1962	2201	2464
45	1297	1818	1938	2081	2344	2584
50	1364	1913	2033	2177	2464	2727
55	1430	2009	2153	2297	2584	2871
60	1498	2105	2249	2392	2703	2990

Dept. of Health Dietary reference values for food energy and nutrients for the United Kingdom (1991) London: HMSO to have a faster stride frequency when running) – again, raising the energy cost of any given activity. However, the energy cost decreases as children become more proficient at performing the activity. Exactly how much active children should eat is difficult to predict, but for children who are not overweight or underweight, you can use their appetite as a guide to portion sizes. Be guided, too, by their energy levels. If children are not eating enough, then their energy levels will be persistently low, they will feel lethargic and under-perform at sports. On the other hand, if they appear to have plenty of energy and get-up-and-go, then they are probably eating enough.

DO YOUNG ATHLETES BURN FUEL DIFFERENTLY FROM ADULTS?

Studies suggest that during exercise children use relatively more fat and less carbohydrate than do adolescents or adults (Martinez & Haymes, 1992; Berg & Keul, 1988). This applies to both endurance and short higher intensity activities, where

Table 12.3	Physical Activity Level (PAL)
1.4	Mostly sitting, little physical activity
1.5	Mostly sitting, some walking, low levels of exercise
1.6	Daily moderate exercise
1.8	Daily moderate – high exercise level
2.0	Daily high exercise level

Table 12.4	Calories expended in various activities

Activity	Calories in 30 minutes
Cycling (11.2 km/h)	88
Running (12 km/h)	248
Sitting	24
Standing	26
Swimming (crawl, 4.8 km/h)	353
Tennis	125
Walking	88

Values are based on measurements made on adults, scaled down to the body weight of 33 kg, with an added margin of 25%. Heavier children will burn slightly more calories; lighter children will burn less.

they tend to rely more on aerobic metabolism (in which fat is a major fuel). The nutritional implications are not clear, but there is no reason to recommend they should consume more than 35% of their total energy as fat.

HOW MUCH PROTEIN SHOULD YOUNG ATHLETES CONSUME?

Because children are growing and developing, they need more protein relative to their weight than adults. The reference nutrient intakes for protein published by the Department of Health give a general guideline for boys and girls of different ages. These are given in Table 12.5. Most children need about 1 g per kg body weight (adults need 0.75 g/ kg BW). For example, a child who weighs 40 kg should eat about 40 g of protein daily. However, the published values do not take account of exercise, so active children may need a little more protein, around 1.1–1.2 g/ kg body weight/day (Ziegler *et al.*, 1998).

Young athletes can meet their protein needs by including 2–4 portions of protein-rich foods in their daily diet (lean meat, fish, poultry, eggs, beans, lentils, nuts, tofu and quorn) as well as balanced amounts of grains (bread, pasta, cereals) and dairy foods (milk, yoghurt, cheese), all of which also supply smaller amounts of protein.

Vegetarian children should eat a wide variety of plant proteins: beans, lentils, grains, nuts, seeds, soya and quorn (see Chapter 13 'The Vegetarian Athlete').

SHOULD YOUNG ATHLETES USE PROTEIN SUPPLEMENTS?

Protein supplements, such as protein shakes and bars, are unnecessary for children. Even the very active should be able to get enough protein from their diet. While such supplements may have a role to play in the diets of some adult athletes, there is no justification for giving them to children. It is more important that children learn how to plan a balanced diet from ordinary foods and how to get protein from the right food combinations.

HOW MUCH CARBOHYDRATE SHOULD YOUNG ATHLETES CONSUME?

It is recommended that children obtain at least 50% of their energy from carbohydrate (National Heart Forum; Caroline Walker Trust, 2005). For example, a 13-year-old boy who consumes 2220 calories per day would need to eat a minimum 296 g carbohydrate.

Table 12.5 Daily protein requirements of children		
Age	Boys	Girls
4–6 years	19.7 g	19.7 g
7–10 years	28.3 g	28.3 g
11–14 years	42.1 g	41.2 g
15–18 years	55.2 g	45.0 g

Dept. of Health Dietary reference values for food energy and nutrients for the United Kingdom, London: HMSO (1991)

As a rough guide, young athletes should aim for 4–6 portions from the grains/potato group, as well as 2–4 portions from the fruit group and 2–4 portions from the calcium-rich food group, both of which also provide some carbohydrate. The exact portion size depends on their energy need. Generally, older, heavier and more active children need bigger portions. Be guided by their appetite but don't get too prescriptive about the exact amount they should eat. Check the carbohydrate content of foods in the table in Appendix One: Glycaemic Index and Glycaemic Load (pp. 289–291).

WHAT SHOULD YOUNG ATHLETES EAT BEFORE TRAINING OR COMPETITION?

Most of the energy needed for exercise is provided by whatever the athlete has eaten several hours or even days before. Carbohydrate in their food will have been converted into glycogen and stored in their muscles and liver. If they have eaten the right amount of carbohydrate, they will have high levels of glycogen in their muscles, ready to fuel their activity. If they have not eaten enough carbohydrate, they will have low stocks of glycogen, putting them at risk of early fatigue during exercise.

Food eaten before exercise needs to stop children feeling hungry during training, be easily digested and have a moderate to low GI. Such a snack or meal provides sustained energy and will help the athlete keep going longer during exercise. But don't let them eat lots of sugary foods such as sweets and soft drinks just before exercising. This may cause a surge of blood glucose and insulin followed by a rapid fall, resulting in hypoglycaemia, early fatigue and reduced performance.

Pre-exercise snacks

Eaten approximately 1 hour before exercise with a drink of water:

- Fresh fruit and glass of milk
- Small wholemeal sandwich filled with honey, peanut butter or hummus
- Cereal bar or dried fruit bar
- Pot of fruit yoghurt and a banana or apple
- Small packet or pot of dried fruit, e.g. apricots, raisins
- Breakfast cereal with milk
- Yoghurt drink or flavoured milk
- Wholemeal crackers or rice cakes with a little cheese
- Homemade muffins and cakes (see recipes on pages 284–288).

The boxes above and overleaf give some ideas for suitable pre-exercise meals and snacks. It takes a certain amount of trial and error to find out which foods and what amounts suit an individual best. Adjust the quantities according to their appetite, how they feel and what they like. It's important that they feel comfortable with the types and amounts of foods. Don't offer anything new before a competition, as it may not agree with them.

TIMING THE PRE-EXERCISE MEAL

The exact timing of the pre-exercise meal will probably depend on practical constraints – for example, the training session may be straight after school, leaving very little time to eat. If there is less than one hour between eating and training, give them a light snack (see box 'Pre-exercise snacks').

Pre-exercise meals

Eaten 2–3 hours before exercise with a drink of water:

- Sandwich/roll/bagel/wrap filled with tuna, cheese, chicken or peanut butter
- Jacket potato with cheese, tuna or baked beans
- Pasta with tomato-based sauce and cheese or a lean bolognese sauce
- Rice or noodles with chicken or lentils
- Breakfast cereal with milk and banana
- Porridge with raisins
- Lentil/vegetable or chicken soup with wholemeal bread.

If they have more than two hours between eating and training, their normal balanced meal will be suitable. This should be based around a carbo-hydrate food such as bread or potatoes together with a little protein such as chicken or beans, as well as a portion of vegetables and a drink (see box 'Pre-exercise meals').

WHAT SHOULD YOUNG ATHLETES EAT BEFORE AN EVENT?

If they are competing, you need to make sure that the young athletes have access to the right kinds of food. It's definitely a good idea to pack a supply of food because suitable foods and drinks may not be available at the event venue. Young athletes should have their normal meal about 2–3 hours before the event – enough time to digest the food and for the stomach to empty. For example, if the event is in the morning, schedule breakfast 2–3 hours before the event start time. Similarly,

if the event is in the afternoon, adjust the timing of lunch to 2–3 hours before the event.

Like adults, children may feel too nervous or excited to eat on the day of the event. So, offer nutritious drinks (such as diluted fruit juice, sports drinks, milk-based drinks or yoghurt drinks), or light snacks. If they skip meals, children may become light-headed or nauseous during the event and will not perform at their best. Here are some simple rules to follow on the day of the event:

- Do not eat or drink anything new
- Stick to familiar foods and drinks
- Take your own foods and drinks wherever possible
- Drink plenty of water or diluted juice before and after the event
- Have high-carbohydrate snacks (see box 'Pre-exercise snacks')
- Avoid high fat foods before the event
- Avoid eating sweets and chocolate during the hour before the event
- Avoid soft drinks (containing more than 6 g sugar/100 ml) an hour before the event
- Encourage children to go to the toilet just before the event.

WHAT SHOULD YOUNG ATHLETES EAT DURING EXERCISE?

If young athletes will be exercising continually for less than 90 minutes, they won't need to eat anything during exercise. They should, however, be encouraged to take regular drink breaks, ideally every 15–20 minutes or whenever there is a suit-able break in training or play. Make sure they take a water bottle and keep it within easy reach – for example, at the poolside, at the side of the football pitch or by the track.

During an all-day training session or competition, have food and drink available during the short breaks. For example, make opportunities to refuel between swimming heats, tennis games, and gymnastic events. During matches or tournaments lasting more than an hour (e.g. football, cricket or hockey), offer them food and drink during the half-time interval. High carbohydrate, low fat foods and drinks are the obvious choice because these will help to keep energy levels high, maintain their blood glucose level, delay the onset of fatigue and prevent hypoglycaemia. As you will almost certainly need to take them with you, they should also be non-perishable, portable and quick and easy to eat. Sometimes food is provided at events, but you will need to check exactly what will be available beforehand – it may be crisps, chocolate bars, biscuits and soft drinks, all of which are unhelpful for good performance! Check the box opposite for suitable snacks.

WHAT SHOULD YOUNG ATHLETES EAT AFTER EXERCISE?

After exercise, the priority is to replenish fluid losses. So give young athletes a drink straightaway – water or diluted fruit juice are the best drinks.

They also need to replace the energy they have just used. The post-exercise snack or meal is perhaps the most important meal, as it determines how fast athletes will recover before the next training session. Unless they will be eating a meal within half an hour, give them a snack to stave off hunger and promote recovery. The exact amounts you should provide will depend on their appetite and body size. As a guide, give just enough to alleviate their hunger and keep them going until their mealtime. Studies with adult athletes have shown that 1 g of carbohydrate per

Snacks for short breaks during training or competition

- Water, diluted fruit juice or sports drinks
- Bananas
- Fresh fruit – grapes, apples, satsumas, pears
- Dried fruit – raisins, apricots, mango
- Crackers and rice cakes with bananas or honey
- Rolls, sandwiches, English muffins, mini-bagels, mini-pancakes
- Fruit, cereal and energy bars.

kg body weight eaten within two hours of exercise speeds recovery.

Opt for foods with a moderate or high GI, which will raise blood glucose levels fairly rapidly and then be converted into glycogen in the muscles. Studies with adult athletes have found that including a little protein (in a ratio of about 3:1) enhances recovery further. Check the box below for suitable recovery snacks and meals. In practice, many of the snacks on offer in the canteen or vending machines at leisure clubs and sports centres are unsuitable. Foods like crisps, chocolate bars, sweets and fizzy drinks will not promote good recovery after exercise. They are little more than concentrated forms of sugar, fat or salt, and actually slow down rehydration. Because they provide a lot of calories too, these foods can take away the young athlete's appetite for healthier foods at the next meal.

So what can you do? Let your leisure centre know that you are unhappy with the choice of snacks on offer to children, ask other parents and coaches to do the same and suggest that they replace these 'junk' snacks with healthier foods. Any of the suggestions in the box ('Suitable recovery snacks') would be appropriate. Encourage children to take their own drinks and snacks.

Suitable recovery snacks

Accompany all snacks with a drink of water or diluted fruit juice:

- Fresh fruit e.g. bananas, grapes, and apples
- Dried fruit
- Nuts and raisins
- Fruit yoghurt
- Yoghurt drink
- Smoothie (bought or homemade)
- Roll or bagel with jam or honey
- Mini-pancakes
- Homemade muffins, bar, biscuits (see recipes on pages 284–288)
- Homemade apple, carrot or fruit cake
- Flavoured milk or yoghurt drink.

Suitable recovery meals

Accompany all meals with a drink of water or diluted fruit juice, and 1–2 portions of vegetables or salad:

- Jacket potatoes with beans, tuna or cheese
- Pasta with tomato sauce and cheese
- Rice with chicken and stir-fried vegetables
- Fish pie
- Baked beans on toast
- Fish cakes or bean burgers or falafel with jacket potatoes.

WHAT SHOULD YOUNG ATHLETES EAT WHEN TRAVELLING OR COMPETING AWAY?

When young athletes are travelling to compete away from home, organise their food and drink in advance and take these with you. They may need snacks for the journey so take a supply of suitable foods – use any of the suggestions in the box 'Snacks for eating on the move'. Do not rely on roadside cafés, fast food restaurants, railway or airport catering outlets – healthy choices are often limited at these places. Make sure you take plenty of drinks, in case of delays. Air-conditioned travel in cars, coaches and planes can quickly make children dehydrated.

Try to find out what catering arrangements have been made at the venue. Check the local restaurants and takeaways. Encourage children to choose dishes that are high in carbohydrate, such as pasta, pizza or rice dishes. And warn them against trying anything unfamiliar or unusual – the last thing they need is an upset stomach before the event! When travelling abroad, it's best to avoid common food poisoning culprits – chicken, seafood and meat dishes – unless you are sure they have been properly cooked and heated to a high temperature. Be wary of such foods served lukewarm. Check the box below for suitable meals when travelling away.

Remember, too, that young athletes will probably be feeling nervous or apprehensive when travelling away. They may not feel like eating much food. In this case, encourage them to have plenty of nutritious drinks instead, such as fruit juice, smoothies, yoghurt drinks and milkshakes. Pack their favourite foods – of the non-perishable variety – to tempt their appetite. Sometimes it's a case of simply getting them to eat something

Snacks for eating on the move

- Sandwiches filled with chicken or tuna or cheese with salad; banana and peanut butter; Marmite
- Rice cakes, oatcakes and wholemeal crackers
- Bottles of water
- Cartons of fruit juice
- Yoghurt drinks
- Individual cheese portions
- Small bags of nuts – peanuts, cashews, almonds
- Fresh fruit – apples, bananas, grapes
- Miniboxes of raisins
- Fruit bar or liquorice bar
- Sesame snaps
- Prepared vegetable crudités e.g. carrots, peppers, cucumber and celery.

Suitable restaurant meals and fast foods when travelling to an event

- Simple pasta dishes with tomato sauce
- Rice and stir-fried vegetable dishes
- Pizza with tomato and vegetable toppings
- Simple noodle dishes
- Jacket potatoes with cheese
- Pancakes with syrup.

Restaurant meals and fast foods to avoid

- Burgers and chips
- Chicken nuggets
- Pasta with creamy or oily sauces
- Takeaway curries
- Takeaway kebabs
- Battered fish and chips
- Lukewarm chicken, turkey, meat, fish or seafood dishes
- Hot dogs
- Fried chicken meals.

rather than nothing. If they stop eating they will run down their energy reserves, putting them at a disadvantage for competition.

ARE YOUNG ATHLETES MORE SUSCEPTIBLE TO DEHYDRATION THAN ADULTS?

Young athletes are much more susceptible to dehydration and overheating than adults for the following reasons:

- they sweat less than adults (sweat helps to keep the body's temperature stable)
- they cannot cope with very hot conditions as well as adults
- they get hotter during exercise
- they have a greater surface area for their body weight
- they often fail to recognise or respond to feelings of thirst.

The increase in core temperature at any given level of dehydration is quite a bit greater in young athletes than in adults. Encourage young athletes to check their hydration status with a 'pee test' (*see* p. 107).

On average, young athletes lose between 350–700 ml of body fluid per hour's exercise. If it's hot and humid or they are wearing lots of layers of clothing, they will sweat more and lose even more fluid. Encourage them to drink plenty of fluid before, during and after exercise. As for adults, fluid losses depend on:

- The temperature and humidity of the surroundings – the warmer and higher the humidity, the greater their sweat losses, so they will need to drink more.
- How hard they are exercising – the harder they exercise, the more they sweat, so they will need to drink more.
- How long they are exercising – the longer they exercise, the greater the sweat losses, so they will need to drink accordingly.
- Their size – the bigger they are, the greater the sweat loss, so the more they need to drink.
- Their fitness – the fitter they are, the earlier and more profusely they sweat (it's a sign of good body temperature control), so they will need to drink more than their less fit friends.

In some sports where body weight is a factor in performance (e.g. gymnastics), coaches (hopefully a minority) restrict fluids during training, in the misguided belief that the human body will eventually adapt to low fluid intakes, or perhaps this is simply to remove the hassle and distraction of drinking itself! However, even if children manage to exercise, they will be performing below par. They will also be at risk of developing heat cramps and heat exhaustion.

The risks of dehydration in young athletes are similar to those in adults. Here's a reminder:

- Exercise feels much harder
- Heart rate increases more than usual
- May develop cramps, headaches and nausea

Warning signs of dehydration

Children can become dehydrated more easily than adults. Here are some of the signs to look out for.

Early symptoms:
- Unusually lacking in energy
- Fatiguing early during exercise
- Complaining of feeling too hot
- Skin appears flushed and feels clammy
- Passing only small volumes of dark coloured urine
- Nausea.

Action: Drink 100–200 ml water or sports drink every 10–15 minutes.

Advanced symptoms:
- A bad headache
- Becomes dizzy or light-headed
- Appears disorientated
- Short of breath.

Action: Drink 100–200 ml sports drink every 10–15 minutes. Seek professional help.

- Concentration is reduced
- Ability to perform sports skills drops
- Fatigues sooner and loses stamina.

HOW MUCH SHOULD YOUNG ATHLETES DRINK BEFORE EXERCISE?

Like adults, young athletes should aim to be well-hydrated before exercise. If they are slightly dehydrated at this stage, there is a bigger risk of overheating once they start exercising. Encourage them to drink 6–8 cups (1–1.5 litres) of fluid during the day and, as a final measure, top up with 150–200 ml (a large glass) of water 45 minutes before exercise.

HOW MUCH SHOULD YOUNG ATHLETES DRINK DURING EXERCISE?

Use the following guidelines, in conjunction with the considerations below, to plan a drinking strategy:

Before exercise
150–200 ml 45 mins before activity

During exercise
75–100 ml every 15–20 mins

After exercise
Drink freely until no longer thirsty, plus an extra glass, or drink 300 ml for every 0.2 kg weight loss.

You can estimate how much fluid young athletes have lost during exercise by weighing them before and after training. For each 1 kg lost, they should drink 1.5 litres of fluid. This accounts for the fact that they continue to sweat after exercise and lose more fluid through urine during this time. For example, if the young athlete weighs 0.3 kg less after exercise, he has lost 0.3 litres (300 ml) of fluid. To replace 300 ml of fluid, he needs to drink 450 ml of fluid during and after training. But don't expect young athletes to drink large volumes after exercising. Divide their drinks into manageable amounts to be taken during and after exercise. A good strategy would be to drink, say, 100 ml at three regular intervals during exercise, then 150 ml afterwards.

How can young athletes be encouraged to drink enough while exercising?

- Make drinking more fun with a squeezy bottle or a novelty water bottle.
- Make sure they place the bottle within easy access, e.g. at one end of the pool or by the side of the track, court, gym or pitch.
- Allow drinking time during training/play – encourage them to take regular sips, ideally every 10–20 mins. This may take practice.
- Tell them not to wait until they are thirsty – plan a drink during the first 20 minutes of exercise, then at regular intervals during the session, even if they are not thirsty.
- If they are playing in a team, work out suitable drink breaks, e.g. half-time during a match, or while listening to the coach during practice sessions.
- If they don't like water, offer a flavoured drink such as diluted fruit juice, dilute squash or a sports drink (see 'What should young athletes drink?').
- Slightly chilling the drink (to around 8–10ºC) usually encourages children to drink more.

What should young athletes drink?

As with adults, plain water is best for most activities lasting less than 90 minutes. It replaces lost fluids rapidly and so makes a perfectly good drink for sport. But there are two potential problems with drinking water. Firstly, many young athletes are not very keen on drinking water, so they may not drink enough. Secondly, water tends to quench one's thirst even if the body is still dehydrated. Encourage water whenever possible, but if young athletes find it difficult to drink enough water, give them a flavoured drink. Diluted pure fruit juice (diluted one or two parts water to one part juice), sugar-free squash or ordinary diluted squash are less expensive alternatives. But bear in mind that most brands are laden with additives, including artificial sweeteners, colours and flavourings, which you may prefer to avoid. Organic squashes are better options, although they are more expensive.

Although commercial sports drinks may not benefit young athletes' performance for activities lasting less than 90 mins (compared with water or flavoured drinks), they will encourage them to drink larger volumes of fluid (Wilk & Bar-Or, 1996; Rivera-Brown *et al.*, 1999). But a word of caution with commercial sports drinks: in practice, many children find that sports drinks sit 'heavily' in their stomachs. So, you may either

What young athletes shouldn't drink!

- Fizzy drinks – the bubbles in fizzy drinks may cause a burning sensation in the mouth, especially if drunk quickly and will certainly stop children from drinking enough fluid. Fizzy drinks can also upset the stomach and make them feel bloated and uncomfortable during exercise.
- Ready-to-drink soft drinks – these are too concentrated in sugar and will tend to sit in the stomach too long during exercise. They may make children feel nauseous and uncomfortable.
- Drinks containing caffeine – caffeinated soft drinks, cola, coffee and tea increase the heart rate and may cause trembling and restlessness at night – children are more sensitive to caffeine than adults.

Choosing the best drink for exercise

Exercise lasting less than 90 minutes

- Water
- Fruit juice diluted 2 parts water to 1 part juice
- Sports drink alternated with water.

Exercise lasting more than 90 minutes

- Sports drink (4–6 g sugars/100 ml)
- Fruit juice diluted 1–2 parts water to 1 part juice
- Squash (ideally organic), diluted 6 parts water to 1 part squash.

dilute the sports drink down with water (if making up from powder, add a little extra water) or alternate sports drinks with water.

If children will be exercising hard and continuously for more than 90 minutes, sports drinks containing around 4–6 g of sugars per 100 ml may benefit their performance. This is because the sugars in these drinks help fuel the exercising muscles and postpone fatigue. The electrolytes (sodium and potassium) in the drinks are designed to stimulate thirst and make them drink more (see Chapter 7: Hydration). On the downside, sports drinks are relatively expensive. It's cheaper to make your own version by diluting fruit juice (one part juice to one or two parts of water) or organic squash (diluted one part squash to six parts water). Both would also help maintain energy (blood glucose) levels during prolonged exercise. The most important thing is that children drink enough. Therefore, the taste is important. If they don't like it, they won't drink it! So, experiment with different flavours until you find the ones they like. A little trial and error may be needed to find the best strength drink, too. If it's too concentrated, it will sit in their stomachs and make them feel uncomfortable.

Six ways to keep cool

1. Provide extra water during hot and humid weather.
2. Schedule exercise for the cooler times of the day during hot weather.
3. Schedule regular drink breaks during sessions, ideally in the shade during hot weather.
4. Encourage young athletes to wear loose fitting, natural-fibre clothing during exercise, which allows them to sweat freely and permits moisture to evaporate.
5. Let them acclimatise gradually to hot or humid weather conditions – allow two weeks.
6. Make sure they drink extra water 24 hours before a competition.

How to choose a supplement

1. Choose a comprehensive formula designed for your children's age range; ideally the following nutrients should be there: vitamin A, vitamin C, vitamin D, vitamin E, thiamin, riboflavin, niacin, vitamin B6, folic acid, vitamin B12, biotin, pantothenic acid, beta carotene, calcium, phosphorus, iron, magnesium, zinc, iodine.
2. Check that the quantities of each nutrient are no more than 100% of the RDA stated on the label.
3. Avoid supplements with added colours.
4. Try to choose brands that have been produced by established manufacturers with a good reputation for quality control and clinical research.

SHOULD YOUNG ATHLETES TAKE VITAMIN SUPPLEMENTS?

In theory, young athletes should not need supplements if they are eating a well-balanced diet and eating a wide variety of foods. But, in practice, not many children manage to do this. Reliance on fast foods, ready-meals and processed snacks as well as peer pressure and time pressure make this very difficult to achieve. The National Diet and Nutrition Survey of British Schoolchildren revealed that the most commonly eaten foods among 4–18 year olds, eaten by 80% of children, are white bread, crisps, biscuits, potatoes and chocolate bars (Gregory *et al.*, 2000). On average, they ate only 2 portions of fruit and vegetables a day and less than half ever ate green leafy vegetables. Intakes of zinc, magnesium, calcium and iron were below the RNI among 15–18 year olds.

A well-formulated children's multivitamin and mineral supplement can help ensure they get enough vitamins and minerals so that their growth, physical and mental development and physical performance will not be impaired. Low intakes of certain vitamins and minerals have been linked with lower IQ, reasoning ability, physical performance, poor attention and behavioural problems.

It is possible that supplementation can help correct deficiencies and produce a significant improvement in these aspects in children. However, extra vitamins and minerals won't make children more brainy or sporty if they are already well nourished.

SHOULD YOUNG ATHLETES TAKE CREATINE?

There is no research to support the use of sports supplements in young athletes and the long-term risks are unknown (Unnithan *et al.*, 2001). One of the most popular supplements is creatine. No sports organisation has recommended its use in people under 18. The American College of Sports Medicine and American Academy of Paediatrics position statements advise against the use of creatine for athletes under 18 years of age. Because dietary supplements are not regulated, there is a possibility that creatine supplements may contain impurities that would cause a positive drug test.

Creatine would in any case have little benefit in young athletes. Firstly, they rely more on aerobic than anaerobic metabolism, so any attempt to enhance anaerobic energy production through creatine supplementation would be of limited effect. Secondly, the biggest improvement to performance comes from training at this stage of development. Hard training and a balanced diet, not supplements, are the keys to optimal performance.

WHEN SHOULD YOUNG ATHLETES LOSE WEIGHT FOR THEIR SPORT?

Some young athletes may feel pressurised to lose weight to improve their performance in sport. Low body weights or fat percentages are often correlated with improved running speed, jumping ability, endurance and performance in many sports. Whether they are overweight or not, unfortunately, young athletes are often influenced to lose weight by the successes of thinner teammates or by the remarks of a well-meaning coach.

So what should you do? Young athletes who are a healthy weight or body fat percentage (*see* Figures 12.1 and 12.2) should not be encouraged to lose weight. If they are unhappy about their weight, the problem may be one of poor self-esteem or being ill-matched to their sport. For example, children with a naturally large build would not be well-matched to sports requiring a naturally slim physique such as long-distance running, ballet, or gymnastics.

If you feel that a young athlete has a genuine weight problem and that reducing body fat would benefit their performance, health and self-esteem, follow the advice on p. 202 ('The healthy way to tackle weight'), or consult a registered nutritionist or dietitian (see www.senr.org.uk). Usually a strategy that increases their daily activity level and training intensity, together with a healthier diet, is all that is needed. Allow plenty of time – months rather than weeks – for fat loss. Under professional guidance, young athletes should lose no more than 1–2 kg per month, depending on their age and weight. Weight loss goals must be realistic and achievable for their build and degree of maturity. They should reach this goal at least three or four weeks before competition. This will allow them to compete at their best. You should discourage strict dieting, diuretics, excessive exercise, and use of saunas as weight loss methods, as they can be very dangerous for growing athletes. In the short term, these methods could result in an excessive loss of water, low muscle glycogen stores, fatigue and poor performance. Long-term, they could lead to yo-yo dieting, eating disorders, poor health and impaired development.

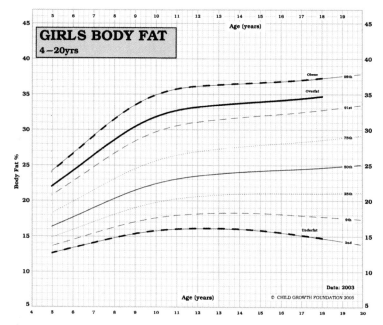

Figure 12.1 Healthy body fat for girls

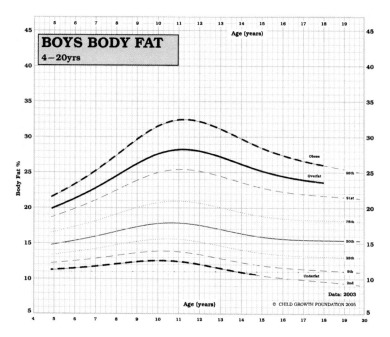

Figure 12.2 Healthy body fat for boys

How to assess overweight and body fatness in children and adolescents

Body mass index (BMI = weight (kg)/height (m)^2) (see Table 12.6) is commonly used in adults to define overweight. There are also international standards, which define cut-off points related to age to define overweight and obesity in children (Figures 12.1 and 12.2). A BMI higher than the normal limit for their age means they are overweight; a BMI higher than the obese value suggests their health is at risk. However, as with adults, using BMIs with athletic children can be misleading and lead to a misclassification of overweight, as they do not distinguish between weight in the form of fat or lean tissue.

Body fat centile charts provide more accurate information for assessing children and young athletes. The simplest way to measure body fat percentage is with a body composition analyser based on bioelectrical impedance and calibrated for children (e.g. Tanita Innerscan Family Health).

THE HEALTHY WAY TO TACKLE WEIGHT

The best thing you can do is to encourage a balanced diet and regular physical activity. Talk to young athletes about healthy eating and exercise, teach by example and let them make their own decisions about food.

- **Don't** tell a young athlete that they are 'greedy' or 'lazy'.
- **Do** tell them that you recognise how hard it is to make healthy choices at times.
- **Don't** make a young athlete feel guilty about their eating habits.
- **Do** praise them lavishly when you see them eating healthily.

Table 12.6	BMIs for overweight or obesity in children			
Age	**Overweight**		**Obese**	
	Boys	**Girls**	**Boys**	**Girls**
5	17.4	17.1	19.3	19.2
6	17.6	17.3	19.8	19.7
7	17.9	17.8	20.6	20.5
8	18.4	18.3	21.6	21.6
9	19.1	19.1	22.8	22.8
10	19.8	19.9	24.0	24.1
11	20.6	20.7	25.1	25.4
12	21.2	21.7	26.0	26.7
13	21.9	22.6	26.8	27.8

Source: Cole et al., (2000)

Build self-esteem

If you can build young athletes' self-esteem and help them feel more positive about themselves, they are more likely to make healthier food choices. Make a point of praising their accomplishments, emphasising their strengths, and encouraging them to try new skills to foster success. Never call them fat or tell them to lose weight. Let them know that its what's inside that matters and play down your concerns about their weight – or even your own weight.

Don't say diet

You shouldn't restrict a young athlete's calorie intake without the advice of a nutritionist dietitian. Nutritional needs during childhood are

Table 12.7	Dietary reference values for boys 4–18 years+				
	Dietary Reference Value (DRV)	**4–6**	**7–10**	**11–14**	**15–18**
Energy	EAR	1715 kcal	1979 kcal	2220 kcal	2755 kcal
Fat	Max 35% energy	67 g	77 g	86 g	107 g
Saturated fat	Max 11% energy	21 g	24 g	27 g	34 g
Carbohydrate	Min 50% energy	229 g	263 g	296 g	367 g
Added sugars*	Max 11% energy	50 g	58 g	65 g	81 g
Fibre **	8 g per 1000 kcal	14 g	16 g	18 g	22 g
Protein		19.7 g	28 g	42 g	55 g
Iron		6.1 mg	8.7 mg	11.3 mg	11.3 mg
Zinc		6.5 mg	7.0 mg	9.0 mg	9.5 mg
Calcium		450 mg	550 mg	1000 mg	1000 mg
Vitamin A		500 ug	500 ug	600 ug	700 ug
Vitamin C		30 mg	30 mg	35 mg	40 mg
Folate		100 ug	150 ug	200 ug	200 ug
Salt***		3 g	5 g	6 g	6 g

+ Department of Health (1991) Dietary reference values for food energy and nutrients for the United Kingdom. London: HMSO
EAR = Estimated Average Requirement
* Non-milk extrinsic sugars
** Proportion of adult DRV (18 g) i.e. 8 g/ 1000 kcal
*** Scientific Advisory Committee on Nutrition (2003) Salt and Health. London: HMSO

Source: S Jebb et al., 2004

Table 12.8 Dietary reference values for girls 4–18 years+

	Dietary Reference Value (DRV)	4–6	7–10	11–14	15–18
Energy	EAR	1545 kcal	1740 kcal	1845 kcal	2110 kcal
Fat	Max 35% energy	60 g	68 g	72 g	82 g
Saturated fat	Max 11% energy	19 g	21 g	23 g	26 g
Carbohydrate	Min 50% energy	206 g	232 g	246 g	281 g
Added sugars*	Max 11% energy	45 g	51 g	54 g	62 g
Fibre **	8 g per 1000 kcal	12 g	14 g	15 g	17 g
Protein		19.7 g	28 g	41 g	45 g
Iron		6.1 mg	8.7 mg	14.8 mg	14.8 mg
Zinc		6.5 mg	7.0 mg	9.0 mg	7.0 mg
Calcium		450 mg	550 mg	800 mg	800 mg
Vitamin A		500 ug	500 ug	600 ug	600 ug
Vitamin C		30 mg	30 mg	35 mg	40 mg
Folate		100 ug	150 ug	200 ug	200 ug
Salt***		3 g	5 g	6 g	6 g

+Department of Health (1991) Dietary reference values for food energy and nutrients for the United Kingdom, London: HMSO
EAR = Estimated Average Requirement
* Non-milk extrinsic sugars
** Proportion of adult DRV (18 g) i.e. 8 g/ 1000 kcal
*** Scientific Advisory Committee on Nutrition (2003) Salt and Health. London: HMSO

Source: S Jebb *et al.*, 2004

high and important nutrients essential to a child's health could be missed out. Instead, make healthy changes to what they eat.

Set a good example
Young athletes are more likely to copy what you do than what you say. They learn a lot about food and activity by watching their parents. They should see that you exercise and eat a balanced diet. Share mealtimes as often as possible and eat the same meals.

Don't use food as a reward
Rewarding good behaviour with sweet treats only reinforces the idea that they are a special treat and makes children crave them more. Allow them in

Let them eat fruit... and other healthy snacks

- Fresh fruit e.g. apple slices, satsumas, clementines, grapes, strawberries
- Wholemeal toast with Marmite
- Grilled tomatoes on wholemeal toast
- Low fat yoghurt
- Low fat milk
- Nuts e.g. cashews, peanuts, almonds, brazils
- Wholegrain breakfast cereal with milk
- Plain popcorn
- Vegetable crudités (carrot, pepper and cucumber sticks)
- Rice cake with sliced bananas or cottage cheese.

moderation, say, on one day of the week and at the end of a meal.

Don't ban any foods

Allow all foods, but explain that certain ones should be eaten only occasionally or kept as occasional treats. Banning a food increases children's desire for it and makes it more likely that they will eat it in secret.

Provide healthy snacks

Instead of biscuits, crisps and chocolate, make sure there are healthier alternatives to hand. Fresh fruit, low fat yoghurt, wholemeal toast, and wholegrain breakfast cereals are good choices. Keep them in a place where your child can easily get them – for example, a fruit bowl on the table, yoghurts at the front of the fridge.

Get them moving more

Although a young athlete trains and plays sport, they may be very inactive the rest of the time. Look for opportunities to increase their daily activity. For example, encourage them to walk or cycle to and from school. Try to increase the amount of exercise you do together as a family – swimming, playing football, a family walk or bike ride.

Limit time spent watching television

Plan and agree exactly what they will watch on television and agree on a defined time period. Once the programmes have finished, switch off the television, no matter how much they protest. Don't place a television in your children's bedrooms.

Balance activity and viewing time

Let the number of hours they have exercised equal the number of hours they are allowed to watch television. If they have done an hour's physical activity during the day, you could allocate an hour's television watching.

How much exercise should children get?

Current advice (Department of Health, 2011) is: To maintain a basic level of health, children and young people aged 5–18 need to do:

- At least 60 minutes (1 hour) of physical activity every day, which should be a mix of moderate-intensity aerobic activity, such as fast walking, and vigorous-intensity aerobic activity, such as running.
- On three days a week, these activities should involve muscle-strengthening activities, such as push-ups, and bone-strengthening activities, such as running.

Don't snack and view

Discourage eating meals or unhealthy snacks while watching television. Because their mind will be on the television and not on the food, they won't notice when they are full up.

TOP TIPS TO MAINTAIN A HEALTHY WEIGHT

- Aim for five portions of fruit and vegetables a day.
- Follow the one-third rule – vegetables should fill at least one third of the plate. This will help satisfy hunger as well as providing protective nutrients.
- Always eat food sitting at a table – eating in front of the TV or eating on the run makes you eat more because you don't concentrate fully.
- Give them fruit to take to school for break times – apples, satsumas and grapes are all suitable.
- Don't ditch dairy products in a bid to save calories: switch to low-fat or skimmed versions. They contain just as much calcium.
- Give brown rather than white – wholegrain bread, bran cereals and wholewheat pasta are rich in fibre, which makes your child feel fuller. Switch gradually, though, to avoid stomach upsets.
- Don't ban chocolate – for treats, offer a fun-sized chocolate bar.
- Have soup made with lots of veggies more often – it's filling, low in calories, and nutritious. Your child can help make it, or you can buy ready-made fresh versions.
- Make healthier chips by thickly slicing potatoes, tossing in a little olive oil and baking in the oven.
- Include fruit for desserts – fresh fruit, stewed apples or pears with custard, baked apples, and fruit crumble.

- Encourage them to eat slowly and enjoy every mouthful. Teach by example.
- Start the day with porridge – oats keep your child fuller for longer and keep cravings at bay.
- Include baked beans and lentils in meals – they are filling, nutritious and don't cause a rapid rise in blood sugar.
- Encourage them to drink at least 6 glasses of fluid a day. Thirst is sometimes mistaken for hunger.

HOW CAN YOUNG ATHLETES PUT ON WEIGHT?

Many young athletes struggle to keep up their weight or put on any weight, because they burn a lot of energy in sport. Encourage them to eat more frequent meals and snacks – six or seven times a day. They may not be able to meet their daily energy demands for growth and activity from three meals.

Aim to add in three or four snacks or mini meals a day. To gain weight, children need to consume more calories than they use for growth and exercise. Make the energy and nutrient content of the food more concentrated. Here are some suggestions:

- Serve bigger portions, particularly of pasta, potatoes, rice, cereals, dairy products and protein-rich foods.
- Provide three to four nutritious energy-giving snacks between meals – see the box for suggestions.
- Include nutritious drinks, e.g. milk, homemade milkshakes, yoghurt drinks, fruit smoothies and fruit juice.
- Scatter grated cheese on vegetables, soups, potatoes, pasta dishes and hotpots.

- Add dried fruit to breakfast cereals, porridge and yoghurt.
- Spread bread, toast or crackers with peanut butter or nut butter.
- Serve vegetables and main courses with a sauce, such as cheese sauce.
- Avoid filling up on stodgy puddings, biscuits and cakes as they supply calories but few essential nutrients (and are usually loaded with saturated or hydrogenated fat).
- Try milk-based or yoghurt-based puddings, e.g. rice pudding, banana custard, fruit crumble with yoghurt, fruit salad with yoghurt or custard, bread pudding, fruit pancakes.

High energy snacks for weight gain

- Nuts – peanuts, almonds, cashews, brazils, pistachios
- Dried fruit – raisins, sultanas, apricots, dates
- Wholemeal sandwiches with cheese, chicken, ham, tuna, peanut butter or banana
- Yoghurt and fromage frais
- Milk, milkshakes, flavoured milk, and yoghurt drinks
- Breakfast cereal or porridge with milk and dried fruit
- Cheese – slices, cubes or novelty cheese snacks
- Cheese on toast
- Scones, fruit buns, malt loaf
- Small pancakes
- English muffins, rolls or bagels
- Cereal or breakfast bars (check they contain no hydrogenated fat)
- Bread or toast spread with jam or honey

IS STRENGTH TRAINING APPROPRIATE FOR YOUNG ATHLETES?

A well-designed strength training or weight training programme will improve a young athlete's strength, reduce their risk of sports injuries and improve their sports performance. Contrary to the belief that strength training can damage the growth cartilage or stunt their growth, recent studies suggest that it can actually make bones stronger. In fact, there are no reported cases of bone damage in relation to strength training. Children who strength train tend to feel better about themselves as they get stronger, and have higher self-esteem. But strength training is not the same as power lifting, weightlifting or body-building, none of which are recommended for children under 18 years old.

Bulking up should not be the goal of a strength training programme. Children and teenagers should tone their muscles using a light weight (or body weight) and a high number of repetitions, rather than lifting heavy weights. Only after they have passed puberty should children consider adding muscle bulk. Younger children should begin with body weight exercises such as push ups and sit ups. More experienced trainees may use free weights and machines.

Sports scientists say that a well-designed strength training programme can bring many fitness benefits for children and can complement an existing training programme. Indeed the American Academy of Paediatrics Committee on Sports Medicine endorses it. Here are some guidelines:

- Children should be properly supervised during training sessions.

- They should use an age-appropriate routine (adult routines are not suitable) – typically 30 second intervals with breaks in between, with a thorough warm-up and cool-down period.
- Ensure the exercises are performed using proper form and technique.
- Children should start with a relatively light weight and a high number of repetitions.
- No heavy lifts should be included.
- The programme should form part of a total fitness programme.
- The sessions should be varied and fun.

Note: children should complete a medical examination before beginning a strength training programme.

SUMMARY OF KEY POINTS

- Young athletes expend approximately 25% more calories for any given activity compared with adults.
- Young athletes need more protein relative to their weight than adults – about 1 g per kg body weight (adults need 0.75 g/kg). Protein supplements are not necessary.
- It is recommended that young athletes obtain at least 50% of their energy from carbohydrate.
- If young athletes will be exercising continually for less than 90 minutes, they won't need to eat anything during exercise but should be encouraged to take regular drink breaks, ideally every 15–20 minutes.
- After exercise, give young athletes a drink straightaway – water or diluted fruit juice are the best drinks – followed by a high carbohydrate high GI snack to stave off hunger and promote recovery.

- Young athletes are more susceptible to dehydration and overheating than adults.
- Encourage them to drink 6–8 cups (1–1.5 litres) of fluid during the day, then top up with 150–200 ml (a large glass) of water 45 minutes before exercise.
- During exercise, they should aim to drink 75–100 ml every 15–20 mins.
- After exercise, they should drink freely until no longer thirsty, plus an extra glass, or drink 300 ml for every 0.2 kg weight loss.
- As with adults, plain water is best for most activities lasting less than 90 minutes, otherwise a flavoured drink will encourage them to drink enough fluid (examples above).
- Young athletes should not need supplements if they are eating a well-balanced diet and eating a wide variety of foods, but a children's multivitamin and mineral supplement may provide assurance.
- There is no research to support the use of sports supplements in young athletes and the long term risks are unknown. The ACSM specifically warn against the use of creatine in athletes under 18.
- If an athlete has a genuine weight problem, seek professional advice. Talk to young athletes about healthy eating and exercise, teach by example and let them make their own decisions about food.
- Young athletes who struggle to keep up their weight or put on any weight should be encouraged to eat more frequent meals and snacks and focus on energy and nutrient-rich foods (examples above).

THE VEGETARIAN ATHLETE

13

Many athletes choose to follow a vegetarian diet or avoid red meat either for ethical reasons or in the belief that such a diet is healthier. Indeed, large-scale prospective dietary surveys have found that vegetarians have higher intakes of fruit and vegetables, fibre, antioxidant nutrients and phyto-nutrients, and lower intakes of saturated fat and cholesterol than do meat-eaters (Davey *et al.*, 2003; Keys *et al.*, 1996). It is estimated that one in twenty people in the UK are vegetarian (National Diet and Nutrition Survey 2001) and one in three eat meat only occasionally (Gallup, 2001). The question is whether the benefits of a vegetarian diet extend to enhanced physical fitness and performance. This chapter considers the research in this area and covers the key nutritional considerations for vegetarian athletes. It also provides practical advice to help vegetarian athletes meet their requirements.

IS A VEGETARIAN DIET SUITABLE FOR ATHLETES?

Many people imagine that a plant-based diet cannot fulfil an athlete's nutritional requirements, that meat is necessary for building strength and endurance, and that vegetarian athletes are smaller, weaker, less muscular and less powerful than their meat-eating counterparts. There is no truth to support these misconceptions. On the contrary, the American Dietetic Association and Dietitians of Canada's 1997 position paper on vegetarian diets states that the needs of competitive athletes can be met through a vegetarian diet (ADA, 1997). This view is echoed in the 2000 ADA and American College of Sports Medicine joint position paper on physical fitness

What is the definition of a vegetarian?

A vegetarian diet is defined as one that does not include meat, poultry, game, fish, shellfish or crustacea, or slaughter by-products such as gelatine or animal fats. It includes grains, pulses, nuts, seeds, vegetables and fruits with or without the use of dairy products and eggs. A lacto-ovo-vegetarian eats both dairy products and eggs. This is the most common type of vegetarian diet. A lacto-vegetarian eats dairy products but not eggs.

A vegan does not eat dairy products, eggs, or any other animal product.

and athletic performance which states 'foods of animal origin are not essential to ensure optimal athletic performance' (ADA/DC/ACSM, 2000).

CAN A VEGETARIAN DIET BENEFIT ATHLETIC PERFORMANCE?

Researchers at the University of British Columbia, Vancouver, Canada, addressed this question when they carried out a review of studies on vegetarian athletes. They concluded that well-planned and varied vegetarian diets don't hinder athletic potential and do indeed support athletic performance (Barr & Rideout, 2004). However, a vegetarian diet *per se* is not associated with improved aerobic performance (Nieman, 1999).

Several studies have found no significant differences in performance, physical fitness (aerobic or anaerobic capacities), limb circumference, and strength between vegetarian and non-vegetarian athletes (Williams, 1985; Hanne *et al.*, 1986). Even among female athletes consuming a semi-vegetarian diet (less than 100 g red meat per week), there was no difference in their maximum aerobic capacity – or aerobic fitness – compared with meat-eaters (Snyder, 1989). And long-term vegetarian women (average duration of vegetarianism 46 years) had equal health status to non-vegetarian women, according to another study (Nieman, 1989).

Danish researchers tested athletes after they had consumed either a vegetarian or non-vegetarian diet for 6 weeks alternately (Richter *et al.*, 1991). The carbohydrate content of each diet was kept the same (57% energy). Whichever diet they ate, the athletes experienced no change in aerobic capacity, endurance, muscle glycogen concentration or strength.

In a German study, runners completed a 1000 km race after consuming either a vegetarian or non-vegetarian diet containing similar amounts of carbohydrate (60% energy) (Eisinger, 1994). The finishing times were not influenced by the diet; the running times of the vegetarians were not significantly different from those of the non-vegetarians.

Together, these studies suggest that a vegetarian diet, even when followed for several decades, is compatible with successful athletic performance.

What are the health benefits of a vegetarian diet?

In 2005, the British Dietetic Association stated that, 'a well-balanced vegetarian diet can provide all of the key nutrients needed in the body at all ages' (BDA, 2005). The diets of people who follow a varied, well-balanced vegetarian diet are in line with the current nutritional recommendations for a low fat, high fibre diet. Medical studies have shown that vegetarians are less likely to suffer from such illnesses as heart disease, cancer, diet-related diabetes, obesity and high blood pressure (Appleby *et al.*, 1999).

CAN A VEGETARIAN DIET PROVIDE ENOUGH PROTEIN FOR ATHLETES?

In general, vegetarian diets are lower in protein than non-vegetarian diets but, nevertheless, they tend to meet or exceed the RNI for protein (Janelle & Barr, 1995). But since athletes need more protein than the RNI for the general population (0.75 g/ kg body weight/ day) – endurance athletes need 1.2–1.4 g per kg body weight/ day (ADA/DC/ACSM; Lemon, 1998) and strength training athletes need 1.4–1.8 g per kg of body weight per day (Lemon, 1998; Tarnopolsky & MacLennan, 1992) – the question is whether vegetarians can consume enough protein without taking supplements.

Researchers have concluded that most athletes are able to meet these extra demands from a vegetarian diet as long as a variety of protein-rich foods are consumed and energy intakes are adequate (Nielson, 1999; Lemon, 1995; Barr & Rideout, 2004; Nielson, 1999). Good sources of vegetarian proteins are detailed below.

Contrary to popular belief, even strength athletes can obtain enough protein from a vegetarian diet – the limiting factor for muscle mass gains appears to be total caloric intake, not protein intake.

WHICH FOODS ARE THE BEST PROTEIN SOURCES FOR VEGETARIANS?

Most foods contain at least some protein. Good protein sources for vegetarians include pulses, nuts, seeds, dairy products, eggs, soya products (tofu, soya milk, soya 'yoghurt' and soya mince), cereals, and quorn. The protein content of various foods is shown in Table 13.1.

Single plant foods do not contain all the essential amino acids you need in the right proportions, but when you mix plant foods together, any deficiency in one is cancelled out by any excess in the other. This is known as protein complementing. Many plant proteins are low in one of the essential amino acids (the 'limiting amino acid'). For example, grains are short of lysine while pulses are short of methionine. Combining grains and pulses leads to a high quality protein that is just as good, if not better, than protein from animal foods. A few examples are beans on toast, muesli, or rice and lentils. Adding dairy products or eggs

Vegetarians may benefit more from creatine supplements

Meat is a major source of creatine in the diet – it typically supplies around 1 g per day for non-vegetarians – so vegetarians tend to have lower muscle creatine concentrations than do non-vegetarians (Maughan, 1995). Because initial muscle creatine levels are lower, vegetarians have an increased capacity to load creatine into muscle following supplementation and are likely to gain greater performance benefits in activities that rely on the ATP–PC system (see pages 17–19), i.e. sports involving repeated bouts of anaerobic activity (Watt et al., 2004).

also adds the missing amino acids, e.g. macaroni cheese, quiche, porridge.

Other examples of other protein combinations include:

- Tortilla or wrap filled with re-fried beans
- Bean and vegetable hotpot with rice or pasta
- Quorn chilli with rice
- Peanut butter sandwich
- Lentil soup with a roll
- Quorn korma with naan bread
- Stir-fried tofu and vegetables with rice
- Tofu burger in a roll.

In essence, you can achieve protein complementation by combining plant foods from two or more of the following categories:

1. pulses: beans, lentils, and peas
2. grains: bread, pasta, rice, oats, breakfast cereals, corn, rye

3. nuts and seeds: peanuts, cashews, almonds, sunflower seeds, sesame seeds, and pumpkin seeds

4. quorn and soya products: soya milk, tofu, tempeh (fermented soya curd similar to tofu but with a stronger flavour), soya mince, soya burgers, quorn mince, quorn fillets, and quorn sausages.

It is now known that the body has a pool of amino acids, so that if one meal is deficient, it can be made up from the body's own stores. Because of this, you don't have to worry about complementing amino acids all the time, as long as your diet is generally varied and well balanced. Even those foods not considered high in protein are adding some amino acids to this pool.

WHAT ARE THE PITFALLS OF A VEGETARIAN DIET FOR ATHLETES?

Some athletes may struggle on a vegetarian diet if they give up meat and increase their training at the same time. That's likely to be the case if you start training for an event or race but don't step up your calorie intake or pay attention to protein and carbohydrate intake. Tiredness or weight loss are often blamed on the vegetarian diet rather than a failure to eat enough calories. If you fail

Table 13.1		The protein content of various foods included in a vegetarian diet	
Sources of protein			
Good sources	**(g)**	**Fair sources**	**(g)**
Chickpeas or red kidney beans (140 g)	12 g	Pasta, wholemeal or white (230 g boiled)	7 g
Milk (1 glass/ 200 ml)	7 g	Rice, brown or white (180 g boiled)	5 g
Egg (1, size 2)	8 g	Bread, wholemeal or white (1 slice)	3 g
Lentils (120 g)	9 g	Porridge made with water (200 g)	3 g
Yoghurt (1 carton, 150 g)	6–8 g	Potatoes, boiled (200 g)	4 g
Tofu (100 g)	8 g	Broccoli (100 g)	3 g
Quorn mince (100 g)	12 g		
Peanuts (50 g)	12 g		
Pumpkin seeds (50 g)	12 g		

Table 13.2	The iron content of various foods included in a vegetarian diet		
Sources of iron			
Good sources	**Iron, mg**	**Fair sources**	**Iron, mg**
Chickpeas or red kidney beans (140 g)	4.3 mg	Boiled egg (1)	1.3 mg
Bran flakes (45 g or 1½ oz)	5.3 mg	Cashews (25 g or 4 oz)	1.5 mg
Spinach, boiled (100 g or 3½ oz)	4.0 mg	Avocado (75 g or 3 oz)	1.1 mg
Baked beans (225 g or 8 oz)	3.2 mg	Asparagus (125 g or 4 oz)	1.1 mg
Black treacle (35 g or 1¼ oz)	3.2 mg	1 slice wholemeal bread (40 g)	1.0 mg
Muesli (60 g or 2¼ oz)	2.76 mg	Broccoli, boiled (100 g or 3½ oz)	1.0 mg
4 dried figs (60 g or 2¼ oz)	2.1 mg	Brown rice (200 g or 7 oz)	0.9 mg
8 dried apricots (50 g or 2 oz)	2.1 mg	Peanut butter (20 g or ⅔ oz)	0.5 mg

to adjust your diet when you add extra training, you will lose excessive weight, feel very tired and find recovery takes longer.

As with any dietary change, it is important to plan your diet well and gain as much knowledge about vegetarian diets as possible. Some athletes adopt a vegetarian or vegan diet in order to lose body fat in the belief that such diets are automatically lower in calories. Many do not substitute suitable foods in place of meat and fail to consume enough protein and other nutrients to support their training. Athletes with disordered eating may omit meat – as well as other food groups – from their diet but disordered eating is certainly not a consequence of vegetarianism!

A very bulky vegetarian diet that includes lots of high-fibre foods (e.g. beans, wholegrains) may be too filling if you have high energy needs. To ensure you eat enough calories, you may need to include more compact sources of carbohydrate (e.g. dried fruit, fruit juice) or include a mixture of both wholegrain and refined grain products (e.g. wholemeal and white bread) in your diet.

SPECIAL CONSIDERATIONS ON A VEGETARIAN DIET

Iron and zinc

Omitting meat may result in lower intakes of iron and zinc and, theoretically, an increased risk of iron deficiency anaemia. However, there is evidence that the body adapts over time by increasing the percentage of minerals it absorbs from food. Lowered levels of iron and zinc in the diet result in increased absorption.

Despite iron from plants being less readily absorbed, research has shown that iron-deficiency anaemia is no more common in vegetarians than meat eaters (Alexander *et al.*, 1994; Janelle & Barr, 1995). Even among female endurance athletes, vegetarians are not at greater risk of iron deficiency. Researchers have found that blood levels of haemoglobin and running performance are very similar between non-vegetarian and vegetarian female runners (Snyder, 1989; Seiler, 1989).

Eating vitamin C-rich food (e.g. fruit and vegetables) at the same time as iron-rich foods greatly improves iron absorption. Citric acid (found naturally in fruit and vegetables) and amino acids also promote iron absorption. Good sources of iron for vegetarians include wholegrain cereals, wholemeal bread, nuts, pulses, green vegetables (broccoli, watercress and spinach), fortified cereals, seeds and dried fruit. Table 13.2 shows the iron content of various vegetarian foods.

Table 13.3 The zinc content of various foods included in a vegetarian diet

Sources of zinc			
Good sources	**Zinc, mg**	**Fair sources**	**Zinc, mg**
Chickpeas (200 g or 7 oz)	2.8 mg	Peanut butter (20 g or ⅔ oz)	0.6 mg
Baked beans (225 g or 8 oz)	1.6 mg	Peas, frozen/canned (80 g or 3⅓ oz)	0.6 mg
1 Vegeburger (100 g or 3½ oz)	1.6 mg	3 dried figs (60 g or 2¼ oz)	0.5 mg
Pumpkin seeds (20 g or ⅔ oz)	1.3 mg	3 Brazil nuts (10 g or ⅓ oz)	0.4 mg
Muesli (60 g or 2¼ oz)	1.3 mg	Potatoes, boiled (200 g or 7 oz)	0.4 mg
Cheddar cheese (30 g or 1 oz)	1.2 mg	1 orange (140 g or 5 oz)	0.3 mg
Tahini paste (20 g or ⅔ oz)	1.1 mg	6 almonds (10 g or ⅓ oz)	0.3 mg
1 fruit yoghurt (150 g or 5 oz)	0.9 mg	Peanut butter (20 g or ⅔ oz)	0.6 mg

Table 13.4 The omega-3 content of various foods included in a vegetarian diet

Sources of Omega-3 fatty acids

Good sources	g per 100 g	Portion	g per portion
Flaxseed oil	57 g	1 tablespoon (14 g)	8.0 g
Flaxseeds (ground)	16 g	1 tablespoon (24 g)	3.8 g
Rapeseed oil	9.6 g	1 tablespoon (14 g)	1.3 g
Walnuts	7.5 g	1 tablespoon (28 g)	2.6 g
Walnut oil	11.5 g	1 tablespoon (14 g)	1.6 g
Sweet potatoes	0.03 g	Medium (130 g)	1.3 g
Peanuts	0.4 g	Handful (50 g)	0.2 g
Broccoli	0.1 g	3 tablespoons (125 g)	1.3 g
Pumpkin seeds	8.5 g	2 tablespoons (25 g)	2.1 g
Omega-3 eggs	0.8 g	One egg	0.4 g

Source: MAFF/ RSC (1991); British Nutrition Foundation (1999)

The absorption of zinc and other trace minerals such as copper, manganese and selenium, can be reduced by bran and other plant compounds (phytates, oxalic acid), but most studies have failed to show that vegetarians have lower blood levels of these minerals (Fogelholm, 1995). However, it is advisable to avoid eating too many bran-enriched foods. Whole grains, pulses, nuts, seeds and eggs are good sources of zinc. Table 13.3 shows the zinc content of various vegetarian foods.

Omega 3s

Oily fish are rich in long chain omega-3 fatty acids, so vegetarians who don't eat fish will need to obtain them from other foods. One of the main omega-3 fatty acids, alpha-linolenic acid (ALA), is found in certain plant foods such as pumpkin seeds and flaxseed oil (*see* Table 13.4, which gives the omega-3 fatty acid content of various foods). In the body it is converted to eicosapentanoic acid (EPA) and docosapentanoic acid (DPA) – the two fatty acids which are found in plentiful amounts in oily fish but not other foods and which offer greater cardio protective benefits than the parent ALA.

The Vegetarian Society recommends an ALA intake of 1.5% of energy, or roughly 4 g a day. This should provide enough of the parent omega-3 fatty acid to ensure enough EPA and DHA are formed by the body (conversion rates are around 5–10% for EPA and 2–5% for DHA). Include some of the foods listed in table 13.4 in your daily diet.

You should also aim to achieve a LA to ALA ratio of around 4:1 or slightly lower since a high intake of LA interferes with the conversion process of ALA to EPA and DHA. Replace fat high in omega-6 oils (such as sunflower or corn oil) with fats higher in monounsaturated oils (such as olive oil and nuts), which do not disrupt the formation of EPA and DHA.

EASY MENU PLANNER

Plan your vegetarian diet around the following five food groups to ensure you get the right balance of amino acids and other nutrients.

Fruit and vegetables

5 or more servings a day

- Serving size = approx 80 g, equivalent to 1 medium fruit e.g. apple; 2 small fruit e.g. kiwi fruit; 1 cupful berries e.g. strawberries; 3 heaped tablespoons of cooked vegetables.

Pulses and other protein-rich foods

2–4 servings a day (4–5 if dairy products are excluded).

This group includes beans, lentils, eggs, nuts, seeds, soya milk, soya mince, quorn, tofu, and tempeh.

- Serving size = 4 oz (110 g) cooked pulses; tofu, soya mince; 2 eggs; 1 oz (25 g) nuts or seeds.

Cereals and starchy vegetables

4–6 servings a day depending on activity level

This group includes bread, rice, pasta, breakfast cereals and potatoes. At least half of your servings should be whole grains.

- Serving size = 2 slices of bread; 60 g (uncooked weight) grains or breakfast cereal; 175 g potato.

Milk and dairy products

2–4 servings a day

This group includes milk, yogurt, and cheese. Choose the low fat versions wherever possible.

- Serving size = 200 ml (1/3 pint) milk; 1 carton (150 ml) yogurt/fromage frais; 40 g hard cheese; 125 g cottage cheese

Healthy fats and oils

2–4 portions a day.

This group includes all vegetable oils (try to include at least one source of omega-3 rich oil daily), nuts, seeds, and avocados.

- Serving size = 2 tsp (10 ml) oil, 25 g nuts or seeds, ½ avocado.

SUMMARY OF KEY POINTS

- Overall, vegetarians have higher intakes of fruit and vegetables, fibre, antioxidant nutrients and phytonutrients, and lower intakes of saturated fat and cholesterol compared with meat-eaters.
- Vegetarians suffer less heart disease, hypertension, obesity, diabetes and certain cancers than meat-eaters.
- The nutritional needs of competitive athletes can be fully met through a vegetarian diet.
- Studies have shown that well-planned and varied vegetarian diets don't hinder athletic potential and do indeed support athletic performance.
- There are no significant differences in performance, physical fitness (aerobic or anaerobic capacities), limb circumference, and strength

between vegetarian and non-vegetarian athletes.

- Vegetarian diets are lower in protein than non-vegetarian diets but, nevertheless, most athletes are able to meet these extra demands from a vegetarian diet as long as a variety of protein-rich foods are consumed and energy intakes are adequate.
- Vegetarian athletes are likely to gain greater performance benefits from creatine supple-mentation than meat-eaters, due to their initially lower muscle creatine levels.
- Vegetarians risk low intakes of iron, zinc and omega-3 fatty acids but studies show that iron-deficiency anaemia is no more common in vegetarians than meat eaters.
- Vegetarians can obtain omega-3 fatty acids from foods rich in alpha-linolenic acid (ALA) and should aim for an ALA intake of 1.5% of energy, or roughly 4 g a day.

COMPETITION NUTRITION

14

Your diet before a competition will have a big impact on your performance, and could provide you with that winning edge. In addition, what you eat and drink on the day of the event can affect your ability to recover between heats and your performance in subsequent heats. This chapter covers the whole of the competition period, including the week before the event, during, and after the event. It consolidates much of the information presented in preceding chapters, in particular Chapter 3 on carbohydrate intake and Chapter 7 on fluid intake, and provides specific guidelines for arriving at your competition well-hydrated and with full glycogen stores. It gives pre-competition sample eating plans, which you can use as a basis for developing your personal programme, suitable pre-competition meals and snacks that can be eaten between heats and events. For those athletes who need to make weight for their competition, this chapter gives a simple step-by-step nutrition strategy that will help you lose body fat safely and effectively.

THE WEEK BEFORE

During the week before a competition, your two main aims are:

1. to fill your muscle and liver glycogen stores so that you compete with a 'full' fuel supply
2. to keep well hydrated.

Your preparation will be dictated by the kind of event that you are competing in, the importance of the event and how frequently you compete.

Short duration events lasting less than 4 minutes

Short duration, all-out events lasting less than 4 minutes are fuelled by ATP, PC and muscle glycogen. If you are competing in a sprint event, it is important to allow enough recovery time after your last training session, and to make sure your muscle glycogen stores are replenished. The presence of muscle damage will delay the recovery process. Training which may cause muscle fibre damage should either be scheduled earlier in the week to allow for recovery or avoided altogether. Such training includes plyometrics, heavy weight training and hard running. Reduce your training over the pre-competition week and rest during the three days prior to the competition. Aim to consume 7–8 g carbohydrate/kg body weight/day. Use Table 14.1 as a guide to the amount of carbohydrate you should be eating during the final 3 days.

Endurance events lasting more than 90 minutes

If you are competing in an endurance event lasting longer than 90 minutes, you may benefit from carbohydrate loading. This is detailed in Chapter 3, 'Carbohydrate loading', pp. 50–52. In summary, you should consume a moderate carbohydrate diet (5–7 g/kg body weight/day) for the first three days (this should be less than you are used to eating), followed by a high carbohydrate intake (8–10 g/kg body weight/day) for the final 3 days. Use Table 14.1 as a guide to the amount of carbohydrate you should be eating during the pre-competition week. Your last hard training session should be completed one week before your competition. Then taper your training during the final week so that you perform only very light exercise and rest the day prior to your competition.

Endurance events lasting less than 90 minutes; or multiple heats

If your event lasts less than 90 minutes, or if your competition schedule includes several short heats in one day, your muscle glycogen stores can become depleted. Examples of events with multiple heats include swimming, track cycling and track and field athletics. You can fill your muscle glycogen stores by tapering your training during the final week and maintaining or increasing your carbohydrate intake to about 7–8 g/kg body weight/day during the 3 days prior to your competition. Use Table 14.1 as a guide to the amount of carbohydrate you should be eating during the final 3 days.

Weekly events

If you compete weekly or even more frequently (e.g. in seasonal competitions such as football, netball and cycling), it may not be possible to rest for 3 days prior to each match or race. You would end up with virtually no training time. Perform lower intensity training or technical training during the 2 days before the match and taper only for the most important matches or races. Increase your carbohydrate intake during the final 2 days to 8–10 g/kg body weight/day. Use Table

Table 14.1	Recommended carbohydrate intake for athletes of different body weights	
Body weight (kg)	**Daily carbohydrate intake equivalent to 7–8 g/kg body weight**	**Daily carbohydrate intake equivalent to 8–10 g/kg body weight**
65	455–520 g	520–650 g
70	490–560 g	560–700 g
75	525–600 g	600–750 g
80	560–640 g	640–800 g
85	595–680 g	680–850 g
90	630–720 g	720–900 g

14.1 as a guide to the amount of carbohydrate you should be eating during the final 3 days.

For all events, your total calorie intake should remain about the same as usual during the pre-competition week, but the proportions of carbohydrate, fat and protein will change. Eat larger amounts of carbohydrate-rich foods (e.g. potatoes, bread, rice, dried fruit) and carbohydrate drinks, and smaller amounts of fats and proteins. However, if you are performing a week-long taper, you may need to reduce your calories slightly to match your reduced training needs. You can do this by reducing your fat intake; otherwise you may experience fat gain.

In practice, eat at least 6 small meals a day, avoid gaps longer than 3 hours, and base all your meals on low GI foods. Use the sample eating plans in Table 14.2 as a basis for developing your own plan during the pre-competition week. While they provide the requirements for carbohydrate prior to competition, they are low in fat and protein and are not ideal for the rest of the season.

Check:

- Make sure that you rehydrate fully after training. *See* pp. 108–112 to calculate how much fluid you should consume before and after training. Check your hydration status by monitoring the frequency, volume and colour of your urine during the pre-competition week.
- Avoid any new, or untried foods or food combinations during the pre-competition week.
- If you will be travelling or staying away from home, be prepared to take food with you. Try to find out beforehand what type of food will be available at the event venue and predict any nutritional shortfalls.

WHAT IS THE BEST WAY TO MAKE WEIGHT FOR MY COMPETITION?

For weight-class sports such as boxing, judo, lightweight rowing and bodybuilding, it is an advantage to be as close as possible to the upper limit of your weight category. However, this should not be achieved at the expense of losing lean tissue (by rapid and severe dieting), depleting your glycogen stores (by starving) or dehydration (by fluid restriction, saunas, sweatsuits, diuretics). The principles for making weight for competition are similar to those for weight loss. In summary:

- Set a realistic and achievable goal.
- Allow enough time – aim to lose 0.5 kg body fat per week. This is crucial to your strategy and *cannot be overemphasised*. You must plan to 'make weight' many weeks before your event and *not* at the last minute, as is often the case.
- Monitor your weight and body composition by skinfold thickness measurements and girth measurements (*see* Chapter 8, p. 149).
- Reduce your calorie intake by 15% and never eat less than your resting metabolic rate (*see* Chapter 9, 'Calculating calorie, carbohydrate protein and fat requirements on a fat-loss programme', pp. 146–147).
- Increase the amount and frequency of aerobic training.
- Maintain carbohydrate intake at 5–7 g/kg body weight/day.
- Reduce fat intake to 15–25% of calories.
- Minimise muscle loss by consuming approximately 1.6 g protein/kg body weight/day.
- Eat at frequent and regular intervals (5–6 times a day).

Table 14.2 Pre-competition sample eating plans

Providing 500 g carbohydrate

Breakfast
- 1 large bowl (85 g) breakfast cereal
- 200 ml skimmed milk
- 2 tbsp (60 g) raisins
- 1 glass (200 ml) fruit juice

Morning snack
- 1 banana sandwich (2 slices bread and 1 banana)

Lunch
- 1 large jacket potato (300 g)
- 3 tbsp (90 g) sweetcorn and 1 tbsp (50 g) tuna or cottage cheese
- 2 pieces fresh fruit
- 1 carton low-fat fromage frais

Pre-workout snack
- 1 energy bar

Workout
- 1 L sports drink

Post-workout snack
- 1 serving of a meal replacement product

Dinner
- 1 bowl (85 g uncooked weight) pasta
- 125 g stir-fried vegetables
- 60 g stir-fried chicken or tofu
- 2 slices bread and butter
- 1 large bowl (200 g) fruit salad

Snack
- 2 slices toast with honey
- 1 carton low-fat yoghurt

Providing 700 g carbohydrate

Breakfast
- 4 thick slices toast with honey
- 1 glass (200 ml) fruit juice
- 1 banana

Morning snack
- 2 scotch pancakes
- 2 apples

Lunch
- 1 large bowl (125 g uncooked weight) rice salad with 60 g turkey or 125 g beans and vegetables
- 2 slices bread
- 2 pieces fruit

Pre-workout snack
- 2 bananas

Workout
- 1 L sports drink

Post-workout snack
- 2 cereal bars
- 1 carton (500 ml) flavoured milk

Dinner
- 2 large (2 × 300 g) jacket potatoes
- 1 carton (115 g) cottage cheese or fromage frais
- Broccoli or other vegetable
- 1 piece fresh fruit

Snack
- 1 carton (200 g) low-fat rice pudding

Avoid losing weight at the last minute by starvation or dehydration, as this can be dangerous. Starvation leads to depleted glycogen stores, so you will be unable to perform at your best. Dehydration leads to electrolyte disturbances, cramp and heartbeat irregularities. It is doubtful whether you can refuel and rehydrate sufficiently between the weigh-in and your competition, so aim to be at or within your weight category at least a day before the weigh-in. If you find it very difficult to make weight without resorting to these dangerous methods, consider competing in the next weight category.

A major problem with increasing the carbohydrate content of your diet in the pre-competition week is that the extra carbohydrate, stored with an amount of water equivalent to 3 times its

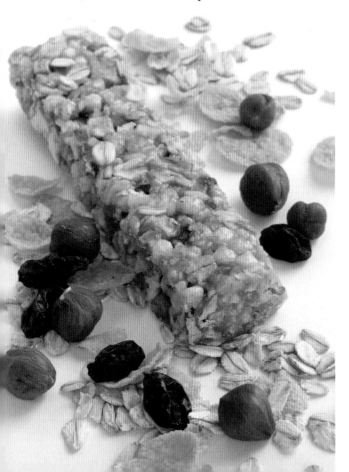

weight, can result in weight gain. While this extra glycogen is advantageous in most sports, it can be a disadvantage in weight-class sports where the cut-off weight is often reached by a whisker. Ideally, you should allow for an extra weight gain of up to 1 kg during the final week. In other words, make weight in advance – aim to attain a weight at least 1 kg below your competing weight.

THE DAY BEFORE

The day before your competition your main aims are:

1. to top up muscle glycogen levels
2. to ensure you are well hydrated.

Continue eating meals high in carbohydrate that have a low GI throughout the day and drinking plenty of fluids. To maximise muscle glycogen replenishment, perform only very light exercise or rest completely. Do not skip your evening meal, even if you experience pre-competition 'nerves', as this is an important time for topping up muscle glycogen. However, stick to familiar and simple foods, avoid fatty or oily foods and avoid alcohol, as it is a diuretic.

WHAT SHOULD I EAT WHEN I AM NERVOUS BEFORE COMPETITION?

Most athletes get pre-competition 'nerves' and this can reduce your appetite and result in problems such as nausea, diarrhoea and stomach cramps. If you find it difficult to eat solid food during this time, consume liquid meals such as meal replacement products (protein-carbohydrate sports supplements), sports drinks, milkshakes, yoghurt drinks and fruit smoothies. Try smooth,

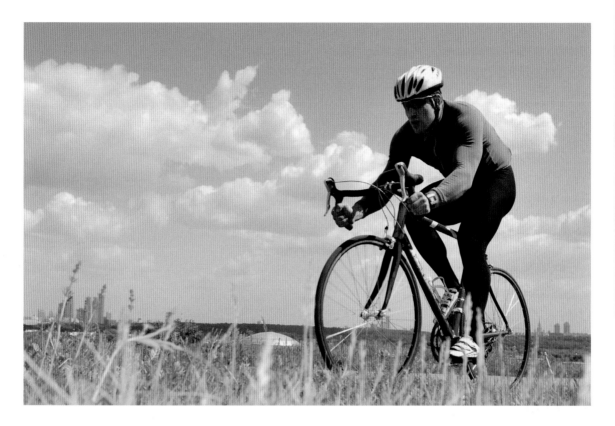

semi-liquid foods such as puréed fruit (e.g. apple purée, mashed banana, apple and apricot purée), yoghurt, porridge, custard and rice pudding. Bland foods such as semolina, mashed potato, or a porridge made from cornmeal or ground rice may agree with your digestive system better. To reduce problems, avoid high-fibre foods such as bran cereals, dried fruit, and pulses. You may wish to avoid vegetables that cause flatulence such as the brassica vegetables (cabbage, cauliflower, Brussel sprouts, broccoli). Caffeine can cause anxiety and problems such as diarrhoea when combined with 'nerves'. In essence, avoid anything that is new or unfamiliar. The golden rule with pre-competition eating is stick with tried and tested foods, which you know agree with you!

ON THE DAY

On the day of your competition, your aims are to:

1. top up liver glycogen stores following the over-night fast
2. maintain blood sugar levels
3. keep hunger at bay
4. keep well hydrated.

Plan to have your main pre-competition meal 2–4 hours before the event. This will allow enough time for your stomach to empty sufficiently and for blood sugar and insulin levels to normalise. It will also top up liver glycogen levels. Nervousness can slow down your digestion rate, so if you have pre-competition nerves you may need to leave a little longer than usual between eating and competing.

The actual timing of your pre-competition meal and the quantity of food eaten depends on

---

Pre-competition meals

Pre-competition breakfast
(2–4 hrs before event)

- Breakfast cereal or porridge with low-fat milk and fresh fruit
- Toast or bread with jam/honey; low-fat yoghurt
- English muffins with honey
- Meal replacement shake

Pre-competition lunches
(2–4 hrs before event)

- Sandwiches or rolls with tuna, cottage cheese or chicken; fresh fruit
- Pasta or rice with tomato-based sauce; fresh fruit
- Baked potato with low-fat filling; fresh fruit

Pre-competition snacks
(1 hr before event)

- Smoothie
- Yoghurt drink
- Fruit, e.g. apples, bananas, oranges, grapes, kiwi
- Tinned fruit
- Meal replacement or energy bar
- Sports drink
- Dried apricots
- Low-fat fruit yoghurt
- Rice pudding
- Mini or Scotch pancakes.

---

the individual, despite the fact that studies recommend consuming 200–300 g carbohydrate during the 4 hours prior to exercise. Pre-competition nerves often slow down digestion, so you may find 200–300 g carbohydrate too filling. The key is to find out what works for you and stick with it.

So, for example, if you are competing in the morning, you may need to get up a little earlier to eat your pre-competition breakfast. If your event is at 10.00 a.m., have your breakfast at 7.00 a.m. Some athletes skip breakfast, preferring to feel 'light' when they compete. However, it is not a good strategy to compete on an empty stomach, particularly if your event lasts longer than 1 hour, or you will be competing in a number of heats. Low liver glycogen and blood sugar levels may reduce your endurance and result in early fatigue. As explained in Chapter 3, liver glycogen is important for maintaining blood sugar levels and supplying fuel to the exercising muscles when muscle glycogen is depleted.

If you are competing in the afternoon, have a substantial breakfast and schedule lunch approximately 2–4 hours before the competition. If you are competing in the evening, eat your meals at 3-hourly intervals during the day, again scheduling your last meal approximately 2–4 hours before competition.

WHAT SHOULD I EAT ON THE DAY OF MY COMPETITION?

Your pre-competition meal should be:

- based on low GI carbohydrates
- low in fat
- low in protein
- low or moderate in fibre
- not too bulky or filling

- not salty or spicy
- enjoyable and familiar
- easy to digest
- include a drink – approx. 500 ml 2 hours before the event.

Suitable types of meals are given in the box, 'Pre-competition meals'. Remember, you can reduce the GI of a meal by adding protein. If you really do not feel like eating, have a liquid meal or semi-liquid foods (*see* 'What should I eat when I am nervous before competition?' on p. 222).

SHOULD I EAT OR DRINK JUST BEFORE MY COMPETITION?

Consume your pre-event meal 2–4 hours before the start of the event. This will provide a sustained supply of energy, maintain blood sugar levels during the event (particularly during the latter stages), and delay fatigue. Aim to consume about 2.5 g carbohydrate/kg body weight (*see* pp. 38–39, Chapter 3.) Most athletes find that low GI foods avoid any risk of hypoglycaemia at the start of the competition. However, make sure that you have rehearsed your eating programme plenty of times during training before the event. Do not try anything new on the day of competition. The timing is fairly individual, so experiment in training first!

You should also make sure that you are well hydrated before the competition (check the colour of your urine!) and aim to drink a further 125–250 ml fluid about 15–30 minutes before the event. Carry a drink bottle with you at all times.

SHOULD I EAT OR DRINK DURING MY COMPETITION?

If you are competing for more than about 60 minutes, you may find that extra carbohydrate will help delay fatigue and maintain your performance, particularly in the latter stages. Depending on your exercise intensity and duration, aim to take in 30–60 g carbohydrate per hour. Start consuming the food or drink after about 30 minutes and continue at regular intervals, as it takes approximately 30 minutes for digestion and absorption.

If your glycogen stores are low at the start of the event (which hopefully they are not!), then consuming additional carbohydrate during the event will have a fairly immediate effect on your performance.

Any carbohydrate with a high or moderate GI would be suitable, but you may find liquids easier to consume than solids. Isotonic sports drinks or carbohydrate (glucose polymer) drinks are popular because they serve to replenish fluid losses and prevent dehydration as well as supplying carbohydrate. Avoid high fructose drinks because they are not absorbed as fast as sucrose, glucose and glucose polymers. They may also cause stomach

Table 14.3	Recommended quantity of a 6% isotonic drink during exercise (60 g glucose/sucrose/glucose polymer dissolved in 1 L water)		
Moderate intensity (30 g carbohydrate/h)	Moderate–high intensity (45 g carbohydrate/h)	High intensity (60 g carbohydrate/h)
500 ml/h	750 ml/h	1000 ml/h

cramps or diarrhoea! Recommended quantities of isotonic drinks for different types of events are given in Table 14.3.

If you are competing in certain events such as cycling, sailing, distance canoeing or running, you may be able to take solid foods with you or arrange pick-up points. Suitable foods include energy bars, dried-fruit bars, cereal bars, bananas, breakfast bars, or raisins. If you are competing in matches and tournaments (e.g. football, tennis), take suitable snacks and drinks for the intervals and position them close by. Make use of every available opportunity to consume some fluid.

Table 14.4	Foods suitable to eat between heats or immediately after events

- Sports drinks (home made or commercial)
- Meal replacement shake
- Bananas
- Breakfast cereal
- Meal replacement bars or energy bar
- Fruit bars
- Cereal bars or breakfast bars
- Sandwiches or rolls filled with honey, jam or bananas
- Oatmeal biscuits; fig rolls
- Dried fruit
- Home-made muffins and bars – see recipes pp. 284–288
- Rice cakes or low-fat crackers with bananas or jam
- Smoothie
- Yoghurt drink

(Accompany solid foods with sufficient water to replace fluid losses)

If you are competing for more than 60 minutes, avoid or delay dehydration by drinking 125–250 ml every 10–20 minutes during exercise. Clearly, the more you sweat, the more you need to drink. However, do not be guided by thirst because this is not a good indicator of your hydration status. Studies have shown that you can maintain optimal performance if you can replace at least 80% of your sweat loss during exercise or keep within 1% of your body weight.

WHAT TO EAT BETWEEN HEATS OR EVENTS?

If you compete in several heats or matches during the day, it's important to refuel and rehydrate as fast as possible so that you have a good chance of performing well in your next competition. Consume at least 1 g carbohydrate/kg body weight during the 2-hour post-exercise period (muscle glycogen replenishment is faster during this time). If you've only a few hours between heats, you may prefer liquid meals such as meal replacement products, sports drinks and glucose polymer drinks. These will help replace both glycogen and fluid. If you are able to eat solid food, choose carbohydrates with a high GI that you find easy to digest and that are not too filling. Suitable foods are listed in Table 14.4. Take these with you in your kit bag. Drink at least 500 ml fluid immediately after competing and continue drinking at regular intervals to replace fluid losses.

WHAT TO EAT AFTER COMPETITION?

After your competition, your immediate aims are to replenish glycogen stores and fluid losses. If you are competing the following day or within the next few days, your post-event food intake is crucial. Again, choose foods with a moderate or high GI to ensure rapid refuelling, and aim for 1 g carbohydrate per kg body weight during the 2-hour post exercise period. Any of the foods listed in Table 14.4 would be suitable. Drink at least 500 ml fluid immediately after competing and continue drinking at regular intervals to replace fluid losses.

Your immediate post-event food should be followed by a carbohydrate-rich meal approximately 2 hours later. Suitable post-event meals include pasta dishes, noodle dishes, thick-base pizzas (with vegetable toppings), and baked potatoes. Avoid rich or fatty meals (e.g. oily curries, chips, burgers), as these will delay refuelling and can make you feel bloated after competing. Don't forget to drink plenty of rehydrating fluid before embarking on that celebratory alcoholic drink!

SUMMARY OF KEY POINTS
See Table 14.5

Table 14.5	Summary of key points		
Timing	**Aims**	**Food and drink recommendations**	**Examples**
The week before	1 Fill muscle glycogen stores 2 Maintain hydration	• Taper training • 7–8 g/kg body weight/day for 3 days before event • Low GI meals • Monitor fluid intake and urine	• Pasta with fish or beans • Rice with chicken or tofu • Jacket potatoes with tuna or cottage cheese
The night before	1 Top up muscle glycogen 2 Maintain hydration	• High carbohydrate meal (low GI) • Plenty of fluid • Moderate–low fibre • Low fat • Familiar foods	• Pasta dish with tomato-based sauce • Rice dishes
2–4 hours before	1 Top up liver glycogen 2 Maintain hydration 3 Prevent hunger	• Low GI meal • High carbohydrate, low fat and low protein • Easily digestible • 400–600 ml fluid	• Cereal and low-fat milk • Bread, toast, sandwiches, rolls • Potato with tuna or cottage cheese

Table 14.5 Summary of key points – continued

Timing	Aims	Food and drink recommendations	Examples
1 hour before	1 Maintain blood sugar 2 Maintain hydration	• 1 g carbohydrate/kg body weight • Easy to digest	• Sports drink • Smoothie • Energy or meal replacement bar • Dried apricots
15–30 min before	1 Maintain hydration	• Up to 150 ml fluid	• Water • Sports drink
During events lasting more than 60 min	1 Maintain blood sugar 2 Offset fluid losses	• 30–60 g carbohydrate/hour • High or moderate GI • 150–350 ml fluid every 15–20 min	• Sports drinks • Glucose polymer drinks • Energy bars with water
Between heats or events	1 Replenish muscle and liver glycogen 2 Replace fluid	• 1 g/kg body weight within 2 hours • High GI carbohydrate • 500 ml fluid immediately after • Continue fluids	• Sports drinks • Meal replacement products • Rice cakes, energy bars, rolls • Bananas
Post-competition	1 Replenish muscle and liver glycogen 2 Replace fluid	• 1 g/kg body weight within 2 hours • High GI carbohydrate • 500 ml fluid immediately after • Continue fluids	• Sports drinks • Energy bars • Pasta dishes • Rice dishes • Pizza

YOUR PERSONAL NUTRITION PROGRAMME

15

Nutrition scientists have provided general guidelines as to the proportion of nutrients athletes should consume to optimise their performance. Tailoring this information to suit your specific needs is the next critical step. Your nutritional requirements depend on many factors, including your body weight, your body composition, the energy demands of your training programme, your daily activity levels, your health status and your individual metabolism. In a nutshell, your diet should comprise:

Carbohydrate:
- 3–5 g/kg body weight during low intensity training
- 5–7 g/kg body weight during moderate intensity training
- 7–12 g/kg body weight during moderate to heavy endurance training or fuelling up for an endurance event

Protein:
- 1.2–1.7 g/kg from protein

Fat:
- 20–33% fat.

These recommendations cover your needs whether you are aiming to maintain, lose or gain weight. The main difference will be your total calorie intake.

This chapter gives a step-by-step guide to calculating your calorie, carbohydrate, protein and fat needs. The rationale for calculating your calorie requirements to lose body fat as well as the initial steps on calculating your resting metabolic rate (RMR) and your maintenance calorie needs are detailed in Chapter 9, pp.145–147 'Calculating calorie, carbohydrate, protein and fat requirements on a weight-loss programme'. The rationale for calculating your calorie needs in a weight-gain programme is given in Chapter 10, 'How much should I eat?', pp. 166–167.

Sample daily menu plans that fit in with these nutrition recommendations are also given and can be used as a basis for developing your personal nutrition programme.

This chapter also addresses some of the most common problems faced by athletes and those leading an active lifestyle: eating on the run, in a hurry, on a budget, and adapting family meals. If you lead a busy lifestyle, it may be tempting to skip meals or rely on snacks that are high in fat or sugar. This chapter gives you plenty of practical ideas for healthy snacks that you can take with you. It also provides useful suggestions on overcoming the difficulties of putting theory into practice.

STEP 1: ESTIMATE YOUR CALORIE NEEDS

First, calculate your maintenance calorie intake by following steps 1–4 in Chapter 9, pp. 145–147. Then, if your programme aim is to:

a) lose body fat/weight: reduce your calorie intake by 15% – i.e. multiply your maintenance calories by 0.85 (85%).

b) increase lean body weight/muscle: increase your calorie intake by 20% – i.e. multiply your maintenance calories by 1.2 (120%).

Below is a sample of calculations for a 70 kg male athlete aged 18–30 years who is sedentary during the day, and performs 2 hours weight training (900 kcal) and 1 hour swimming (385 kcal) per week.

- Body weight in kg: = 70
- RMR ((70 × 15.3) + 679): = 1750
- Daily energy expenditure (1750 × 1.4): = 2450
- Weekly exercise calories (900 + 385): = 1285
- Daily exercise calories (1285 ÷ 7): = 184
- Maintenance calorie intake (2450 + 184): = 2634

Calorie requirements to meet weight goal:

a) to lose weight (2634 × 0.85) = 2239
b) to gain weight (2634 × 1.2) = 3160

STEP 2: CALCULATE YOUR CARBOHYDRATE INTAKE

Calculate your carbohydrate needs according to your activity level and body weight, using Table 3.1, p. 29. In a 24-hour period during moderate intensity training days, you should consume 5–7 g/kg body weight. During moder-

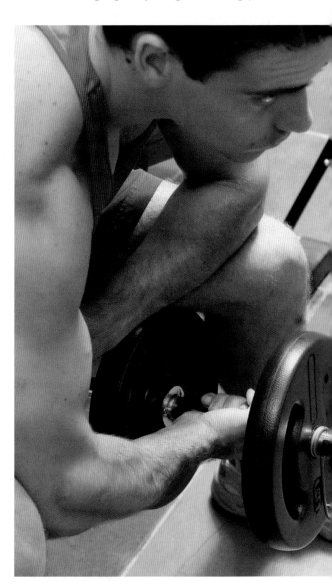

Table 15.1 Estimating calorie and carbohydrate requirements for weight maintenance, fat loss and muscle gain for a 70 kg athlete during low or moderate training.

	Weight maintenance	Weight loss	Weight gain
Calorie requirement (calculated in Step 1)	2634	2239	3160
Carbohydrate needs g/kg BW	5–7 g	5–7 g	5–7 g
Carbohydrate needs/day	350–490 g	298–417 g	420–588 g

Table 15.2 Estimating protein requirements for weight maintenance, weight loss and weight gain

	Weight maintenance	Weight loss	Weight gain
Body weight, kg	70	70	70
Protein needs, g/kg BW	1.2–1.7	1.6	1.4–1.7
Protein needs/day	84–119 g	112 g	98–119 g

ate to heavy endurance training 7–12 g/ kg is recommended.

- For weight loss: your calorie needs decrease by 15%, and so should your usual carbohydrate intake.
- For weight gain: your calorie needs increase by 20%, and so should your usual carbohydrate intake.

Table 15.1 shows a sample of calculations for weight maintenance, fat loss and muscle gain for a 70 kg male athlete aged 18–30 years who exercises for 1 hour per day.

Step 3: Calculate your protein intake

Your protein requirement is based on the following recommendations:
- Endurance athletes: 1.2–1.4 g/kg body weight/ day
- Power and strength athletes: 1.4–1.7 g/kg body weight/day
- Weight loss programme: 1.6 g/kg body weight/ day
- Weight gain programme: 1.4–1.7 g/kg body weight/ day.

Table 15.2 shows the calculations for estimating the protein requirements for different goals.

STEP 4: CALCULATE YOUR FAT INTAKE

This is the balance left once you have calculated your carbohydrate and protein requirements. Use the following calculation:

- Carbohydrate calories = grams carbohydrate x 4
- Protein calories = grams protein x 4
- Fat calories = Total daily calories − carbohydrate calories − protein calories
- Grams fat = fat calories ÷ 9

Table 15.3 shows the calculations for estimating the fat requirements for different goals.

STEP 5: FLUID INTAKE.

Follow these guidelines, which are based on the IOC (2011) and IAAF (2007) recommendations and those of the ACSM, ADA and DC (2009):

- Ensure you are fully hydrated before exercise.
- Drink little and often according to thirst during exercise.
- For most exercise lasting 1 hour or less, water is fine for replacing fluid losses.
- For high-intensity exercise lasting more than 1 hour, a hypotonic or isotonic sports drink containing 4–8% carbohydrate may reduce fatigue and improve performance. The general recommendation is to consume 30–60 g carbohydrate per hour.
- After exercise, drink 1.2–1.5 l for every 1 kg body weight lost as sweat during exercise.

MEAL PLANS

To help you plan your personal diet, here are some detailed sample meal plans, which are in line with the nutritional recommendations outlined in the first section of this chapter. There are 3 sets of

Table 15.3	Estimating fat requirements	Weight maintenance	Weight loss	Weight gain
A	Total daily calories	2634	2239	3162
B	Carbohydrate intake	350–490 g	298–417 g	420–588 g
C	Carbohydrate calories (B × 4)	1400–1960	1192–1668	1680–2352
D	Protein intake	84–119 g	112 g	98–119 g
E	Protein calories (D × 4)	336–476	448	392–476
F	Fat calories (A − C − E)	198–898	123–599	334–1090
	Fat intake (F × 9)	22–99 g	14–66 g	37–121 g

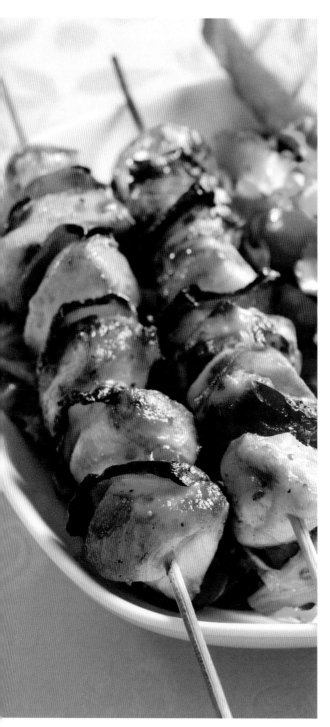

daily menu plans providing 2500 kcal, 3000 kcal and 3500 kcal. In addition, there are 3 similar sets of daily menu plans that exclude meat and fish, which are suitable for vegetarians. For each set, there are 5 daily menus designed to give you plenty of variety and plenty of ideas upon which to base your own diet. For more menu ideas, *see* Chapter 16, which includes more than 50 recipes for all types of diets.

The nutritional composition of each food has been listed to show its relative contribution of calories, protein, carbohydrate and fat to the daily totals. Both the total grams and the total percentage of energy contributed by protein, carbohydrate and fat are given for each daily menu. If you wish to carry out similar calculations for other foods when constructing your own menu, you may use a reputable set of food composition tables such as McCance & Widdowson (1991) or a dietary analysis software program, both detailed in the Further Reading section on p. 324.

Notes to all menus:

- Use an oil that is rich in linolenic acid, e.g. rapeseed, flax, soya, walnut.
- Use a spread high in monounsaturates or poly-unsaturates, containing no hydrogenated or trans fatty acids.

Daily menu plans providing approx 2500 kcal per day

Menu 1 (2500 kcal)

	Kcal	Protein (g)	Carbohydrate (g)	Fat (g)
Breakfast				
1 average bowl (60 g) muesli	220	6	40	5
2 tbsp (80 g) low-fat yoghurt	34	3	5	0
200 ml skimmed milk	66	7	10	0
1 glass (150 ml) orange juice	54	1	13	0
Mid-morning				
2 apples	94	1	24	0
1 carton (150 g) low-fat fruit yoghurt	135	6	27	1
Lunch				
1 large (225 g) baked potato	306	9	71	0
1 tbsp (5 g) olive oil spread	85	0	0	9
1 small tin (100 g) tuna in brine	99	24	0	1
1 bowl (125 g) salad	15	1	2	0
1 tbsp (11 g) oil/vinegar dressing	99	0	0	11
2 kiwi fruit	59	1	13	1
Mid-afternoon				
1 orange	59	2	14	0
1 carton (150 g) low-fat fruit yoghurt	135	6	27	1
Workout				
500 ml juice 500 ml water	180	3	44	1
Post-workout				
2 bananas	190	2	46	1
Dinner				
1 portion (120 g) grilled chicken	176	36	0	4
⅓ plate (85 g uncooked weight) pasta with:	296	10	64	2
1 tbsp (11 g) olive oil	99	0	0	11
1 large portion (125 g) broccoli	30	4	1	1
1 large portion (125 g) carrots	30	1	6	1
1 tbsp (30 g) pasta sauce/tomato salsa	14	1	2	0
Evening				
1 portion (85 g) red grapes	48	0	12	0
Total	**2523**	**124**	**428**	**50**
% energy		**19%**	**63%**	**18%**

Menu 2 (2500 kcal)

	Kcal	Protein (g)	Carbohydrate (g)	Fat (g)
Breakfast				
2 slices wholegrain toast	174	7	34	2
2 tsp (10 g) olive oil spread	57	0	0	6
2 heaped tsp (30 g) honey	86	0	23	0
1 carton (150 g) low-fat fruit yoghurt	135	6	27	1
Mid-morning				
2 apples	94	1	24	0
1 cereal or energy bar (33 g)	154	3	20	7
Lunch				
1 large (225 g) baked potato	306	9	71	0
Chopped cooked chicken (70 g)	103	21	0	2
Sweetcorn (125 g)	153	4	33	2
1 bowl (125 g) salad	15	1	2	0
1 tbsp (11 g) oil/vinegar dressing	99	0	0	11
Mid-afternoon				
2 portions (200 g) berries e.g. strawberries	54	2	12	0
Workout				
500 ml juice 500 ml water	180	3	44	1
Post-workout				
1 serving meal replacement product	174	18	26	0
Dinner				
1 average portion (175 g) grilled salmon	308	35	0	19
⅓ plate (85 g uncooked weight) brown rice	303	6	69	2
1 large portion (125 g) spinach	24	3	1	1
Evening				
1 carton (150 g) low-fat fruit yoghurt	135	6	27	1
Total	**2554**	**123**	**413**	**59**
% energy		**19%**	**60%**	**21%**

Menu 3   (2500 kcal)

	Kcal	Protein (g)	Carbohydrate (g)	Fat (g)
Breakfast				
1 cup (60 g) porridge oats	241	7	44	5
300 ml skimmed milk	99	10	15	0
1 tbsp (30 g) raisins	82	1	21	0
1 glass (200 ml) orange juice	72	1	18	0
Mid-morning				
1 cereal or fruit bar (33 g)	154	3	20	7
Lunch				
1 bagel (90 g)	241	8	46	4
spread with 2 tsp (10 g) olive oil spread	57	0	0	6
Half a carton (100 g) low-fat soft cheese	98	14	2	4
1 bowl (125 g) salad	15	1	2	0
1 tbsp (11 g) oil/vinegar dressing	99	0	0	11
Mid-afternoon				
1 large handful (60 g) dried fruit, e.g. dates, apricots	162	2	41	0
Workout				
500 ml juice 500 ml water	180	3	44	1
Post-workout				
4 rice cakes	129	2	29	1
1 carton (150 g) low-fat fruit yoghurt	135	6	27	1
Dinner				
Spicy chicken with rice (recipe p. 266)	610	58	74	11
1 portion (85 g) green cabbage	14	1	2	0
1 portion (85 g) peas	64	0	16	0
Evening				
1 pear	57	0	0	6
Total	**2509**	**123**	**409**	**53**
% energy		**20%**	**61%**	**19%**

Menu 4   (2500 kcal)

	Kcal	Protein (g)	Carbohydrate (g)	Fat (g)
Breakfast				
1 glass (150 ml) orange juice	54	1	13	0
2 slices (80 g) wholegrain toast	174	7	34	2
2 tsp (10 g) olive oil spread	57	0	0	6
2 scrambled or poached eggs	160	14	0	12
Mid-morning				
1 banana	95	1	23	0
1 portion (100 g) berries	27	1	6	0
Lunch				
Pasta salad made with:				
pasta (100 g uncooked weight)	348	12	76	2
2 tbsp (85 g) tuna in brine	84	20	0	1
1 large handful (100 g) chopped peppers	32	1	6	0
1 tbsp (11 g) oil dressing	99	0	0	11
1 orange	59	2	14	0
Mid-afternoon				
1 small cereal or protein bar (33 g)	154	3	20	7
Workout				
500 ml juice 500 ml water	180	3	44	1
Post-workout				
1 serving meal replacement product	174	18	26	0
Dinner				
1 portion (100 g) turkey breast (baked/grilled)	105	23	0	2
1 portion noodles (100 g uncooked weight)	388	12	76	6
1 portion (85 g) curly kale	20	2	1	1
1 portion (85 g) cauliflower	24	2	2	1
Evening				
½ mango (150 g)	86	1	21	0
2 Weetabix and 150 ml skimmed milk	191	9	37	1
Total	**2511**	**133**	**400**	**53**
% energy		**21%**	**60%**	**19%**

Menu 5 (2500 kcal)

	Kcal	Protein (g)	Carbohydrate (g)	Fat (g)
Breakfast				
3 Shredded Wheat (70 g)	228	7	48	2
200 ml skimmed milk	66	7	10	0
2 tbsp (60 g) raisins	163	1	42	0
1 glass (150 ml) orange juice	54	1	13	0
Mid-morning				
Peanut butter sandwich with:				
2 slices (80 g) wholegrain bread	174	7	34	2
and 1 tbsp (40 g) peanut butter	242	10	3	21
Lunch				
1 wholewheat pitta bread (80 g)	174	7	34	2
2 tsp (14 g) olive oil spread	80	0	0	9
2 slices (70 g) turkey	74	17	0	1
1 bowl (125 g) salad	15	1	2	0
Mid-afternoon				
125 g berries	27	1	6	0
1 carton (150 g) low-fat fruit yoghurt	135	6	27	1
Workout				
500 ml juice 500 ml water	180	3	44	1
Post-workout				
2 cereal or energy bars	308	6	40	14
Dinner				
1 portion (175 g) grilled white fish	168	37	0	2
1 large (300 g) sweet potato	345	5	84	1
1 portion (85 g) carrots	20	1	4	0
1 portion (85 g) courgettes	16	2	2	0
Evening				
2 oranges	118	4	28	0
Total	2587	121	399	58
% energy		19%	60%	21%

Daily menu plans providing approx 3000 kcal per day

Menu 1   **(3000 kcal)**

	Kcal	Protein (g)	Carbohydrate (g)	Fat (g)
Breakfast				
1 average bowl (60 g) muesli	220	6	40	5
2 tbsp (80 g) low-fat yoghurt	34	3	5	0
200 ml skimmed milk	66	7	10	0
1 glass (150 ml) orange juice	54	1	13	0
1 slice (40 g) wholegrain toast	87	4	17	1
1 heaped tsp (7 g) olive oil spread	40	0	0	4
Mid-morning				
2 apples	94	1	24	0
1 carton (150 g) low-fat fruit yoghurt	135	6	27	1
Lunch				
1 large (225 g) baked potato	306	9	71	0
1 tbsp (5 g) olive oil spread	85	0	0	9
1 small tin (100 g) tuna in brine	99	24	0	1
1 bowl (125 g) salad	15	1	2	0
1 tbsp (11 g) oil/vinegar dressing	99	0	0	11
2 kiwi fruit	59	1	13	1
Mid-afternoon				
1 orange	59	2	14	0
1 carton (150 g) low-fat fruit yoghurt	135	6	27	1
Workout				
500 ml juice 500 ml water	180	3	44	1
Post-workout				
2 bananas	190	2	46	1
Dinner				
1 portion (120 g) grilled chicken	176	36	0	4
½ plate (125 g uncooked weight) pasta with:	435	15	95	2
1 tbsp (11 g) olive oil	99	0	0	11
1 large portion (125 g) broccoli	30	4	1	1
1 large portion (125 g) carrots	30	1	6	1
1 tbsp (30 g) pasta sauce/tomato salsa	14	1	2	0
Evening				
1 portion (85 g) red grapes	48	0	12	0
1 slice (40 g) wholegrain toast	87	4	17	1
1 heaped tsp (7 g) olive oil spread	40	0	0	4
Total	**2916**	**138**	**505**	**63**
% energy		**18%**	**63%**	**19%**

Menu 2 (3000 kcal)

	Kcal	Protein (g)	Carbohydrate (g)	Fat (g)
Breakfast				
4 slices wholegrain toast	347	14	67	4
4 tsp (20 g) olive oil spread	114	0	0	13
4 heaped tsp (60 g) honey	173	0	46	0
1 carton (150 g) low-fat fruit yoghurt	135	6	27	1
Mid-morning				
2 apples	94	1	24	0
1 cereal or energy bar (33 g)	154	3	20	7
Lunch				
1 large (225 g) baked potato	306	9	71	0
Chopped cooked chicken (70 g)	103	21	0	2
Sweetcorn (125 g)	153	4	33	2
1 bowl (125 g) salad	15	1	2	0
1 tbsp (11 g) oil/vinegar dressing	99	0	0	11
Mid-afternoon				
2 portions (200 g) berries e.g. strawberries	54	2	12	0
Workout				
500 ml juice 500 ml water	180	3	44	1
Post-workout				
1 serving meal replacement product	174	18	26	0
Dinner				
1 average portion (175 g) grilled salmon	308	35	0	19
½ plate (115 g uncooked weight) boiled brown rice	411	8	93	3
1 large portion (125 g) spinach	24	3	1	1
Evening				
1 carton (150 g) low-fat fruit yoghurt	135	6	27	1
Total	2979	133	494	71
% energy		18%	61%	21%

Menu 3 (3000 kcal)

	Kcal	Protein (g)	Carbohydrate (g)	Fat (g)
Breakfast				
1½ cups (100 g) porridge oats	401	12	73	9
500 ml skimmed milk	165	16	25	1
2 tbsp (60 g) raisins	163	1	42	0
1 glass (200 ml) orange juice	72	1	18	0
Mid-morning				
1 cereal or fruit bar (33 g)	154	3	20	7
Lunch				
1 bagel (90 g)	241	8	46	4
with 2 tsp (10 g) olive oil spread	57	0	0	6
Half a carton (100 g) low-fat soft cheese	98	14	2	4
1 bowl (125 g) salad	15	1	2	0
1 tbsp (11 g) oil/vinegar dressing	99	0	0	11
Mid-afternoon				
2 large handfuls (120 g) dried fruit, e.g. dates, apricots	162	2	41	0
Workout				
500 ml juice 500 ml water	180	3	44	1
Post-workout				
4 rice cakes	129	2	29	1
1 carton (150 g) low-fat fruit yoghurt	135	6	27	1
Dinner				
Spicy chicken with rice (recipe p. 266)	610	58	74	11
1 portion (85 g) green cabbage	14	1	2	0
1 portion (85 g) peas	64	0	16	0
Evening				
1 pear	57	0	0	6
Total	**2816**	**138**	**510**	**57**
% energy		**18%**	**64%**	**17%**

Menu 4	(3000 kcal)			
	Kcal	**Protein (g)**	**Carbohydrate (g)**	**Fat (g)**
Breakfast				
1 glass (150 ml) orange juice	54	1	13	0
3 slices (120 g) wholegrain toast	260	11	50	3
3 tsp (15 g) olive oil spread	85	0	0	9
2 scrambled or poached eggs	160	14	0	12
Mid-morning				
2 bananas	190	2	46	1
1 portion (100 g) berries	27	1	6	0
Lunch				
Pasta salad made with:				
(150 g uncooked weight) pasta	522	18	114	3
2 tbsp (85 g) tuna in brine	84	20	0	1
1 large handful (100 g) chopped peppers	32	1	6	0
1 tbsp (11 g) oil dressing	99	0	0	11
1 orange	59	2	14	0
Mid-afternoon				
1 small cereal or protein bar (33 g)	154	3	20	7
Workout				
500 ml juice 500 ml water	180	3	44	1
Post-workout				
1 serving meal replacement product	174	18	26	0
Dinner				
1 portion (100 g) turkey breast (baked/grilled)	105	23	0	2
1 large portion (125 g uncooked weight) noodles	485	15	95	8
1 portion (85 g) curly kale	20	2	1	1
1 portion (85 g) cauliflower	24	2	2	1
Evening				
½ mango (150 g)	86	1	21	0
2 Weetabix and 150 ml skimmed milk	191	9	37	1
Total	**2991**	**147**	**497**	**60**
% energy		**20%**	**62%**	**18%**

Menu 5 (3000 kcal)

	Kcal	Protein (g)	Carbohydrate (g)	Fat (g)
Breakfast				
4 Shredded Wheat (100 g)	325	11	68	3
300 ml skimmed milk	99	10	15	0
2 tbsp (60 g) raisins	163	1	42	0
1 glass (150 ml) orange juice	54	1	13	0
Mid-morning				
Peanut butter sandwich with:				
2 slices (80 g) wholegrain bread	174	7	34	2
and 1 tbsp (40 g) peanut butter	242	10	3	21
Lunch				
2 wholewheat pitta bread (160 g)	348	14	68	4
2 heaped tsp (14 g) olive oil spread	80	0	0	9
3 slices (100 g) turkey	105	24	0	1
1 bowl (125 g) salad	15	1	2	0
Mid-afternoon				
125 g berries	27	1	6	0
1 carton (150 g) low-fat fruit yoghurt	135	6	27	1
Workout				
500 ml juice 500 ml water	180	3	44	1
Post-workout				
2 cereal or energy bars	308	6	40	14
Dinner				
1 portion (175 g) grilled white fish	168	37	0	2
2 large (450 g total weight) sweet potato	518	7	126	2
1 portion (85 g) carrots	20	1	4	0
1 portion (85 g) courgettes	16	2	2	0
Evening				
2 oranges	118	4	28	0
Total	**3095**	**144**	**500**	**62**
% energy		**19%**	**62%**	**19%**

Daily menu plans providing approx 3500 kcal per day

Menu 1   (3500 kcal)

	Kcal	Protein (g)	Carbohydrate (g)	Fat (g)
Breakfast				
1 average bowl (60 g) muesli	220	6	40	5
2 tbsp (80 g) low-fat yoghurt	34	3	5	0
200 ml skimmed milk	66	7	10	0
1 glass (150 ml) orange juice	54	1	13	0
2 slices (80 g) wholegrain toast	174	7	34	2
2 heaped tsp (14 g) olive oil spread	80	0	0	9
Mid-morning				
2 apples	94	1	24	0
1 carton (150 g) low-fat fruit yoghurt	135	6	27	1
Lunch				
2 average (350 g total weight) baked potatoes	476	14	111	1
2 tbsp (10 g) olive oil spread	170	0	0	18
1 small tin (100 g) tuna in brine	99	24	0	1
1 bowl (125 g) mixed salad	15	1	2	0
1 tbsp (11 g) oil/vinegar dressing	99	0	0	11
2 kiwi fruit	59	1	13	1
Mid-afternoon				
1 orange	59	2	14	0
1 carton (150 g) low-fat fruit yoghurt	135	6	27	1
Workout				
500 ml juice 500 ml water	180	3	44	1
Post-workout				
2 bananas	190	2	46	1
Dinner				
1 large portion (150 g) grilled chicken	221	45	0	5
½ plate (125 g uncooked weight) pasta with:	435	15	95	2
1 tbsp (11 g) olive oil	99	0	0	11
1 large portion (125 g) broccoli	30	4	1	1
1 large portion (125 g) carrots	30	1	6	1
1 tbsp (30 g) pasta sauce/tomato salsa	14	1	2	0
Evening				
1 portion (85 g) red grapes	48	0	12	0
2 slices (80 g) wholegrain toast	174	7	34	2
2 heaped tsp (14 g) olive oil spread	80	0	0	9
Total	**3470**	**159**	**579**	**85**
% energy		**18%**	**61%**	**21%**

Menu 2 (3500 kcal)

	Kcal	Protein (g)	Carbohydrate (g)	Fat (g)
Breakfast				
4 slices wholegrain toast	347	14	67	4
4 tsp (20 g) olive oil spread	114	0	0	13
4 heaped tsp (60 g) honey	173	0	46	0
1 carton (150 g) low-fat fruit yoghurt	135	6	27	1
Mid-morning				
2 apples	94	1	24	0
1 cereal or energy bar (33 g)	154	3	20	7
Lunch				
1 very large (300 g) baked potato	408	12	95	1
Chopped cooked chicken (100 g)	147	30	0	3
Sweetcorn (150 g)	183	4	40	2
1 bowl (125 g) salad	15	1	2	0
1 tbsp (11 g) oil/vinegar dressing	99	0	0	11
Mid-afternoon				
1 wholegrain roll	121	5	24	1
2 tsp (10 g) olive oil spread	57	0	0	6
2 portions (200 g) berries e.g. strawberries	54	2	12	0
Workout				
500 ml juice 500 ml water	180	3	44	1
Post-workout				
1 serving meal replacement product	174	18	26	0
Dinner				
1 average portion (175 g) grilled salmon	308	35	0	19
½ plate (150 g uncooked weight) boiled brown rice	536	10	122	4
1 large portion (125 g) spinach	24	3	1	1
Evening				
1 carton (150 g) low-fat fruit yoghurt	135	6	27	1
Total	**3458**	**152**	**577**	**81**
% energy		**17%**	**62%**	**21%**

Menu 3 (3500 kcal)

	Kcal	Protein (g)	Carbohydrate (g)	Fat (g)
Breakfast				
1½ cups (100 g) porridge oats	401	12	73	9
500 ml skimmed milk	165	16	25	1
2 tbsp (60 g) raisins	163	1	42	0
1 glass (200 ml) orange juice	72	1	18	0
Mid-morning				
2 energy or cereal bars (66 g)	309	7	40	15
Lunch				
2 bagels (180 g) with:	482	17	93	8
4 tsp (20 g) olive oil spread	114	0	0	13
1 carton (200 g) low-fat soft cheese	196	28	4	8
1 bowl (125 g) salad	15	1	2	0
1 tbsp (11 g) oil/vinegar dressing	99	0	0	11
Mid-afternoon				
2 large handfuls (120 g) dried fruit, e.g. dates, apricots	162	2	41	0
Workout				
500 ml juice 500 ml water	180	3	44	1
Post-workout				
4 rice cakes	129	2	29	1
1 carton (150 g) low-fat fruit yoghurt	135	6	27	1
Dinner				
Spicy chicken with rice (recipe p. 266)	610	58	74	11
1 portion (85 g) green cabbage	14	1	2	0
1 portion (85 g) peas	64	0	16	0
Evening				
1 pear	57	0	0	6
Total	**3367**	**163**	**578**	**79**
% energy		**18%**	**61%**	**20%**

Menu 4 (3500 kcal)

	Kcal	Protein (g)	Carbohydrate (g)	Fat (g)
Breakfast				
1 glass (150 ml) orange juice	54	1	13	0
4 slices (160 g) wholegrain toast	347	14	67	4
4 tsp (20 g) olive oil spread	114	0	0	13
2 scrambled or poached eggs	160	14	0	12
Mid-morning				
2 banana	190	2	46	1
1 portion (100 g) berries	27	1	6	0
Lunch				
Pasta salad made with:				
pasta (175 g uncooked weight)	609	21	133	3
2 tbsp (85 g) tuna in brine	84	20	0	1
1 large handful (100 g) chopped peppers	32	1	6	0
1½ tbsp (16 g) oil dressing	144	0	0	16
1 orange	59	2	14	0
Mid-afternoon				
2 energy or cereal bars	309	7	40	15
Workout				
500 ml juice 500 ml water	180	3	44	1
Post-workout				
1 serving meal replacement product	174	18	26	0
Dinner				
1 large portion (125 g) turkey breast (baked/grilled)	131	28	0	2
1 large portion noodles (150 g uncooked weight)	582	18	114	9
1 portion (85 g) curly kale	20	2	1	1
1 portion (85 g) cauliflower	24	2	2	1
Evening				
½ mango (150 g)	86	1	21	0
2 Weetabix and 150 ml skimmed milk	191	9	37	1
Total	**3517**	**166**	**572**	**78**
% energy		**19%**	**61%**	**20%**

Menu 5 (3500 kcal)

	Kcal	Protein (g)	Carbohydrate (g)	Fat (g)
Breakfast				
4 Shredded Wheat (100 g)	325	11	68	3
300 ml skimmed milk	99	10	15	0
4 tbsp (120 g) raisins	326	3	83	0
1 glass (150 ml) orange juice	54	1	13	0
Mid-morning				
Peanut butter sandwich with:				
2 slices (80 g) wholegrain bread	174	7	34	2
and 1 tbsp (40 g) peanut butter	242	10	3	21
Lunch				
2 wholewheat pitta bread (160 g)	348	14	68	4
2 heaped tsp (14 g) olive oil spread	80	0	0	9
3 slices (100 g) turkey	105	24	0	1
1 bowl (125 g) salad	15	1	2	0
Mid-afternoon				
125 g berries	27	1	6	0
1 carton (150 g) low-fat fruit yoghurt	135	6	27	1
Workout				
500 ml juice 500 ml water	180	3	44	1
Post-workout				
2 cereal or energy bars	308	6	40	14
Dinner				
1 portion (175 g) grilled white fish	168	37	0	2
2 large (450 g total weight) sweet potato	518	7	126	2
1 portion (85 g) carrots	20	1	4	0
1 portion (85 g) courgettes	16	2	2	0
Evening				
3 small (scotch) pancakes (90 g)	263	5	39	11
2 oranges	118	4	28	0
Total	**3521**	**167**	**560**	**73**
% energy		**20%**	**61%**	**19%**

Daily menu plans providing approx 2500 kcal per day

Menu I Vegetarian – (2500 kcal)

	Kcal	Protein (g)	Carbohydrate (g)	Fat (g)
Breakfast				
I average bowl (60 g) muesli	220	6	40	5
2 tbsp (80 g) low-fat yoghurt	34	3	5	0
200 ml skimmed milk	66	7	10	0
I glass (150 ml) orange juice	54	1	13	0
Mid-morning				
2 apples	94	1	24	0
I carton (150 g) low-fat fruit yoghurt	135	6	27	1
Lunch				
I large (225 g) baked potato	306	9	71	0
I tbsp (5 g) olive oil spread	85	0	0	9
½ carton (125 g) cottage cheese	123	17	3	5
I bowl (125 g) salad	15	1	2	0
I tbsp (11 g) oil/vinegar dressing	99	0	0	11
2 kiwi fruit	59	1	13	1
Mid-afternoon				
I orange	59	2	14	0
I carton (150 g) low-fat fruit yoghurt	135	6	27	1
Workout				
500 ml juice 500 ml water	180	3	44	1
Post-workout				
2 bananas	190	2	46	1
Dinner				
Mixed bean hotpot (without potatoes) (recipe p. 279)	234	16	41	1
¼ plate (65 g uncooked weight) pasta with:	226	8	49	1
I tbsp (11 g) olive oil	99	0	0	11
I large portion (125 g) broccoli	30	4	1	1
I large portion (125 g) carrots	30	1	6	1
I tbsp (30 g) pasta sauce/tomato salsa	14	1	2	0
Evening				
I portion (85 g) red grapes	48	0	12	0
Total	**2535**	**96**	**457**	**52**
% energy		**15%**	**67%**	**18%**

V Menu 2 Vegetarian – (2500 kcal)

	Kcal	Protein (g)	Carbohydrate (g)	Fat (g)
Breakfast				
2 slices wholegrain toast	174	7	34	2
2 tsp (10 g) olive oil spread	57	0	0	6
2 heaped tsp (30 g) honey	86	0	23	0
1 carton (150 g) low-fat fruit yoghurt	135	6	27	1
Mid-morning				
2 apples	94	1	24	0
1 cereal or energy bar (33 g)	154	3	20	7
Lunch				
1 large (225 g) baked potato	306	9	71	0
2 tbsp (60 g) hummus	112	5	7	8
Sweetcorn (125 g)	153	4	33	2
1 bowl (125 g) salad	15	1	2	0
1 tbsp (11 g) oil/vinegar dressing	99	0	0	11
Mid-afternoon				
2 portions (200 g) berries e.g. strawberries	54	2	12	0
Workout				
500 ml juice 500 ml water	180	3	44	1
Post-workout				
1 serving meal replacement product	174	18	26	0
Dinner				
1 wheat tortilla filled with:	144	4	33	1
¾ pack (150 g) marinated tofu	110	12	1	6
Shredded mixed vegetables (90 g)	38	3	6	0
⅓ plate (85 g uncooked weight) boiled brown rice	303	6	69	2
1 large portion (125 g) spinach	24	3	1	1
Evening				
1 carton (150 g) low-fat fruit yoghurt	135	6	27	1
Total	**2547**	**91**	**460**	**53**
% energy		14%	67%	19%

V Menu 3   Vegetarian – (2500 kcal)

	Kcal	Protein (g)	Carbohydrate (g)	Fat (g)
Breakfast				
I cup (60 g) porridge oats	241	7	44	5
300 ml skimmed milk	99	10	15	0
I tbsp (30 g) raisins	82	1	21	0
I glass (200 ml) orange juice	72	1	18	0
Mid-morning				
I cereal or fruit bar (33 g)	154	3	20	7
Lunch				
I bagel (90 g) with:	241	8	46	4
2 tsp (10 g) olive oil spread	57	0	0	6
Half a carton (100 g) low-fat soft cheese	98	14	2	4
I bowl (125 g) salad	15	1	2	0
I tbsp (11 g) oil/vinegar dressing	99	0	0	11
Mid-afternoon				
I large handful (60 g) dried fruit, e.g. dates, apricots	162	2	41	0
Workout				
500 ml juice 500 ml water	180	3	44	1
Post-workout				
4 rice cakes	129	2	29	1
I carton (150 g) low-fat fruit yoghurt	135	6	27	1
Dinner				
Rice, bean and vegetable stir-fry (recipe p. 278)	526	18	94	11
I portion (85 g) green cabbage	14	1	2	0
I portion (85 g) peas	64	0	16	0
Evening				
I pear	57	0	0	6
Total	**2425**	**88**	**450**	**52**
% energy		**14%**	**67%**	**19%**

V Menu 4 Vegetarian – (2500 kcal)

	Kcal	Protein (g)	Carbohydrate (g)	Fat (g)
Breakfast				
1 glass (150 ml) orange juice	54	1	13	0
2 slices (80 g) wholegrain toast	174	7	34	2
2 tsp (10 g) olive oil spread	57	0	0	6
2 scrambled or poached eggs	160	14	0	12
Mid-morning				
1 banana	95	1	23	0
1 portion (100 g) berries	27	1	6	0
Lunch				
Pasta salad made with:				
pasta (100 g uncooked weight)	348	12	76	2
2 tbsp (85 g) kidney beans	85	6	15	1
1 large handful (100 g) chopped peppers	32	1	6	0
1 tbsp (11 g) oil dressing	99	0	0	11
1 orange	59	2	14	0
Mid-afternoon				
1 small cereal or protein bar (33 g)	154	3	20	7
Workout				
500 ml juice 500 ml water	180	3	44	1
Post-workout				
1 serving meal replacement product	174	18	26	0
Dinner				
Tofu with noodles (recipe p. 273)	533	21	75	19
1 portion (85 g) curly kale	20	2	1	1
1 portion (85 g) cauliflower	24	2	2	1
Evening				
½ mango (150 g)	86	1	21	0
2 Weetabix and 150 ml skimmed milk	191	9	37	1
Total	**2552**	**107**	**415**	**64**
% energy		**17%**	**60%**	**23%**

	Kcal	Protein (g)	Carbohydrate (g)	Fat (g)
Breakfast				
3 Shredded Wheat (70 g)	228	7	48	2
200 ml skimmed milk	66	7	10	0
2 tbsp (60 g) raisins	163	1	42	0
1 glass (150 ml) orange juice	54	1	13	0
Mid-morning				
Peanut butter sandwich with:				
2 slices (80 g) wholegrain bread	174	7	34	2
and 1 tbsp (40 g) peanut butter	242	10	3	21
Lunch				
1 wholewheat pitta bread (80 g)	174	7	34	2
2 heaped tsp (14 g) olive oil spread	80	0	0	9
2 heaped tbsp (85 g) cottage cheese	83	12	2	3
1 bowl (125 g) salad	15	1	2	0
Mid-afternoon				
125 g berries	27	1	6	0
1 carton (150 g) low-fat fruit yoghurt	135	6	27	1
Workout				
500 ml juice 500 ml water	180	3	44	1
Post-workout				
2 cereal or energy bars (66 g)	308	6	40	14
Dinner				
1 beanburger (100 g)	193	11	14	11
1 large (300 g) sweet potato	345	5	84	1
1 portion (85 g) carrots	20	1	4	0
1 portion (85 g) courgettes	16	2	2	0
Evening				
2 oranges	118	4	28	0
Total	**2621**	**90**	**415**	**70**
% energy		**14%**	**61%**	**25%**

Daily menu plans providing approx 3000 kcal per day

V Menu I	Vegetarian – (3000 kcal)			
	Kcal	**Protein (g)**	**Carbohydrate (g)**	**Fat (g)**
Breakfast				
I average bowl (60 g) muesli	220	6	40	5
2 tbsp (80 g) low-fat yoghurt	34	3	5	0
200 ml skimmed milk	66	7	10	0
I glass (150 ml) orange juice	54	I	13	0
I slice (40 g) wholegrain toast	87	4	17	I
I heaped tsp (7 g) olive oil spread	40	0	0	4
Mid-morning				
2 apples	94	I	24	0
I carton (150 g) low-fat fruit yoghurt	135	6	27	I
Lunch				
I large (225 g) baked potato	306	9	71	0
I tbsp (15 g) olive oil spread	85	0	0	9
½ carton (125 g) cottage cheese	123	17	3	5
I bowl (125 g) mixed salad	15	I	2	0
I tbsp (11 g) oil/vinegar dressing	99	0	0	11
2 kiwi fruit	59	I	13	I
Mid-afternoon				
I orange	59	2	14	0
I carton (150 g) low-fat fruit yoghurt	135	6	27	I
Workout				
500 ml juice 500 ml water	180	3	44	I
Post-workout				
2 bananas	190	2	46	I
Dinner				
Mixed bean hotpot (without potatoes) (recipe p. 279)	234	16	41	I
½ plate (100 g uncooked weight) pasta with:	348	12	76	2
I tbsp (11 g) olive oil	99	0	0	11
I large portion (125 g) broccoli	30	4	I	I
I large portion (125 g) carrots	30	I	6	I
I tbsp (30 g) pasta sauce/tomato salsa	14	I	2	0
Evening				
I portion (85 g) red grapes	48	0	12	0
I slice (40 g) wholegrain toast	87	4	17	I
I heaped tsp (7 g) olive oil spread	40	0	0	4
Total	**2911**	**109**	**530**	**65**
% energy		**14%**	**66%**	**19%**

	Kcal	Protein (g)	Carbohydrate (g)	Fat (g)
Breakfast				
4 slices wholegrain toast	347	14	67	4
4 tsp (20 g) olive oil spread	114	0	0	13
4 heaped tsp (60 g) honey	173	0	46	0
1 carton (150 g) low-fat fruit yoghurt	135	6	27	1
Mid-morning				
2 apples	94	1	24	0
1 cereal or energy bar (33 g)	154	3	20	7
Lunch				
1 large (225 g) baked potato	306	9	71	0
2 tbsp (60 g) hummus	112	5	7	8
Sweetcorn (125 g)	153	4	33	2
1 bowl (125 g) salad	15	1	2	0
1 tbsp (11 g) oil/vinegar dressing	99	0	0	11
Mid-afternoon				
2 portions (200 g) berries, e.g. strawberries	54	2	12	0
Workout				
500 ml juice 500 ml water	180	3	44	1
Post-workout				
1 serving meal replacement product	174	18	26	0
Dinner				
1 wheat tortilla filled with:	144	4	33	1
¾ pack (150 g) marinated tofu	110	12	1	6
Shredded mixed vegetables (90 g)	38	3	6	0
½ plate (115 g uncooked weight) boiled brown rice	411	8	93	3
1 large portion (125 g) spinach	24	3	1	1
Evening				
1 carton (150 g) low-fat fruit yoghurt	135	6	27	1
Total	**2972**	**101**	**541**	**65**
% energy		**13%**	**67%**	**19%**

V   Menu 3   Vegetarian – (3000 kcal)

	Kcal	Protein (g)	Carbohydrate (g)	Fat (g)
Breakfast				
1½ cup (100 g) porridge oats	401	12	73	9
500 ml skimmed milk	165	16	25	1
2 tbsp (60 g) raisins	163	1	42	0
1 glass (200 ml) orange juice	72	1	18	0
Mid-morning				
1 cereal or fruit bar (33 g)	154	3	20	7
Lunch				
1 bagel (90 g) with:	241	8	46	4
2 tsp (10 g) olive oil spread	57	0	0	6
Half a carton (100 g) low-fat soft cheese	98	14	2	4
1 bowl (125 g) salad	15	1	2	0
1 tbsp (11 g) oil/vinegar dressing	99	0	0	11
Mid-afternoon				
2 large handfuls (120 g) dried fruit, e.g. dates, apricots	162	2	41	0
Workout				
500 ml juice 500 ml water	180	3	44	1
Post-workout				
4 rice cakes	129	2	29	1
1 carton (150 g) low-fat fruit yoghurt	135	6	27	1
Dinner				
Rice, bean and vegetable stir-fry (recipe p. 278)	526	18	94	11
1 portion (85 g) green cabbage	14	1	2	0
1 portion (85 g) peas	64	0	16	0
Evening				
1 pear	57	0	0	6
Total	**2732**	**102**	**550**	**61**
% energy		14%	68%	18%

	Kcal	Protein (g)	Carbohydrate (g)	Fat (g)
Breakfast				
1 glass (150 ml) orange juice	54	1	13	0
3 slices (120 g) wholegrain toast	260	11	50	3
3 tsp (15 g) olive oil spread	85	0	0	9
2 scrambled or poached eggs	160	14	0	12
Mid-morning				
2 banana	190	2	46	1
1 portion (100 g) berries	27	1	6	0
Lunch				
Pasta salad made with pasta (150 g uncooked weight)	522	18	114	3
2 tbsp (85 g) kidney beans	85	6	15	1
1 large handful (100 g) chopped peppers	32	1	6	0
1 tbsp (11 g) oil dressing	99	0	0	11
1 orange	59	2	14	0
Mid-afternoon				
1 small cereal or protein bar (33 g)	154	3	20	7
Workout				
500 ml juice 500 ml water	180	3	44	1
Post-workout				
1 serving meal replacement product	174	18	26	0
Dinner				
1 large portion Tofu with noodles (recipe p. 273) (use 100 g noodles)	591	23	86	20
1 portion (85 g) curly kale	20	2	1	1
1 portion (85 g) cauliflower	24	2	2	1
Evening				
½ mango (150 g)	86	1	21	0
2 Weetabix and 150 ml skimmed milk	191	9	37	1
Total	**2993**	**119**	**501**	**70**
% energy		**16%**	**63%**	**21%**

V Menu 5 Vegetarian – (3000 kcal)

	Kcal	Protein (g)	Carbohydrate (g)	Fat (g)
Breakfast				
4 Shredded Wheat (100 g)	325	11	68	3
300 ml skimmed milk	99	10	15	0
2 tbsp (60 g) raisins	163	1	42	0
1 glass (150 ml) orange juice	54	1	13	0
Mid-morning				
Peanut butter sandwich with:				
2 slices (80 g) wholegrain bread	174	7	34	2
and 1 tbsp (40 g) peanut butter	242	10	3	21
Lunch				
2 wholewheat pitta bread (160 g)	348	14	68	4
2 heaped tsp (14 g) olive oil spread	80	0	0	9
½ carton (100 g) cottage cheese	98	14	2	4
1 bowl (125 g) salad	15	1	2	0
Mid-afternoon				
125 g berries	27	1	6	0
1 carton (150 g) low-fat fruit yoghurt	135	6	27	1
Workout				
500 ml juice 500 ml water	180	3	44	1
Post-workout				
2 cereal or energy bars (66 g)	308	6	40	14
Dinner				
1 beanburger (100 g)	193	11	14	11
2 large (450 g total weight) sweet potato	518	7	126	2
1 portion (85 g) carrots	20	1	4	0
1 portion (85 g) courgettes	16	2	2	0
Evening				
2 oranges	118	4	28	0
Total	3113	108	516	74
% energy		14%	64%	22%

Daily menu plans providing approx 3500 kcal per day

V Menu I Vegetarian – (3500 kcal)

	Kcal	Protein (g)	Carbohydrate (g)	Fat (g)
Breakfast				
I average bowl (60 g) muesli	220	6	40	5
2 tbsp (80 g) low-fat yoghurt	34	3	5	0
200 ml skimmed milk	66	7	10	0
I glass (150 ml) orange juice	54	I	13	0
2 slices (80 g) wholegrain toast	174	7	34	2
2 heaped tsp (14 g) olive oil spread	80	0	0	9
Mid-morning				
2 apples	94	I	24	0
I carton (150 g) low-fat fruit yoghurt	135	6	27	I
Lunch				
2 average (350 g total weight) baked potatoes	476	14	111	I
2 tbsp (30 g) olive oil spread	170	0	0	18
¾ carton (150 g) cottage cheese	147	21	3	6
I bowl (125 g) mixed salad	15	I	2	0
I tbsp (11 g) oil/vinegar dressing	99	0	0	11
2 kiwi fruit	59	I	13	I
Mid-afternoon				
I orange	59	2	14	0
I carton (150 g) low-fat fruit yoghurt	135	6	27	I
Workout				
500 ml juice 500 ml water	180	3	44	I
Post-workout				
2 bananas	190	2	46	I
Dinner				
Mixed bean hotpot (without potatoes) (recipe p. 279)	234	16	41	I
3 tbsp (50 g) soya mince added to hotpot	132	22	6	3
½ plate (100 g uncooked weight) pasta with:	348	12	76	2
I tbsp (11 g) olive oil	99	0	0	11
I large portion (125 g) broccoli	30	4	I	I
I large portion (125 g) carrots	30	I	6	I
I tbsp (30 g) pasta sauce/tomato salsa	14	I	2	0
Evening				
I portion (85 g) red grapes	48	0	12	0
2 slices (80 g) wholegrain toast	174	7	34	2
I heaped tsp (7 g) olive oil spread	80	0	0	9
Total	**3576**	**126**	**607**	**83**
% energy		**14%**	**64%**	**21%**

V Menu 2   Vegetarian – (3500 kcal)

	Kcal	Protein (g)	Carbohydrate (g)	Fat (g)
Breakfast				
4 slices wholegrain toast	347	14	67	4
4 tsp (20 g) olive oil spread	114	0	0	13
4 heaped tsp (60 g) honey	173	0	46	0
1 carton (150 g) low-fat fruit yoghurt	135	6	27	1
Mid-morning				
2 apples	94	1	24	0
1 cereal or energy bar (33 g)	154	3	20	7
Lunch				
1 very large (300 g) baked potato	408	12	95	1
2 heaped tbsp (100 g) hummus	187	8	12	13
Sweetcorn (150 g)	183	4	40	2
1 bowl (125 g) salad	15	1	2	0
1 tbsp (11 g) oil/vinegar dressing	99	0	0	11
Mid-afternoon				
1 wholegrain roll	121	5	24	1
2 tsp (10 g) olive oil spread	57	0	0	6
2 portions (200 g) berries e.g. strawberries	54	2	12	0
Workout				
500 ml juice 500 ml water	180	3	44	1
Post-workout				
1 serving meal replacement product	174	18	26	0
Dinner				
1 wheat tortilla filled with:	144	4	33	1
1 pack (175 g) marinated tofu	128	14	1	7
Shredded mixed vegetables (90 g)	38	3	6	0
½ plate (125 g uncooked weight) boiled brown rice	446	8	102	3
1 large portion (125 g) spinach	24	3	1	1
Evening				
1 carton (150 g) low-fat fruit yoghurt	135	6	27	1
Total	**3410**	**117**	**612**	**82**
% energy		**13%**	**65%**	**21%**

Menu 3 Vegetarian – (3500 kcal)

	Kcal	Protein (g)	Carbohydrate (g)	Fat (g)
Breakfast				
1½ cups (100 g) porridge oats	401	12	73	9
500 ml skimmed milk	165	16	25	1
2 tbsp (60 g) raisins	163	1	42	0
1 glass (200 ml) orange juice	72	1	18	0
Mid-morning				
2 energy or cereal bars (66 g)	309	7	40	15
Lunch				
2 bagels (180 g) with:	482	17	93	8
4 tsp (20 g) olive oil spread	114	0	0	13
1 carton (200 g) low-fat soft cheese	196	28	4	8
1 bowl (125 g) salad	15	1	2	0
1 tbsp (11 g) oil/vinegar dressing	99	0	0	11
Mid-afternoon				
2 large handfuls (120 g) dried fruit, e.g. dates, apricots	162	2	41	0
Workout				
500 ml juice 500 ml water	180	3	44	1
Post-workout				
4 rice cakes	129	2	29	1
1 carton (150 g) low-fat fruit yoghurt	135	6	27	1
Dinner				
Rice, bean and vegetable stir-fry (recipe p. 278)	526	18	94	11
1 portion (85 g) green cabbage	14	1	2	0
1 portion (85 g) peas	64	0	16	0
Evening				
1 pear	57	0	0	6
Total	**3283**	**128**	**619**	**79**
% energy		**14%**	**65%**	**20%**

	Kcal	Protein (g)	Carbohydrate (g)	Fat (g)
Breakfast				
1 glass (150 ml) orange juice	54	1	13	0
4 slices (160 g) wholegrain toast	347	14	67	4
4 tsp (20 g) olive oil spread	114	0	0	13
2 scrambled or poached eggs	160	14	0	12
Mid-morning				
2 bananas	190	2	46	1
1 portion (100 g) berries	27	1	6	0
Lunch				
Pasta salad made with:				
Pasta (175 g uncooked weight)	609	21	133	3
4 tbsp (150 g) red kidney beans	150	10	27	1
1 large handful (100 g) chopped peppers	32	1	6	0
1½ tbsp (16 g) oil dressing	144	0	0	16
1 orange	59	2	14	0
Mid-afternoon				
2 energy or cereal bars (66 g)	309	7	40	15
Workout				
500 ml juice 500 ml water	180	3	44	1
Post-workout				
1 serving meal replacement product	174	18	26	0
Dinner				
Large portion tofu with noodles (recipe p. 273) (use 100 g noodles)	725	30	105	24
1 portion (85 g) curly kale	20	2	1	1
1 portion (85 g) cauliflower	24	2	2	1
Evening				
½ mango (150 g)	86	1	21	0
2 Weetabix and 150 ml skimmed milk	191	9	37	1
Total	3595	134	550	91
% energy		16%	60%	24%

Menu 5 Vegetarian – (3500 kcal)

	Kcal	Protein (g)	Carbohydrate (g)	Fat (g)
Breakfast				
4 Shredded Wheat (100 g)	325	11	68	3
300 ml skimmed milk	99	10	15	0
4 tbsp (120 g) raisins	326	3	83	0
1 glass (150 ml) orange juice	54	1	13	0
Mid-morning				
Peanut butter sandwich with 2 slices (80 g) wholegrain bread with:	174	7	34	2
1 tbsp (40 g) peanut butter	242	10	3	21
Lunch				
2 wholewheat pitta bread (160 g)	348	14	68	4
2 heaped tsp (14 g) olive oil spread	80	0	0	9
¾ carton (175 g) cottage cheese	172	24	4	7
1 bowl (125 g) salad	15	1	2	0
Mid-afternoon				
125 g berries	27	1	6	0
1 carton (150 g) low-fat fruit yoghurt	135	6	27	1
Workout				
500 ml juice 500 ml water	180	3	44	1
Post-workout				
2 cereal or energy bars (66 g)	308	6	40	14
Dinner				
1 beanburger (100 g)	193	11	14	11
1 portion (175 g) grilled white fish	168	37	0	2
2 large (450 g total weight) sweet potato	518	7	126	2
1 portion (85 g) carrots	20	1	4	0
1 portion (85 g) courgettes	16	2	2	0
Evening				
3 small (scotch) pancakes (90 g)	263	5	39	11
2 oranges	118	4	28	0
Total	**3781**	**124**	**578**	**88**
% energy		14%	63%	23%

16

THE RECIPES

BREAKFASTS

Fruit Muesli

Serves 4

175 g (6 oz) oats
300 ml (½ pint) milk
40 g (1½ oz) sultanas
40 g (1½ oz) toasted flaked almonds, chopped
   hazelnuts or cashews
225 g (8 oz) fresh fruit, e.g. bananas,
   blueberries, strawberries, raspberries
1 apple, peeled and grated
1 tbsp honey

- In a large bowl, mix together the oats, milk, sultanas, and nuts. Cover and leave overnight in the fridge.
- Just before serving, stir in the fruit, grated apple and honey. Spoon into cereal bowls.

Nutritional information (per serving):
Calories = 329; protein = 11 g;
carbohydrate = 52 g; fat = 10 g;
fibre = 5.7 g

Athlete's Porridge

Serves 1

50 g (2 oz) porridge oats
350 ml (12 fl oz) milk
1 banana, sliced
25 g (1 oz) dried fruit e.g. raisins, dates or figs

- Mix the oats and milk in a saucepan. Bring to the boil and simmer for approx 5 minutes, stirring frequently.
- Top with the fresh and dried fruit.

Nutritional information (per serving):
Calories = 476; protein = 20 g;
carbohydrate = 85 g; fat = 5.4 g;
fibre = 5.0 g

Breakfast Muffins

Makes 8 muffins

125 g (4 oz) self-raising flour
125 g (4 oz) oatmeal
25 g (1 oz) butter or margarine
40 g (1½ oz) soft brown sugar
1 egg
150 ml (5 fl oz) milk
50 g (2 oz) chopped dates or raisins

* Preheat the oven to 220°C/425°F/Gas mark 7.
* Mix the flour and oatmeal together in a bowl. Add the butter, sugar, egg and milk. Mix well.
* Stir in the dried fruit.
* Spoon in to a non-stick muffin tray and bake for approx 15 minutes until golden brown.

Yoghurt with dried fruit compote

Serves 4

Zest and juice of 1 orange
2 tbsp (30 ml) acacia honey
300 ml (½ pint) water
150 ml (5 fl oz) orange juice
75 g (3 oz) ready-to-eat dried figs, halved
75 g (3 oz) ready-to-eat dried apricots
75 g (3 oz) ready-to-eat pitted prunes
450 ml (¾ pint) whole milk or Greek-style yoghurt

* Combine the zest, freshly squeezed juice, honey, water and orange juice in a saucepan.
* Bring mixture to the boil, stirring until the honey is dissolved, then add the dried fruit and simmer, covered, for about 15 minutes until they become plump and soft. Allow to cool and keep covered in the fridge until you are ready to serve.
* Divide the yoghurt between 4 bowls. Top with the fruit compote.

Nutritional information (per serving):
Calories = 189; protein = 5.0 g;
carbohydrate = 33 g; fat = 5.0 g fat;
fibre = 1.7 g

Nutritional information (per serving):
Calories = 223 calories; protein = 8.6 g;
carbohydrate = 41 g; fat = 3.9 g;
fibre = 3.6 g

MAIN MEALS

Greek yoghurt with banana and honey

Serves 2

2 bananas
300 g (11 oz) Greek-style bio-yoghurt
1–2 level tbsp (15–30 ml) honey
2 tbsp toasted flaked almonds (or walnuts,
    hazelnuts or pecans)

- Slice the bananas into two bowls. Spoon half the yoghurt on top of each bowl. Drizzle with honey and scatter over the toasted nuts.

Spicy Chicken with Rice

Serves 2

2 tsp (10 ml) sunflower oil
2 chicken breasts (approx. 175 g/6 oz each)
175 g (6 oz) brown rice
1 onion, chopped
2 cloves garlic, crushed
1–2 tsp (5–10 ml) curry powder (to taste)
1 tbsp tomato purée
3 tbsp (45 ml) water

- Cook the chicken breasts under a hot grill for 10–15 mins, turning a few times.
- Boil the rice for 20–25 mins.
- Meanwhile, heat the oil in a large non-stick pan and cook the onion for 5 mins, until golden.
- Add the garlic and curry powder and cook for a further 2 mins.
- Cut the chicken into chunks and add to the pan with tomato purée and water.
- Cover and cook for a further 5–10 mins.
- Serve with rice and green vegetables.

Nutritional information (per serving):
Calories = 368; protein = 12 g;
carbohydrate = 43 g; fat = 18 g fat;
fibre = 2.2 g

Nutritional information (per serving):
Calories = 657; protein = 58 g;
carbohydrate = 74 g; fat = 16.1 g;
fibre = 2.2 g

Chicken with butternut squash

Serves 4

400 g (14 oz) butternut squash
1 tbsp extra virgin olive oil
2 tbsp chopped fresh thyme (or 2 tsp dried thyme)
4 chicken breasts on the bone
A little salt and freshly ground black pepper

- Heat the oven to 200°C/400°F/gas mark 6.
- Peel the butternut squash and cut the flesh into 5mm (¼ inch) slices. Cover the base of a baking tin with the squash slices, drizzle over a little oil, then scatter with thyme and season with black pepper.
- Place the chicken breasts over the squash, drizzle over a little olive oil, turn so that they are well-coated with oil.
- Cook the chicken and the squash in the oven for 20–30 minutes, depending on the size of the chicken breasts, until the chicken is golden. The squash should be soft but not mushy.

Moroccan chicken with rice

Serves 1

1 skinless chicken breast
1 clove garlic, crushed
½ red chilli, deseeded and chopped (use according to taste)
A pinch of paprika
A pinch of ground cumin
1 lemon
1 tbsp (15 ml) fresh mint leaves
75 g (3 oz) wholegrain rice
1 tbsp (15 ml) toasted pumpkin seeds

- Slash the chicken breast 3 or 4 times.
- Place the garlic, chilli, paprika, cumin, the juice of half the lemon and mint leaves in a bowl and mix well. Add the chicken and turn a few times. Leave to marinate for ideally 30 minutes.
- Meanwhile, boil the rice according to packet instructions, approx. 25 minutes. Drain and mix with the toasted pumpkin seeds.
- Preheat the grill. Place the chicken on a baking tray and grill for 6 or 7 minutes each side until cooked through.
- Spoon the rice on to a plate and place the chicken on top. Serve with green vegetables.

Nutritional information (per serving):
Calories = 252; protein = 40 g;
carbohydrate = 8.3 g; fat = 6.9 g;
fibre = 1.6 g

Nutritional information (per serving):
Calories = 545; protein = 48 g;
carbohydrate = 63 g; fat = 13 g;
fibre = 2.3 g

Salmon and bean salad

Serves 4

150 g (5 oz) salad leaves
400 g (14 oz) can mixed beans, drained and
    rinsed
4 tbsp low fat vinaigrette dressing
2 tbsp fresh chopped parsley
200 g (7 oz) can wild red salmon, drained
200 g (7 oz) cherry tomatoes, halved
4 spring onions, chopped

- Arrange the salad leaves on 4 plates.
- Mix the beans with the vinaigrette, parsley and freshly ground black pepper.
- Remove the skin and bones from the salmon and lightly flake the flesh. Mix with the tomatoes, spring onions and the bean mixture. Heap on top of the salad leaves.

> **Nutritional information (per serving):**
> Calories = 250; protein = 16 g;
> carbohydrate = 12 g; fat = 15 g;
> fibre = 4.1 g

Sweet and sour chicken with mango

Serves 4

For the sweet & sour sauce:
4 tbsp (60 ml) water
2 tbsp (30 ml) each dry sherry, sesame oil, and
    white wine vinegar
1 tbsp (15 ml) light soy sauce
2 tsp honey

1 large mango
2 tbsp sunflower oil
4 chicken breast fillets, cut into 1 cm (½ inch)
    pieces
2 onions, sliced
250 g (9 oz) broccoli, divided into small florets
1 tsp grated fresh ginger

- For the sauce, combine the water, sherry, sesame oil, vinegar, soy sauce and honey.

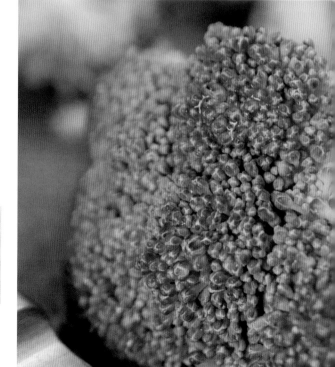

- Slice through the mango either side of the stone. Peel, then cut the flesh into cubes.
- Heat half the sunflower oil in a wok or large frying pan, add the chicken and quickly brown on all sides for 2–3 minutes. Transfer to a warm plate.
- Heat the remaining oil, add the onions and cook for 1–2 minutes until softened. Add the broccoli and ginger followed by the sauce and the mango.
- Bring to the boil and then simmer gently for 3 minutes. Return the chicken to the wok and continue to cook for a further 2–3 minutes until thoroughly cooked. Serve with Basmati rice.

Nutritional information (per serving):
Calories = 255; protein = 23 g; carbohydrate = 8.7 g; fat = 14 g; fibre = 2.6 g

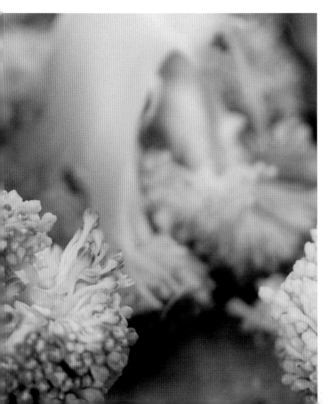

Chicken and lentil salad

Makes 4 servings
2 tbsp olive oil
4 chicken breast fillets, sliced
1 clove garlic, crushed
1 small onion, chopped
400 g (14 oz) can lentils, drained and rinsed
3–4 tomatoes, finely chopped
2 tbsp lemon juice
1 tbsp clear honey
2 tbsp fresh flat-leaf parsley, roughly chopped

- Heat 1 tablespoon of the olive oil in a large frying pan over a high heat and sauté the chicken for 5–6 minutes or until cooked and there is no pink meat.
- Add the garlic, onion, lentils and tomatoes and cook, stirring, for about 2 minutes until heated.
- For the dressing, shake together the remaining olive oil, lemon juice and honey in a bottle or screw top jar.
- Stir the dressing and half the parsley into the lentils in the pan. Transfer to a serving dish, scatter over the remaining parsley and serve warm.

Nutritional information (per serving):
Calories = 347; protein = 45 g; carbohydrate = 20 g; fat = 10 g; fibre = 2.4 g

Pilaff with Plaice

Serves 2

175 g (6 oz) brown rice
600 ml (1 pint) water
1 small onion, chopped
Pinch of turmeric (or mild curry powder)
1 courgette
1 small red pepper
350 g (12 oz) plaice fillets, cut into strips
Salt and freshly ground black pepper
1 tbsp sunflower seeds (optional)

- Place rice, water, onion and turmeric in a large saucepan.
- Bring to the boil, cover and simmer for 20 mins.
- Add courgette, red pepper, plaice and seasoning.
- Cook for a further 5 mins or until fish is cooked and water absorbed.
- Scatter sunflower seeds over before serving.

Noodles with Prawns and Green Beans

Serves 2

225 g (8 oz) frozen or fresh whole green beans
175 g (6 oz) egg noodles
1 tsp (5 ml) oil
175 g (6 oz) peeled prawns
1 tbsp (15 ml) soy sauce

- Cook green beans in a little boiling water for 5 mins, then drain.
- Cook noodles in a large pan for 10 mins.
- Meanwhile, heat oil in a wok or frying pan and stir-fry prawns for 2 mins.
- Add beans, noodles and soy sauce, and heat through.

Nutritional information (per serving):
Calories = 530; protein = 40 g;
carbohydrate = 76 g; fat = 9.5 g;
fibre = 3.1 g

Nutritional information (per serving):
Calories = 483; protein = 32.4 g;
carbohydrate = 66 g; fat =11.8 g;
fibre = 5.2 g

Potato and Fish Pie

Serves 2

450 g (1 lb) potatoes
200 g (7 oz) white fish fillets (e.g. cod or plaice)
3 tbsp (45 ml) skimmed milk
2 eggs
1 tbsp parsley
1 tbsp (15 ml) lemon juice

- Cut potatoes into chunks and boil until tender.
- Drain, then mash with the flaked fish, milk, eggs, parsley and lemon juice.
- Place in a dish, then cook either in microwave at full power for 5 mins, or in oven at 200°C/400°F/gas mark 6 for 20 mins.
- Serve with green vegetables.

Baked eggs with roasted Mediterranean vegetables

Serves 2

½ aubergine, sliced
1 courgette, sliced
½ yellow pepper, sliced
½ red pepper, sliced
½ bulb of fennel, cut into wedges
1 small onion, sliced
1 tbsp (15 ml) olive oil
1 clove garlic, crushed
A few sprigs of rosemary
A handful of black olives
2 large eggs

- Preheat the oven to 200°C/400°F/gas mark 6.
- Place all the vegetables in an ovenproof dish. Drizzle over the olive oil, add the garlic and rosemary, then toss lightly so that the vegetables are well coated in the oil. Roast in the oven for about 20 minutes until the vegetables are just tender.
- Mix in the black olives. Make two wells in the middle of the vegetables. Crack an egg into each indentation. Bake for a further 8–10 minutes or until the eggs are set.
- Serve with crusty bread.

Nutritional information (per serving):
Calories = 352; protein = 33.3 g;
carbohydrate = 39.4 g; fat = 7.9 g;
fibre = 2.8 g

Nutritional information (per serving):
Calories = 201; protein = 10 g;
carbohydrate = 9 g; fat = 14 g fat;
fibre = 4 g

Sweet potato Spanish tortilla

Serves 1

1 small sweet potato (175 g/6 oz), peeled and
  thickly sliced
1 tbsp (15ml) olive oil
1 small onion, chopped
Salt and freshly ground black pepper
2 large eggs, beaten
1 tbsp (15ml) freshly chopped parsley

- Cook the sweet potato in a small pan of boiling water for 5–6 minutes until just tender. Drain and set aside.
- Preheat the grill to medium.
- Heat the oil in an ovenproof frying pan and fry the onion over a medium heat for 3–4 minutes or until softened. Add the sweet potato and season to taste with the salt and pepper.
- Pour in the eggs and cook for 1–2 minutes until the egg starts to set. Transfer to the grill and cook for 3–4 minutes or until the top is golden and the tortilla is cooked through.
- Slide the tortilla onto a plate, scatter over the parsley and cut into wedges. Serve with a simple salad.

Nutritional information (per serving):
Calories = 447; protein = 18 g;
carbohydrate = 42 g; fat = 25 g;
fibre = 5 g

Stir-fried vegetable omelette

Serves 1

2 teaspoons/10ml vegetable oil
1 small onion, sliced
1 garlic clove, crushed
1 teaspoon/5ml chopped fresh root ginger
Vegetables, e.g. carrot, cut into strips; red pepper,
  deseeded and sliced; mangetout, trimmed and
  halved; button mushrooms, sliced
1 tablespoon/15ml soy sauce
Juice of ½ lime
2 large eggs
Salt and freshly ground black pepper
2 teaspoons/10ml vegetable oil

- For the stir-fried vegetables, heat the oil in a wok or heavy-based pan, and then add the onion, garlic and ginger. Cook for two minutes and add the carrot, mangetout and mushrooms. Stir-fry for 3–4 minutes until softened. Stir in the soy sauce and lime juice and set aside.
- For the omelette, beat the eggs in a small bowl and season with salt and pepper. Heat the oil in a medium non-stick frying pan, add the egg mixture and cook for 2–3 minutes over a medium heat until the egg is almost set all the way through.
- Pile the stir-fried vegetables on one half of the omelette and fold the other half over the top. Slide onto a plate and serve with boiled noodles or rice.

Nutritional information (per serving):
Calories = 372; protein = 20 g;
carbohydrate = 16 g; fat = 26 g;
fibre = 4 g

Tofu with Noodles

Serves 2

For the marinade:
2 tbsp (30 ml) soy sauce
2 tbsp (30 ml) dry sherry
1 tbsp (15 ml) wine vinegar

For the dish:
225 g (8 oz) tofu (bean curd), cubed
1 tbsp (15 ml) olive oil
1 clove garlic, crushed
1 piece fresh root ginger, chopped
1 red pepper, sliced
100 g (3½ oz) mange tout
1 tsp cornflour
175 g (6 oz) noodles, cooked in water

- Mix the ingredients for the marinade together. Add the tofu and leave for at least 30 minutes in the fridge (or overnight). Heat the oil in a wok and stir-fry the the garlic, ginger and vegetables for 4 minutes. Remove the tofu from the marinade.
- Blend the marinade with the cornflour, and pour over the vegetables. Stir until the sauce has thickened. Place vegetables and sauce in a serving dish. Stir fry the tofu for 2 minutes, and add to the vegetables. Serve with noodles.

Potato, pea and spinach frittata

Serves 2

1 potato (175 g/6 oz), peeled and sliced
75 g (3 oz) frozen peas
2 tsp (10 ml) olive oil
1 onion, finely sliced
1 clove garlic, crushed
4 large eggs
Salt and freshly ground black pepper
200 g (7 oz) fresh baby leaf spinach

- Cook the potato in a small pan of boiling water for 5–6 minutes or until tender. Add the peas during the last 3 minutes. Drain.
- Heat the olive oil in a frying pan, add the onions and garlic and sauté for 4–5 minutes or until they are softened.
- Beat the eggs in a large bowl and season with salt and freshly ground pepper. Add to the pan, stir in the potatoes, peas and spinach and cook over a medium heat for a few minutes until the eggs are almost set. Place the pan underneath a hot grill to finish cooking. The frittata should be set and golden on top.
- Slide a knife around the edge and slide the frittata on to a large plate. Serve in wedges with a simple salad.

THE RECIPES

Nutritional information (per serving):
Calories = 533; protein = 21 g;
carbohydrate = 75 g; fat = 19 g;
fibre = 3.8 g

Nutritional information (per serving):
Calories = 347; protein = 23 g;
carbohydrate = 27 g; fat = 18 g;
fibre = 6 g

Hummus with pine nuts

Serves 4

400 g (14 oz) tinned chickpeas or 125 g (4 oz)
   dried chickpeas, soaked overnight and then
   boiled for 45 minutes
1–2 cloves garlic, crushed
2 tbsp (30 ml) extra virgin olive oil
1 tbsp (15 ml) tahini (sesame seed paste)
Juice of ½ lemon
2–4 tbsp (30–60 ml) water
Salt and freshly ground black pepper
1–2 tbsp (15–30 ml) pine nuts

- Drain and rinse the chickpeas. Reserve 1–2 tablespoons of chickpeas. Put the remainder in a food processor or blender with the garlic, olive oil, tahini, lemon juice and water. Whizz until smooth, add a little salt and freshly ground black pepper and process again. Taste to check the seasoning. Add extra water if necessary to give the desired consistency.
- Meanwhile lightly toast the pine nuts under a hot grill for 3–4 minutes until they are lightly coloured but not brown (watch carefully because they colour quickly).
- Stir in the reserved whole chickpeas. Spoon into a shallow dish. Scatter over the pine nuts and drizzle over a few drops of olive oil. Chill in the fridge for at least 2 hours before serving.

Nutritional information (per serving):
Calories = 193; protein = 6.8 g;
carbohydrate = 12 g; fat = 13 g;
fibre = 3.5 g

Chickpeas with butternut squash and tomatoes

Serves 4

2 tbsp extra virgin olive oil
2 onions, chopped
1 red pepper, deseeded and chopped
225 g (8 oz) butternut squash, peeled and
   chopped
400 g (14 oz) tinned chopped tomatoes
250 ml (8 fl oz) vegetable stock
2 x 400 g (14 oz) tins chickpeas, drained and
   rinsed
225 g (8 oz) potatoes, peeled and chopped

- Heat the oil in a heavy based pan, add the onion and pepper and cook over a moderate heat for 5 minutes.
- Add the squash, tomatoes, vegetable stock, chickpeas and potatoes, stir and then bring to the boil. Lower the heat and simmer for 20 minutes, stirring occasionally.
- Serve sprinkled with a little grated cheese.

Nutritional information (per serving):
Calories = 331; protein = 15 g;
carbohydrate = 48 g; fat = 10 g;
fibre = 9.8 g

Spicy couscous

Serves 4

250 g (9 oz) couscous
400 ml (14 fl oz) hot vegetable stock or water
½ red pepper
½ yellow pepper
1 red onion, sliced
10–12 cherry tomatoes, halved
2 tbsp (30 ml) extra virgin olive oil
½ tsp cumin seeds
A small handful of fresh coriander, chopped
1 tbsp lemon juice
Salt and freshly ground black pepper

- Put the couscous in a large bowl and cover with the hot stock or water. Stir briefly, cover and allow to stand for 5 minutes until the stock has been absorbed. Fluff up with a fork.
- Remove the seeds from the peppers and cut them into wide strips. Place in a large roasting tin with the onion slices and cherry tomatoes, drizzle over the olive oil, scatter over the cumin seeds and toss lightly so that the vegetables are well coated in the oil.
- Roast in the oven for about 15 minutes until the peppers are slightly charred on the outside and tender in the middle. Allow to cool, then roughly chop the peppers.
- Add the roasted vegetables (with the cumin seeds), coriander and lemon juice to the couscous. Season to taste. Stir well to combine and serve.

Nutritional information (per serving):
Calories = 224; protein = 4.7 g; carbohydrate = 39 g; fat = 6.5 g; fibre = 1.5 g

Roasted vegetables with marinated tofu

Serves 2

1 small red onion, roughly sliced
½ red pepper, cut into strips
½ yellow pepper, cut into strips
½ orange pepper, cut into strips
1 small courgette, trimmed and thickly sliced
¼ aubergine, cut into 2 cm (¾ inch) cubes
2 cloves garlic, crushed
1–2 tbsp (15–30 ml) extra virgin olive oil
200 g (7 oz) marinated tofu pieces
freshly ground black pepper
A small handful of fresh basil, roughly torn

- Preheat the oven to 200°C/400°F/gas mark 6.
- Place the prepared vegetables in a large roasting tin and scatter over the crushed garlic. Pour over the olive oil and toss lightly thoroughly coating the vegetables.
- Roast in the oven for about 25 minutes, turning them occasionally. Scatter the tofu pieces over and continue roasting for 5 minutes until the vegetables are slightly charred on the outside and tender in the middle.
- Remove from the oven and spoon onto a serving dish. Grind over the black pepper and sprinkle with the torn basil.

Nutritional information (per serving):
Calories = 245; protein = 11 g; carbohydrate = 14 g; fat = 16 g; fibre = 4 g

Vegetable risotto with cashew nuts

Serves 2

2 tbsp (30 ml) olive oil
1 onion, chopped
1 red pepper, chopped
1 clove garlic, crushed
1 bay leaf ·
150 g (5 oz) wholegrain rice
500 ml (18 fl oz) hot vegetable stock
75 g (3 oz) green beans, cut into 2 cm (¾ inch)
   lengths
125 g (4 oz) sugar snap peas
2 tomatoes, deseeded and chopped
50 g (2 oz) baby spinach leaves
Freshly ground black pepper
50 g (2 oz) cashew nuts, lightly toasted

- Heat the olive oil in a large heavy-based pan and cook the onion with the red pepper, garlic and bay leaf over a moderate heat, stirring frequently.
- Stir in the rice and cook for 1–2 minutes, stirring constantly until the grains are coated with oil and translucent.
- Add half the hot vegetable stock and bring to the boil. Reduce the heat and simmer gently until the liquid is absorbed. Add the remaining stock, a ladleful at a time, stirring and continue to simmer until the rice is almost tender (about 25–30 minutes). Add the green beans, peas and tomatoes and continue cooking for a further 5 minutes. As a guide, the total cooking time should be around 35 minutes.
- Add the spinach leaves to the hot risotto. Stir until the leaves have wilted. Remove the pan from the heat.
- Season to taste with freshly ground black pepper, then scatter over the cashew nuts.

Nutritional information (per serving):

Calories = 652; protein = 16 g;
carbohydrate = 84 g; fat = 29 g;
fibre = 8.5 g

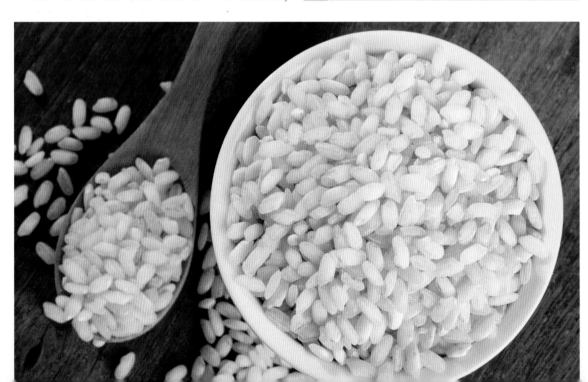

Pasta with chickpeas and spinach

Serves 4

400 g (14 oz) can chickpeas, drained and rinsed
350g (12 oz) tub fresh tomato pasta sauce
400g (14 oz) fresh penne pasta
200g (7 oz) bag fresh spinach
Freshly ground black pepper
25g (1 oz) parmesan shavings
Olive oil, to drizzle

- Place the chickpeas in a medium pan with the tomato sauce and 100 ml (3½ fl oz) cold water. Bring to the boil over a low heat. Turn off the heat and cover.
- Meanwhile, bring a large pan of water to the boil. Add the pasta and return to the boil for 5 minutes or until the pasta is just tender. Drain thoroughly. Stir in the spinach and allow to wilt.
- Place the pasta in a serving dish and pour the hot pasta sauce and chickpea mixture over the top, then toss together and season with black pepper. Top each serving with Parmesan shavings and a drizzle of olive oil.

Vegetable stir-fry with sesame noodles

Serves 4

1 tsp clear honey
Juice of 1 large orange
3 tbsp soy sauce
2 tbsp oil
1 onion, sliced
1 large carrot, peeled and cut into thin strips
225 g (8 oz) pak choi or spring cabbage, shredded
2.5 cm (1 inch) piece root ginger, peeled and grated
1 clove garlic, crushed
225 g (8 oz) ready-cooked egg noodles
3 tbsp sesame seeds, toasted

- In a small bowl, mix together the honey, orange juice and soy sauce and set aside.
- Heat the oil in a wok or large frying pan. Add the onion and carrot and stir-fry for 2–3 minutes. Add the pak choi or cabbage, ginger and garlic and stir-fry for a further 2–3 minutes.
- Add the ready-cooked egg noodles to the wok and pour in the spicy sauce mix. Toss everything together and cook for a further 2– 3 minutes, or until piping hot. Scatter with the toasted sesame seeds and serve at once.

Nutritional information (per serving):
Calories = 434; protein = 20 g;
carbohydrate = 76 g; fat = 7.8 g;
fibre = 6.5 g

Nutritional information (per serving):
Calories = 330; protein = 9.3 g;
carbohydrate = 44 g; fat = 14 g;
fibre = 4.2 g

Rice, Bean and Vegetable Stir Fry

Serves 2

175 g (6 oz) brown rice
1 tbsp (15 ml) olive oil
1 onion, chopped
2 cloves garlic, crushed
1 piece fresh root ginger, chopped
125 g (4 oz) large mushrooms, sliced
2 stalks celery, chopped
125 g (4 oz) peas
½ a 400 g (14 oz) can red kidney beans

- Cover the rice with plenty of boiling water.
- Bring to the boil and simmer for 25–30 mins.
- Meanwhile, heat the oil in a wok over a high heat.
- Add the onion, and stir fry for 1 min.
- Add the garlic, ginger, mushrooms, celery and peas, and stir fry for 3 mins.
- Tip in the red kidney beans and cooked rice.
- Cook for a further 2 mins, until all ingredients are thoroughly heated through.

Vegetarian Chilli

Serves 2

1 clove garlic, crushed
1 onion, chopped
1 green or red pepper, chopped
½ tsp chilli powder (or to taste)
225 g (8 oz) can tomatoes
50 g (2 oz) red lentils
300 ml (½ pint) water
175 g (6 oz) rice
½ a 400 g (14 oz) can red kidney beans

- Place the garlic, onion, pepper, chilli, tomatoes, lentils, water and rice in a large pan.
- Bring to the boil and simmer for 20 mins.
- Add the drained kidney beans and cook for a further 5 mins.
- Season to taste.
- Serve with broccoli or green salad.

Nutritional information (per serving):
Calories = 526; protein = 18.3 g;
carbohydrate = 94.2 g; fat = 11.3 g;
fibre = 11.1 g

Nutritional information (per serving):
Calories = 550; protein = 21 g;
carbohydrate = 119 g; fat = 2.3 g;
fibre = 10.4 g

Mixed Bean Hotpot

Serves 2

400 g (14 oz) can of beans (e.g. red kidney
   beans, chickpeas or haricot beans)
125 g (4 oz) green beans
225 g (8 oz) can tomatoes
1 tbsp tomato puree
1 tsp mixed herbs
450 g (1 lb) potatoes, boiled and cooled

- Place the drained beans in a large casserole dish and mix in the green beans, tomatoes, puree and herbs.
- Thinly slice the potatoes and arrange on top.
- Bake at 170°C/325°F/gas mark 3 for 30 mins until the potatoes are cooked, or microwave on full for 8 mins.
- Serve with green vegetables or salad.

Lentil and Vegetable Lasagne

Serves 2

6 sheets ready-cooked lasagne

For the lentil and vegetable sauce:
100 g (4 oz) red lentils
1 onion, chopped
400 g (14 oz) tin of tomatoes
2 carrots, chopped
1 tsp oregano
150 ml (¼ pint) water

For the topping:
125 g (4 oz) fromage frais
2 eggs
1 tbsp parmesan cheese

- Place all the ingredients for the lentil and vegetable sauce in a saucepan and bring to the boil.
- Simmer for 20 mins or cook in a pressure cooker for 3 mins (release steam slowly).
- Place half of the sauce in a dish, with several lasagne sheets on top. Then add the rest of the sauce, followed by the remaining lasagne sheets. For topping, beat the eggs with fromage frais, then spoon them on top of the lasagne. Sprinkle with parmesan cheese. Bake at 200°C/400°F/ gas mark 6 for 40 mins, until the topping is golden. Serve with a large mixed salad.

Nutritional information (per serving):
Calories = 346; protein = 16.8 g;
carbohydrate = 71 g; fat = 1.5 g;
fibre = 14.2 g

Nutritional information (per serving):
Calories = 513; protein = 33 g;
carbohydrate = 75 g; fat = 10.9 g;
fibre = 6 g

DESSERTS

Bean Burgers

Serves 2

1 small onion, finely chopped
1 clove garlic, crushed
2 tsp (10 ml) oil
400 g (14 oz) tin red kidney beans, drained
1 tbsp parsley
1 tbsp (15 ml) lemon juice
Oats for coating

- Cook the onion and garlic in the oil for 5 mins.
- Mash with a fork or blend in food processor with other ingredients, except the oats, until a coarse puree.
- Add a little flour if necessary for a firmer texture.
- Place oats in a dish.
- In your hands, form mixture into 4 large burgers, coating them with oats.
- Grill for about 2 mins on each side, fry in a small amount of hot oil, or barbecue.
- Serve in a wholemeal bap or pitta bread with lots of salad.

Banana Pancakes

Makes 8 pancakes

100 g (3½ oz) wholemeal flour, or fine oatmeal
300 ml (½ pint) milk
2 eggs
1 tsp (5 ml) oil
3 ripe bananas

- Blend all ingredients, except bananas, in a liquidiser for 30 secs.
- Then heat a non-stick frying pan and add oil.
- Pour in 1 tbsp of batter, tilting the pan to coat evenly.
- Cook until underside of pancake is brown.
- Turn, and cook for a further 10 secs until other side is brown.
- Repeat until batter used up.
- Stack pancakes on an ovenproof plate and keep warm in the oven on a very low heat.
- Then, mix one mashed banana with two sliced bananas.
- Place a spoonful on each pancake and fold into quarters.
- Serve with low-fat yoghurt.

Nutritional information (per serving):
Calories = 234; protein = 11.6 g;
carbohydrate = 34 g; fat = 6.6 g;
fibre = 10.2 g

Nutritional information (per serving):
Calories = 103; protein = 5.1 g;
carbohydrate = 17.1 g; fat = 2 g;
fibre = 1.5 g

Baked Apples

Serves 1

1 large cooking apple
1 tbsp raisins or sultanas
1 tsp honey
1 tsp toasted, chopped hazelnuts (optional)

- Remove core from the apple.
- Score skin lightly around middle. Place in a small dish. Mix together the raisins or sultanas, honey and nuts and fill centre of the apple.
- Cover loosely with foil and bake at 180°C/350°F/gas mark 4 for 45–60 mins or cover with another dish and microwave on medium power for 5–7 mins (depending on the size of the apple).
- Serve with yoghurt, low-fat custard or fromage frais.

Wholemeal Bread and Butter Pudding

Serves 4

8 slices wholemeal bread
40 g (1½ oz) low-fat spread
75 g (3 oz) sultanas
1 tbsp brown sugar
3 eggs
600 ml (1 pint) milk
Nutmeg

- Spread the bread with the low fat spread.
- Cut each slice into 4 squares and place in a 1 litre (2 pint) dish.
- Scatter sultanas between each slice.
- Beat together the sugar, eggs, and milk and pour over the bread.
- Sprinkle with a little grated nutmeg.
- Leave to soak for 30 mins, if time allows.
- Bake at 350°F/180°C/gas mark 4 for 1 hour, until the top is golden.

Nutritional information (per serving):
Calories = 144; protein = 1.2 g;
carbohydrate = 33 g; fat = 1.8 g;
fibre = 0.6 g

Nutritional information (per serving):
Calories = 345; protein = 17 g;
carbohydrate = 49 g; fat = 10.5 g;
fibre = 3.9 g

Oat apple crumble

Serves 6
700 g (1½ lb) cooking apples, peeled and sliced
75 g (3 oz) clear honey
½ tsp cinnamon
4 tbsp (60 ml) water

Topping
125 g (4 oz) plain flour
75 g (3 oz) olive oil margarine
50 g (2 oz) oats
50 g (2 oz) brown sugar

- Preheat the oven to 190°C/ 375°C/ gas mark 5.
- Place the apples, honey and cinnamon in a deep baking dish. Combine well and pour the water over.
- For the crumble topping, put the flour in a bowl and rub in the margarine until the mixture resembles coarse breadcrumbs. Mix in the oats and sugar. Alternatively, mix in a food mixer or processor.
- Sprinkle the crumble mixture over the fruit. Bake for 20–25 minutes until the topping is golden and fruit is tender.

Spiced fruit skewers

Serves 4
50 g (2 oz) clear honey
1 tbsp (15 ml) lemon juice
Juice of 1 orange
8 cardamom pods, lightly crushed
1 cinnamon stick, halved
8 Medjool dates, pitted
8 apricots, halved and stoned
4 plums, halved and stoned

- Place the honey, lemon juice, orange juice, cardamom pods and cinnamon stick in a shallow dish. Add the dates, apricots and plums. Marinate for at least 30 minutes.
- Drain the fruits, reserving the honey syrup, and thread onto 4 long wooden skewers. Cook under a preheated grill (or over a prepared barbecue) for 10–15 minutes, or until beginning to colour.

Nutritional information (per serving):
Calories = 311; protein = 3.4 g;
carbohydrate = 52 g; fat = 11 g;
fibre = 3.1 g

Nutritional information (per serving):
Calories = 147; protein = 1.9 g;
carbohydrate = 37 g; fat = 0.2 g;
fibre = 3.2 g

Exotic fruit with lime

Serves 4

2 tbsp clear honey
100 ml (3½ fl oz) water
Zest of 1 lime
20 g (⅔ oz) pack fresh mint leaves
1 pineapple, skin removed, quartered and cored
3 kiwi fruit, peeled and cut into chunks
1 mango, peeled and sliced

- Place the honey, water and lime zest and half the mint in a jug. Allow to infuse for 1 hour, then strain.
- Cut the pineapple into small wedges and toss gently in a large bowl with the kiwi fruit and mango pieces. Pour the cooled syrup over and combine well.
- Divide the fruit between 4 bowls, decorate with the remaining mint and serve with natural yoghurt.

Roasted Peaches and Plums with yoghurt

Serves 4

4 ripe peaches
4 ripe plums
1 cinnamon stick, broken in half
Zest and juice of 2 oranges
2 tbsp clear honey
400 g (14 oz) Greek-style yoghurt

- Preheat the oven to 200°C/400°F/gas mark 6.
- Halve and stone the peaches and plums and arrange, cut sides up, in a shallow dish large enough to hold them all in one layer.
- Put the cinnamon stick, orange zest and juice and honey in a small pan. Heat gently until the honey has melted. Pour evenly over the fruit. Roast in the oven for 25–30 minutes, basting halfway through the cooking time, until the fruit is tender.
- Cool for 10 minutes, then divide between serving plates. Place a dessertspoonful of yogurt into the cavity of each fruit and drizzle some of the honey syrup over. Serve the rest of the yogurt separately.

Nutritional information (per serving):
Calories = 124; protein = 1.4 g;
carbohydrate = 30 g; fat = 0.6 g;
fibre = 3.7 g

Nutritional information (per serving):
Calories = 179; protein = 6.4 g;
carbohydrate = 26 g; fat = 6.2 g;
fibre = 2.6 g

SNACKS

Fruit Scotch pancakes

Serves 2–4
100 g (3½ oz) plain flour
1 tbsp sugar
1 tsp baking powder
2 medium eggs
75 ml (5 fl oz) semi-skimmed milk
50 g (2 oz) raisins
50 g (2 oz) ready-to-eat dried apricots, chopped
Oil for brushing

- Mix together the dry ingredients in a bowl. Add the eggs and a splash of milk and whisk until smooth. Stir in the raisins and apricots.
- Heat a large griddle or heavy-based non-stick frying pan and brush it lightly with oil. Drop small spoonfuls of the batter on to the griddle to make 8–10 cm (3–4 inch) rounds and cook for about 2 minutes or until air bubbles start to form on the surface. Turn and cook the other side for 1–2 minutes or until golden. You may need to cook in 2 batches.
- Serve with fresh fruit and honey.

Nutritional information (per serving):
For 2 servings:
Calories = 423; protein = 25 g;
carbohydrate = 76 g; fat = 9 g;
fibre = 4 g

For 4 servings:
Calories = 212; protein = 8 g;
carbohydrate = 38 g; fat = 5 g;
fibre = 2 g

Banana Muffins

Makes 10 muffins
50 g (2 oz) butter
75 g (3 oz) brown sugar
1 egg
225 g (8 oz) flour (wholemeal or half wholemeal, half white)
2 mashed bananas
Pinch of salt
1 tsp baking powder
1 tsp (5 ml) vanilla essence
5 tbsp (75 ml) milk

- Combine all ingredients in a large bowl.
- Spoon into 10 non-stick bun tins (or paper cases).
- Bake at 190°C/375°F/gas mark 5 for approx. 20 mins.

Variations:
- Add 50 g (2 oz) chocolate chips to the mixture (recommended!).
- Substitute 225 g (8 oz) fresh blueberries or 75 g (3 oz) dried blueberries for the bananas.
- Substitute 225 g (8 oz) fresh cranberries or 75 g (3 oz) dried cranberries for the bananas.
- Add 50 g (2 oz) chopped walnuts.
- Substitute 100 g (3½ oz) chopped dried apricots for the bananas. Add the grated rind of 1 lemon instead of the vanilla essence.

Nutritional information (per serving):
Calories = 164; protein = 4.1 g;
carbohydrate = 27 g; fat = 5.3 g;
fibre = 2.2 g

Raisin Bread

Makes one loaf (10 slices)

225 g (8 oz) strong flour (half wholemeal, half white)

½ tsp salt

1½ tbsp sugar

1 sachet easy-blend yeast

1 tbsp melted butter

180 ml (6 fl oz) warm water

100 g (3½ oz) raisins

- Mix together the flour, salt, sugar, yeast and butter.
- Add the warm water to form a dough.
- Turn out onto a floured surface and knead for 5–10 mins.
- Knead in the raisins.
- Place in a bowl, cover and leave in warm place or at room temperature to rise until doubled in size (approximately 1 hour).
- Knead for a few mins then shape into a loaf.
- Place on an oiled baking tray and bake at 220°C/425°F/gas mark 7 for 20 mins or until it sounds hollow when tapped underneath.

Variations:

- Add 2 tsp cinnamon to the flour mixture.
- Substitute 100 g (3½ oz) chopped dried apricots for the raisins.
- Substitute 100 g (3½ oz) sultanas for the raisins.
- Add 1 tsp grated orange rind.
- Add 50 g (2 oz) toasted chopped hazelnuts with the raisins.

Nutritional information (per serving):
Calories = 120; protein = 3.0 g; carbohydrate = 25 g; fat = 1.7 g; fibre = 1.6 g

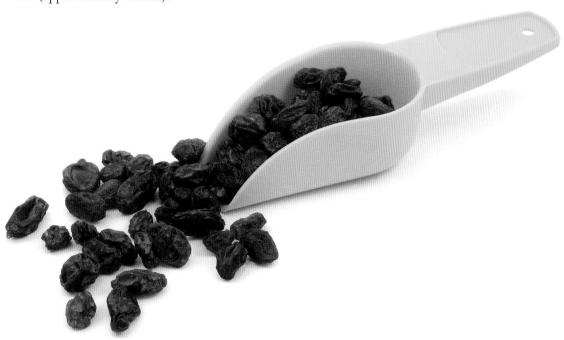

Apple and Cinnamon Oat Bars

Makes 12 bars

2 apples, sliced and cooked, or 175 g (6 oz)
  apple purée
175 g (6 oz) oats
2 tsp cinnamon
4 egg whites
1 tbsp honey
50 g (2 oz) raisins
6 tbsp (90 ml) skimmed milk

- Mix all ingredients together in a bowl.
- Transfer to non-stick baking tin 23 cm × 15 cm (approx. 9" × 6").
- Bake at 200°C/400°F/gas mark 6 for 15 mins.
- When cool, cut into squares.

Sultana flapjacks

Makes 12 slices

200 g (7 oz) butter or margarine
200 g (7 oz) sugar
200 g (7 oz) honey or golden syrup
400 g (14 oz) porridge oats
75 g (3 oz) sultanas

- Preheat the oven to 180°C/350°F/gas mark 4. Butter a 20cm x 30cm cake tin.
- Put the butter, sugar and honey in a saucepan and heat, stirring occasionally, until the butter has melted and the sugar has dissolved. Add the oats and sultanas or cherries and mix well.
- Transfer the oat mixture to the prepared cake tin and spread to about 2cm thick. Smooth the surface with the back of a spoon. Bake in the oven for 15–20 minutes, until lightly golden around the edges, but still slightly soft in the middle. Let cool in the tin, then turn out and cut into squares.

Nutritional information (per serving):
Calories = 87; protein = 3.1 g;
carbohydrate = 17 g; fat = 1.3 g;
fibre = 1.3 g

Nutritional information (per serving):
Calories = 389; protein = 4.5 g;
carbohydrate = 59 g; fat = 17 g;
fibre = 2.4 g

Banana and walnut loaf

Makes 10 slices

Two medium bananas
125 g (4 oz) butter
125 g (4 oz) dark brown sugar
2 eggs
1 tsp vanilla essence
1 tsp ground cinnamon
250 g (9 oz) plain flour
1 tsp baking powder
3 tbsp (45 ml) milk
125 g (4 oz) walnuts

- Preheat the oven to 180°C/350°F/gas mark 4. Butter a 1 kg loaf tin or use 12 large muffin cases.
- Mash the bananas. Cream the butter and sugar until smooth and then beat in the mashed bananas. Add the eggs, vanilla and cinnamon and mix well.
- Add the flour, baking powder and milk, and mix until smooth. Fold in the walnuts.
- Spoon the mixture into the tin and bake for about 50 minutes, until the loaf is crusty on the top and a skewer inserted into the middle comes out clean. Cool in the tin, and then turn out onto a cooling rack. For muffins, cook for 20–25 minutes.

Blueberry muffins

Makes 18

250 g (9 oz) flour
1 tsp baking powder
100 g (3½ oz) caster sugar
2 eggs
50 g (2 oz) melted butter
200 ml (7 fl oz) buttermilk or yoghurt
125 g (4 oz) blueberries

- Preheat oven to 200°C/400°F/gas mark 6. Line 2 x 12-hole muffin trays with paper cases.
- Sift the flour and baking powder into a large bowl and stir in the sugar.
- In another bowl, whisk together the eggs, melted butter and buttermilk. Fold this mixture into the flour and stir the blueberries through. Spoon into paper cases and bake for 20–25 mins until cooked and golden.

Nutritional information (per serving):
Calories = 348; protein = 5.9 g;
carbohydrate = 37 g; fat = 217 g;
fibre = 1.4 g

Nutritional information (per serving):
Calories = 164; protein = 4.0 g;
carbohydrate = 26 g; fat = 5.6 g;
fibre = 1.0 g

Raspberry muffins

Makes 10

4 tbsp (60 ml) sunflower oil
5 tbsp (75 ml) milk
1 large egg
150 g (5 oz) self-raising flour
100 g (4 oz) caster sugar
175 g (6 oz) fresh or frozen raspberries
4 tbsp icing sugar, sifted
2 tsp (10 ml) lemon juice

- Preheat the oven to 200°C/400°F/gas mark 6. Line a six-hole deep muffin tray with paper cases.
- Mix the oil, milk and egg together. Sift the flour and sugar into a bowl. Add the liquid and half the raspberries to the flour and briefly mix until just coming together. Spoon into the muffin cases and scatter over the remaining raspberries. Bake for 25–30 mins.
- Cool the muffins on a wire rack. Sift the icing sugar into a bowl, stir in the lemon juice to make a runny icing. Drizzle the icing over the muffins and leave to set. Pack the muffins into an airtight container. They will keep for 2–3 days.

Nutritional information (per serving):
Calories = 131; protein = 2.7 g;
carbohydrate = 19 g; fat = 5.4 g;
fibre = 0.9 g

Cherry, almond and oat cookies

Makes 15

125 g (4 oz) butter or margarine
125 g (4 oz) granulated or caster sugar
1 tbsp golden syrup
½ tsp vanilla essence
150 g (5 oz) plain white flour
100 g (3½ oz) rolled oats
100 g (3½ oz) ground almonds
100 g (3½ oz) glacé cherries, chopped

- Preheat the oven to 170°C/350°F/gas mark 3 and oil two baking sheets (or use baking parchment).
- Cream together the butter or margarine and the sugar until light and smooth.
- Beat in the golden syrup and vanilla.
- Add the flour, oats and almonds to the mixture, mixing well. Stir in the cherries.
- Place spoonfuls on to the baking sheets, about 2.5 cm (1 inch) apart, then flatten with your hand. Bake for 10–12 minutes or until light golden.

Nutritional information (per serving):
Calories = 216; protein = 3.2 g;
carbohydrate = 27 g; fat = 11 g;
fibre = 1.3 g

APPENDIX ONE:
THE GLYCAEMIC INDEX AND GLYCAEMIC LOAD

Food	Portion size	GI	Carbohydrate (g) per portion	GL per portion
High GI (> 70)				
Dates	6 (60 g)	103	40	42
Glucose	2 tsp (10 g)	99	10	10
French baguette	5 cm slice (30 g)	95	15	15
Lucozade	250 ml bottle	95	42	40
Baked potato	1 average (150 g)	85	30	26
Rice krispies	Small bowl (30 g)	82	26	22
Cornflakes	Small bowl (30 g)	81	26	21
Gatorade	250 ml bottle	78	15	12
Rice cakes	3 (25 g)	78	21	17
Chips	Average portion (150 g)	75	29	22
Shredded wheat	2 (45 g)	75	20	15
Bran flakes	Small bowl (30 g)	74	18	13
Cheerios	Small bowl (30 g)	74	20	15
Mashed potato	4 tbsp (150 g)	74	20	15
Weetabix	2 (40 g)	74	22	16
Bagel	1 (70 g)	72	35	25
Breakfast cereal bar (crunchy nut cornflakes)	1 bar (30 g)	72	26	19
Watermelon	1 slice (120 g)	72	6	4
Golden Grahams	Small bowl (30 g)	71	25	18
Millet	5 tablespoons (150 g)	71	36	25
Water biscuit	3 (25 g)	71	18	13
Wholemeal bread	1 slice (30 g)	71	13	9
Isostar	250 ml can	70	18	13
White bread	1 slice (30 g)	70	14	10
Moderate GI (56–69)				
Fanta	262 ml	68	34	23
Sucrose	2 tsp (10 g)	68	10	7
Croissant	1 (57 g)	67	26	17
Instant porridge	250 g bowl	66	26	17
Cantaloupe melon	1 slice (120 g)	65	6	4
Couscous	5 tbsp (150 g)	65	35	23

Food	Portion size	GI	Carbohydrate (g) per portion	GL per portion
Mars bar	1 bar (60 g)	65	40	26
Raisins	3 tbsp (60 g)	64	44	28
Rye crispbread	2 (25 g)	64	16	11
Shortbread	2 (25 g)	64	16	10
White rice	5 tbsp (150 g)	64	36	23
Tortillas/corn chips	1 bag (50 g)	63	26	17
Ice cream	1 scoop (50 g)	61	13	8
Muesli bar	1 bar (30 g)	61	21	13
Sweet potato	1 medium (150 g)	61	28	17
Just Right cereal	1 small bowl (30 g)	60	22	13
Pizza	1 slice (100 g)	60	35	21
Digestive biscuit	2 (25 g)	59	16	10
Pineapple	2 slices (120 g)	59	13	7
Basmati rice	5 tbsp (150 g)	58	38	22
Porridge	250 g bowl	58	22	13
Squash (diluted)	250 ml glass	58	29	17
Apricots	3 (120 g)	57	9	5
Pitta bread	1 small (30 g)	57	17	10
Power Bar	1 bar (65 g)	56	42	24
Sultanas	3 tbsp (60 g)	56	45	25
Rich tea biscuit	2 (25 g)	55	19	10
Potato – boiled, old	2 medium (150 g)	54	27	15
Oatmeal biscuit	2 (25 g)	54	17	9
Low GI (< 55)				
Brown rice	5 tbsp (150 g)	55	33	18
Honey	1 tablespoon (25 g)	55	18	10
Muesli (Alpen)	1 small bowl (30 g)	55	19	10
Buckwheat	5 tbsp (150 g)	54	30	16
Crisps	1 large packet (50 g)	54	21	11
Sweetcorn	4 tbsp (150 g)	54	17	9
Kiwi fruit	3 (120 g)	53	12	6
Banana	1 (120 g)	52	24	12
Orange juice	1 large glass (250 ml)	52	23	12
Mango	½ (120 g)	51	17	8
Strawberry jam	1 tablespoon (30 g)	51	20	10
Rye bread	1 slice (30 g)	50	12	6
Muesli	1 small bowl (30 g)	49	20	10
Baked beans	1 small tin (150 g)	48	15	7
Bulgar wheat	5 tbsp (150 g)	48	26	12

Food	Portion size	GI	Carbohydrate (g) per portion	GL per portion
Peas	2 tbsp (80 g)	48	7	3
Carrots	2 tbsp (80 g)	47	6	3
Macaroni	5 tbsp (180 g)	47	48	23
Grapes	Small bunch (120 g)	46	18	8
Pineapple juice	1 large glass (250 ml)	46	34	15
Sponge cake	1 slice (63 g)	46	36	17
Muffin, apple	1 (60 g)	44	29	13
Milk chocolate	1 bar (50 g)	43	28	12
All Bran	1 small bowl (30 g)	42	23	9
Orange	1 (120 g)	42	11	5
Peach	1 (120 g)	42	11	5
Apple juice	1 large glass (250 ml)	40	28	11
Strawberries	21 (120 g)	40	3	1
Spaghetti	5 tbsp (180 g)	38	48	18
Plum	3 (120 g)	39	12	5
Apples	1 (120 g)	38	15	6
Pear	1 (120 g)	38	11	4
Protein bar	1 bar (80 g)	38	13	5
Tinned peaches – tinned in fruit juice	½ tin (120 g)	38	11	4
Yoghurt drink	1 glass (200 ml)	38	29	11
Plain yoghurt, low fat	1 large carton (200 g)	36	9	3
Custard	2 tbsp (100 g)	35	17	6
Chocolate milk	1 large glass (250 ml)	34	26	9
Fruit yoghurt, low fat	1 large carton (200 g)	33	31	10
Protein shake	1 carton (250 ml)	32	3	1
Skimmed milk	1 large glass (250 ml)	32	13	4
Apricot (dried)	5 (60 g)	31	28	9
Butter beans	4 tbsp (150 g)	31	20	6
Meal replacement bar	1 bar (40 g)	31	19	6
Lentils (green/ brown)	4 tbsp (150 g)	30	17	5
Chickpeas	4 tbsp (150 g)	28	30	8
Red kidney beans	4 tbsp (150 g)	28	25	7
Whole milk	1 large glass (250 ml)	27	12	3
Lentils (red)	4 tbsp (150 g)	26	18	5
Grapefruit	½ (120 g)	25	11	3
Cherries	Small handful (120 g)	22	12	3
Fructose	2 teaspoon (10 g)	19	10	2
Peanuts	Small handful (50 g)	14	6	1

Adapted with permission from The American Journal of Clinical Nutrition © *Am J Clin Nutr American Society for Nutrition* (Foster-Powell *et al.* 2002)

APPENDIX TWO:
GLOSSARY OF VITAMINS AND MINERALS

Vitamin	Function(s)	Sources	RNI and SUL*
A	Essential for normal colour vision and for the cells in the eye that enable us to see in dim light; promotes healthy skin and mucous membranes lining the mouth, nose, digestive system, etc.	Liver, meat, eggs, whole milk, cheese, oily fish, butter and margarine	Men: 700 µg/day Women: 600 µg/day SUL: 1500 µg/day (800 µg for pregnant women)
Beta-carotene	Converted into vitamin A (6 µg produces 1 µg vitamin A): a powerful antioxidant and free radical scavenger	Brightly coloured fruit and vegetables (e.g. carrots, spinach, apricots, tomatoes)	No official RNI. 15 mg is suggested intake SUL: 7 mg
B$_1$ (Thiamin)	Forms a co-enzyme essential for the conversion of carbohydrates into energy; used for the normal functioning of nerves, brain and muscles	Wholemeal bread and cereals, liver, kidneys, red meat, pulses (beans, lentils and peas)	Men: 0.4 mg/ 1000 calories Women: 0.4 mg/ 1000 calories No SUL. FSA recommends 100 mg

*RNI = Reference nutrient intake
**NV = no value published.
USL = Upper safe levels are guides for self-supplementation. These are maximum levels which should not be exceeded unless advised by a qualified health professional.
SUL = Safe Upper Limit recommended by the Expert Group on Vitamins and Minerals, an independent advisory committee to the Food Standards Agency.

Sources:
Department of Health, 1991.
Food Standards Agency, 2003.

Claim(s) of supplements	The evidence	Possible dangers of high doses
Maintains normal vision, healthy skin, hair and mucous membranes; may help to treat skin problems such as acne and boils; may affect protein manufacture	Not involved in energy production; little evidence to suggest it can improve sporting performance	Liver toxicity from taking supplements: symptoms include liver and bone damage; abdominal pain; dry skin; double vision; vomiting; hair loss; headaches. May also cause birth defects. Pregnant women should avoid liver. Never exceed 9000 µg/day (men), 7500 µg/day (women)
Reduces risk of heart disease, cancer and muscle soreness	As an antioxidant, may help prevent certain cancers. Other carotenoids in food may also be important	Orange tinge to the skin – probably harmless and reversible
May optimise energy production and performance; is usually present within a B-complex or multivitamin	Involved in energy (ATP) production, so the higher the thiamin requirement; increased needs can normally be met in the diet (cereals and other foods high in complex carbohydrates); there is no evidence to suggest that high intakes enhance performance; supplements are probably unnecessary	Cannot be stored – excess is excreted therefore unlikely to be toxic; toxic symptoms (rare) may include insomnia, rapid pulse, weakness and headaches. Avoid taking more than 3 g/day

Vitamin	Function(s)	Sources	RNI and SUL*
B$_2$ (Riboflavin)	Required for the conversion of carbohydrates to energy; promotes healthy skin and eyes and normal nerve functions	Liver, kidneys, red meat, chicken, milk, yoghurt, cheese, eggs	Men: 1.3 mg/day Women: 1.1 mg/day No SUL. FSA recommends 40 mg
Niacin	Helps to convert carbohydrates into energy; promotes healthy skin, normal nerve functions and digestion	Liver, kidneys, red meat, chicken, turkey, nuts, milk, yoghurt and cheese, eggs, bread and cereals	Men: 6.6 mg/ 1000 calories Women: 6.6 mg/ 1000 calories SUL: 17 mg
B$_6$ (Pyridoxine)	Involved in the metabolism of fats, proteins and carbohydrates; promotes healthy skin, hair and normal red blood cell formation; is actively used in many chemical reactions of amino acids and proteins	Liver, nuts, pulses, eggs, bread, cereals, fish, bananas	Men: 1.4 mg/day Women: 1.2 mg/day SUL: 80 mg
Pantothenic acid (B vitamin)	Involved in the metabolism of fats, proteins and carbohydrates; promotes healthy skin, hair and normal growth; helps in the manufacture of hormones and antibodies, which fight infection; helps energy release from food	Liver, wholemeal bread, brown rice, nuts, pulses, eggs, vegetables	No RNI in the UK No SUL

Claim(s) of supplements	The evidence	Possible dangers of high doses
Sportspeople may need more B_2 because they have higher energy needs – supplements may optimise energy production; usually present within a B-complex or multivitamin	Forms part of the enzymes involved in energy production, so exercise may increase the body's requirements; however, these can usually be met by a balanced diet; there is no evidence that supplements improve performance; if you take the contraceptive pill you may need extra B_2	Rarely toxic as it cannot be stored; any excess is excreted in the urine (a bright yellow colour)
Sportspeople need more niacin since it is involved in metabolism; higher doses may help to reduce blood cholesterol levels	Not enough evidence to prove that high doses can help to improve perform-ance; requirements can be met by a balanced diet	Excess is excreted in the urine; doses of more than 200 mg of niacin may cause dilation of the blood vessels near the skin's surface (hot flushes)
Sportspeople may need higher doses to meet their increased energy requirements	Requirements are related to protein intake, so sportspeople on high-protein diets may need extra B_6; endurance work may cause greater-than-normal losses; there is no evidence to suggest that high doses improve performance; extra doses may help to alleviate PMS (pre-menstrual syndrome)	Excess is excreted in the urine; very high doses (over 2 g/day) over months or years may cause numbness and unsteadiness
Since it is involved in protein, fat and carbohydrate metabolism, sportspeople may need higher doses; usually present in a B-complex or multivitamin – for overall wellbeing	No evidence to suggest that high doses improve performance	Excess is excreted in the urine

Vitamin	Function(s)	Sources	RNI and SUL*
Folic acid (B vitamin)	Essential in the formation of DNA; necessary for red blood cell manufacture	Liver and offal, green vegetables, yeast extract, wheatgerm, pulses	Men: 200 µg/day Women: 200 µg/day SUL: 1000 µg (1 mg)
B$_{12}$	Needed for red blood cell manufacture and to prevent some forms of anaemia; used in fat, protein and carbohydrate metabolism; promotes cell growth and development; needed for normal nerve functions	Meat, fish, offal, milk, cheese, yoghurt; vegan sources (fortified foods) are soya protein and milk, yeast extract, breakfast cereals	Men: 1.5 µg/day Women: 1.5 µg/day SUL: 2 mg
Biotin	Involved in the manufacture of fatty acids and glycogen, and in protein metabolism; needed for normal growth and development	Egg yolk, liver and offal, nuts, wholegrain and oats	No RNI in the UK; 10–200 µg/day is thought to be a safe and adequate range SUL: 900 µg
C	Growth and repair of body cells; collagen formation (in connective tissue) and tissue repair; promotes healthy blood vessels, gums and teeth; haemoglobin and red blood cell production; manufacture of adrenalin; powerful antioxidant	Fresh fruit (especially citrus), berries and currants, vegetables (especially dark green, leafy vegetables, tomatoes and peppers)	Men: 40 mg/day Women: 40 mg/day SUL: 1000 mg

Claim(s) of supplements	The evidence	Possible dangers of high doses
Supplements help overall wellbeing, and also prevent folic acid deficiency and anaemia; these would, in theory, hinder aerobic performance	No studies have been carried out on athletic performance and folic acid	Dangers of toxicity are very small, though high doses may reduce zinc absorption and disguise a deficiency of vitamin B_{12}
Since it is involved in the development of red blood cells, the implication is that B_{12} can improve the body's oxygen carrying capacity (and therefore its aerobic performance); athletes have been known to use injections of vitamin B_{12} before competition in the hope that it will improve their endurance; usually present within a B-complex or multivitamin	Extra vitamin B_{12} has no effect on endurance or strength; there is no benefit to be gained from taking supplements (deficiencies are very rare)	Excess is excreted in the urine
Although biotin was once known amongst body builders as the 'dynamite vitamin', no specific role for this vitamin in sporting performance has been claimed; it is usually present within a B-complex or multivitamin	The body can make its own biotin, so supplements are unnecessary	There are no known cases of biotin toxicity
Vitamin C may help to increase oxygen uptake and aerobic energy production; exercise causes an increased loss so extra may be needed; intense exercise tends to cause greater free radical damage, so sportspeople need higher doses	A deficiency reduces physical performance; exercise may increase requirements to approximately 80 mg/day – these can be met by including 5 portions of fresh fruit and vegetables in the diet each day; intakes of 100–150 mg may help prevent heart disease and cancer	Excess is excreted, so toxic symptoms are unlikely; high doses may lead to diarrhoea and increase the risk of kidney stones in people who are prone to them

Vitamin	Function(s)	Sources	RNI and SUL*
D	Controls absorption of calcium from the intestine and helps to regulate calcium metabolism; prevents rickets in children and osteomalacia in adults; helps to regulate bone formation	Sunlight (UV light striking the skin), fresh oils and oily fish, eggs, vitamin-D-fortified cereals, margarines and some yoghurts	No RNI in the UK (5 µg in EU) SUL: 25 µg
E	As an antioxidant, it protects tissues against free radical damage; promotes normal growth and development; helps in normal red blood cell formation	Pure vegetable oils, wheatgerm, wholemeal bread and cereals, egg yolk, nuts, sunflower seeds, avocado	No RNI in the UK; FSA suggests 4 mg (men) 3 mg (women) (10 mg in EU) SUL: 540 mg

Mineral	Function(s)	Sources	RNI and SUL*
Calcium	Important for bone and teeth structure; helps with blood clotting; acts to transmit nerve impulses; helps with muscle contraction	Milk, cheese, yoghurt, soft bones of small fish, seafood, green leafy vegetables, fortified white flour and bread, pulses	700 mg SUL: 1500 mg

Claim(s) of supplements	The evidence	Possible dangers of high doses
No specific claims for athletic performance	So far not shown to be beneficial to performance	Fat-soluble and can be stored in the body; toxicity is rare but symptoms may include high blood pressure, nausea, and irregular heart beat and thirst
Since it is an antioxidant, it may improve oxygen utilisation in the muscle cells; it may also help to protect the cells from the damaging effects of intense exercise; may help to protect against heart disease and cancer	Supplements may have a beneficial effect on performance at high altitudes, and may help reduce heart disease, cancer risk, and post-exercise muscle soreness; requirements are related to intake of polyunsaturated fatty acids	Although it cannot be excreted, toxicity is extremely rare

Claim(s) of supplements	The evidence	Possible dangers of high doses
May help to prevent calcium deficiency and, in some cases, osteoporosis (brittle bone disease)	There is no evidence that extra calcium prevents osteoporosis; exercise (with adequate calcium intake) prevents bone loss, so supplements would seem to be unnecessary; sportspeople who eat few or no dairy products may find calcium supplements useful for meeting basic dietary require-ments; extra calcium may help to reduce the risk of stress fractures in sportswomen with menstrual irregularities	The balance of calcium in the bones and blood is finely controlled by hormones – calcium toxicity is thus virtually unknown. Very high intakes may interfere with the absorption of iron and with kidney function

Mineral	Function(s)	Sources	RNI and SUL*
Sodium	Helps to control body fluid balance; involved in muscle and nerve functions	Table salt, tinned vegetables, fish, meat, ready-made sauces and condiments, processed meats, bread, cheese	Men: 1.6 g/day (= 4 g salt) Women: 1.6 g/day (= 4 g salt) FSA recommends a maximum daily intake of 2.5 g (= 6 g salt)
Potassium	Works with sodium to control fluid balance and muscle and nerve functions	Vegetables, fruit and fruit juices, unprocessed cereals	Men: 3.5 g/day Women: 3.5 g/day SUL: 3.7 g
Iron	Involved in red blood cell formation and oxygen transport and utilisation	Red meat, liver, offal, fortified breakfast cereals, shellfish, wholegrain bread, pasta and cereals, pulses, green leafy vegetables	Men: 6.7 mg/day Women: 16.4 mg/day SUL: 17 mg
Zinc	A component of many enzymes involved in the metabolism of proteins, carbohydrates and fats; helps to heal wounds; assists the immune system; needed for building cells	Meat, eggs, wholegrain cereals, milk and dairy products	Men: 9.5 mg/day Women: 7 mg/day SUL: 25 mg

Claim(s) of supplements	The evidence	Possible dangers of high doses
It has been claimed that extra salt is needed if you sweat a lot or exercise in hot, humid conditions; advocated for treating cramp	Excessive sweating during exercise may cause a marked loss of sodium, but as salt is present in most foods, supplements are usually unnecessary; extra salt is more likely to cause, rather than prevent, cramp – dehydration is normally the cause of cramp (together possibly with a shortage of potassium)	High salt intakes may increase blood pressure, risk of stroke, fluid retention and upset the electrolyte balance of the body
May help to reduce blood pressure and encourage sodium excretion	Extra potassium is not known to enhance performance; may help to prevent cramp	Excess is excreted, therefore toxicity is very rare
Extra iron can improve the oxygen-carrying capacity of red blood cells, and therefore improve aerobic performance; can prevent or treat anaemia	Iron-deficiency anaemia can impair performance especially in aerobic activity; exercise destroys red blood cells and haemoglobin and increases loss of iron, therefore iron requirements of sportspeople may be slightly higher than those of sedentary people; iron is lost through menstruation, so supplements may be sensible for sports-women	High doses may cause constipation and stomach discomfort; they may also interact with zinc, reducing its absorption
Suggest a possible role in high-intensity and strength exercises; may help to boost the immune system	Studies have failed to show that extra zinc is of any benefit to performance; sportspeople with a zinc deficiency may have an impaired immune system, so an adequate intake is important	High doses may cause nausea and vomiting; daily doses of more than 50 mg also interfere with the absorption of iron and other minerals, leading to iron-deficiency anaemia

Mineral	Function(s)	Sources	RNI and SUL*
Magnesium	Involved in the formation of new cells, in muscle contraction and nerve functions; assists with energy production; helps to regulate calcium metabolism; forms part of the mineral structure of bones	Cereals, vegetables, fruit, potatoes, milk	Men: 300 mg/day Women: 270 mg/day SUL: 400 mg
Phosphorus	Assists in bone and teeth formation; involved in energy metabolism as a component of ATP	Cereals, meat, fish, milk and dairy products, green vegetables	550 mg/day SUL: 250 mg from supplements

LIST OF ABBREVIATIONS

ACSM	American College of Sports Medicine	GI	glycaemic index
ADP	adenosine diphosphate	GL	glycaemic load
ALA	alpha-linolenic acid	HDL	high density lipoprotein
ATP	adenosine triphosphate	HMB	beta-hydroxy beta-methylbutyrate
BCAA	branched-chain amino acids	IGF-I	insulin-like growth factor-I
BMI	Body Mass Index	IOC	International Olympic Committee
BMR	basal metabolic rate	LDL	low density lipoprotein
BV	Biological Value	MRP	Meal Replacement Product
EAA	essential amino acid	NEAA	non-essential amino acid
DHA	docosahexanoic acid	PC	phosphocreatine
DHEA	dehydroepiandrosterone	RDA	Recommended Daily Amount
DoH	Department of Health	RMR	resting metabolic rate
DRV	Dietary Reference Value	RNI	Reference Nutrient Intake
EFA	essential fatty acid	ST	slow-twitch (type I) muscle fibres
EPA	eicosapentanoic acid	SUL	safe upper limit
FT	fast-twitch (type II) muscle fibres	VO_2max	maximal aerobic capacity

Claim(s) of supplements	The evidence	Possible dangers of high doses
Magnesium status may be related to aerobic capacity	Studies have failed to show that magnesium supplements are beneficial to performance	May cause diarrhoea
It has been claimed that phosphate loading enhances aerobic performance and delays fatigue	The consensus is that phosphate loading is of little benefit to performance	High intakes over a long period of time may lower blood calcium levels

LIST OF WEIGHTS AND MEASURES

Symbols used:

g	gram
h	hour
kcal	kilocalorie
kJ	kilojoule
L	litre
m	metre
min	minute
mg	milligram (1000 g = 1 g)
ml	millilitre
mmol	millimole
mph	miles per hour
sec	seconds
tbsp	tablespoon
tsp	teaspoon
dl	decilitre (10 dl = 1 L)
µg	microgram (1000 µg = 1 mg)
<	less than
>	greater than
°C	degree Celsius

Conversions:

1 kcal	=	4.2 kJ
25 g	=	1 oz
450 g	=	1 lb
1 kg	=	2.2 lb
5 ml	=	1 tsp
15 ml	=	1 tbsp
25 ml	=	1 fl oz
600 ml	=	1 pint

REFERENCES

Aceto, C. (1997), *Everything You Need to Know about Fat Loss* (Adamsville TN: Fundco).

ACSM (1996), 'Position stand on exercise and fluid replacement'. *Med. Sci. Sports and Ex.*, vol. 28, pp. i–vii.

ACSM/ADA/DC (2000), 'Position of the American Dietetic Association, Dietitians of Canada, and the American College of Sports Medicine: nutrition and athletic performance'. *Med. Sci. Sports and Ex.*, vol. 32 (12), pp. 2130–45.

ADA (American Dietetic Association) (1997), 'Vegetarian diets – ADA position'. *J. Am. Diet. Assoc.*, vol. 97, pp.1317–321.

ADA/DC/ACSM (American Dietetic Association, Dietitians of Canada and the American College of Sports Medicine) (2000), 'Nutrition and athletic performance: position of the American Dietetic Association, Dietitians of Canada, and the American College of Sports Medicine'. *J. Am. Diet. Assoc.*, vol. 100, pp. 1543–1556.

Ahlborg, B. *et al.* (1967), 'Human muscle glycogen content and capacity for prolonged exercise after different diets'. *Forsvarsmedicin*, vol. 3, pp. 85–99.

Albrink, M. J. (1978), 'Dietary fibre, plasma insulin and obesity'. *Am. J. Clin. Nutr.*, vol. 31, S277–9.

Alexander, D., Ball, M. J. and Mann, J., (1994) 'Nutrient intake and hematological status of vegetarians and age-sex matched omnivores'. *Eur. J. Clin. Nutr.*, vol. 48, pp. 538–46.

American Dietetic Association (1993), 'Position of The American Dietetic Association and the Canadian Dietetic Association: nutrition for physical fitness and athletic performance for adults'. *J. Am. Diet. Assoc.*, vol. 93, pp. 691–6.

Anderson, M. *et al.* (2000), 'Improved 2000m rowing performance in competitive oarswomen after caffeine ingestion'. *Int. J. Sport Nutr.*, vol. 10, pp. 464–75.

Antonio, J. and Street, C. (1999), 'Glutamine: a potentially useful supplement for athletes'. *Can. J. Appl. Physiol.*, vol. 24 (1): S69–77.

Appleby, P. N. *et al.* (1999), 'The Oxford Vegetarian Study: an overview'. *Am. J. Clin. Nutr.*, vol. 70 (3 Suppl), pp. 525S–31S.

Armstrong, L. E. *et al.* (2005), 'Fluid, electrolyte and renal indices of hydration during 11 days of controlled caffeine consumption'. *Int. J. Sport Nutr. Exerc. Metab.*, vol 15, pp. 252–65.

Armstrong, L. E. (2002), 'Caffeine, body fluid-electrolyte balance and exercise performance'. *Int. J. Sport Nutr.*, vol. 12, pp. 189–206.

Armstrong, L. E. *et al.* (1985), 'Influence of diuretic-induced dehydration on competitive running performance'. *Med. Sci. Sports Ex.*, vol. 17, pp. 456–61.

Armstrong, L. E. *et al.* (1998), 'Urinary indices during dehydration, exercise and rehydration'. *Int. J. Sport Nutr.*, vol. 8, pp. 345–55.

Ashenden, M. J. *et al.* (1998), 'Serum ferritin and anaemia in trained female athletes'. *Int. J. Sport Nutr.*, vol. 8, pp. 223–9.

Astrand, P. O. (1952), *Experimental studies of physical working capacity in relation to sex and age*, (Copenhagen, Munksgaard).

Bacon, L. *et al.* (2005), 'Size acceptance and intuitive eating improve health for obese, female chronic dieters'. *J. Am. Diet. Assoc.*, vol 105 (6), pp. 929–36.

Barr, S. I. and Costill, D. L. (1989), 'Water. Can the

endurance athlete get too much of a good thing?' *J. Am. Diet. Assoc.*, vol. 89, pp. 1629–32.

Barr, S. I. and Rideout, C. A. (2004), 'Nutritional considerations for vegetarian athletes'. *Nutrition*, vol. 20 (7–8), pp. 696–703.

Barr, T. C. *et al.* (1995), 'Periodic carbohydrate replacement during 50 minutes of high-intensity cycling improves subsequent spring performance'. *Int. J. Sports Nutr.*, vol. 5, pp. 151–8.

Bazzare, T. L. *et al.* (1986), 'Incidence of poor nutritional status among triathletes, endurance athletes and controls'. *Med. Sci. Sports Ex.*, vol. 18, p. 590.

BDA (British Dietetic Association) (2005), *Is vegetarianism as healthy as it is beefed up to be?*, Media Release, May 2005.

Beals, K. A. and Manore, M. M. (1994), 'The prevalence and consequences of subclinical eating disorders in female athletes'. *Int. J. Sport Nutr.*, vol. 4, pp. 157–95.

Beals K. A. and Manore M. M. (2002), 'Disorders of the female athlete triad among collegiate athletes'. *Int. J. Sport Nutr. Exerc. Metab.*, vol. 12, pp. 281–93.

Beals, K. A. and Hill, A. K. (2006), 'The prevalence of disordered eating, menstrual dysfunction and low bone mineral density among US collegiate athletes'. *Int. J. Sports Nutr. Exerc. Metab.*, vol. 16, pp. 1–23.

Beelan, M. *et al.* (2008), Protein coingestion stimulates muscle protein synthesis during resistance type exercise'. *Am. J. Physiol. Endocrinol Metab.*, vol. 295, pp. E70–7.

Beelan, M. *et al.* (2010), 'Nutritional strategies to promote postexercise recovery'. *Int. J. Sport Nutr. Exerc. Metab.*, vol. 20, pp S15–32.

Beis, L. Y. *et al.* (2011), 'Food and macronutrient intake of elite Ethiopian distance runners'. *J. Int. Soc. Sports Nutr.*, vol. 8 pp. 7–11.

Bell, D. G. *et al.* (2001), 'Effect of caffeine and ephedrine ingestion on anaerobic exercise performance'. *Med. Sci. Sport Exerc.*, vol. 33 (8), pp. 1399–1403.

Below, P. R. *et al.* (1995), 'Fluid and carbohydrate ingestion independently improve performance during one hour of intense exercise'. *Med. Sci. Sports Exerc.*, vol. 27, pp. 200–10.

Bennell K. L. *et al.* (1995), 'Risk factors for stress fractures in female track and field athletes: a retrospective anaysis'. *Clin. J. Sports Med.*, vol. 5 pp. 229–35.

Beradi, J. M. *et al.* (2008), 'Recovery from a cycling time trial is enhanced with carbohydrate-protein supplementation vs. isoenergetic carbohydrate supplementation'. *J. Int. Soc. Sports Nutr.* 2008, vol. 5, p. 24.

Berg, A. and Keul, J. (1988), 'Biomechanical changes during exercise in children'. *Young athletes: Biological, psychological and educational perspectives*, ed. R. M. Malina (Champaign, Illinois, Human Kinetics) pp. 61–77.

Bergstrom, J. *et al.* (1976), 'Diet, muscle glycogen and physical performance'. *Acta. Physiol. Scand.*, vol. 71, pp. 140–50.

Bescos, R. *et al.* (2012), 'The effect of nitric oxide related supplements on human performance'. *Sports Med.*, vol. 42(2), pp 99–117.

Betts, J. *et al.* (2007), 'The influence of carbohydrate and protein ingestion during recovery from prolonged exercise on subsequent endurance performance'. *J. Sports Sci.*, vol. 25(13), pp. 1449–1460.

Bishop, N. C. *et al.* (2002), 'Influence of carbohydrate supplementation on plasma cytokine and neutrophil degranulation responses to high intensity intermittent exercise'. *Int. J. Sport Nutr.*, vol. 12, pp. 145–56.

Bledsoe, J. (1999), 'Can taking glutamine boost your immune system?'. *Peak Performance*, vol. 116, pp. 1–4.

Bloomer R. J. *et al.* (2004), 'Effects of antioxidant therapy in women exposed to eccentric exercise'. *Int. J. Sport Nutr. Exerc. Metab.*, vol 14, pp. 377–88.

Bloomer, R. J. *et al.* (2000), 'Effects of meal form and composition on plasma testosterone, cortisol and insulin following resistance exercise'. *Int. J. Sport Nutr.*, vol. 10, pp. 415–24.

Boirie, Y. *et al.* (1997), 'Slow and fast dietary proteins differently modulate postprandial protein accretion'. *Proc. Nat. Acad. Sci. USA.*, vol. 94(26), pp. 14930-5.

Bosch, A. N. *et al.* (1994), 'Influence of carbohydrate ingestion on fuel substrate turnover and oxidation during prolonged exercise'. *J. Appl. Physiol.*, vol. 76, pp. 2364–72.

Borsheim E *et al.* (2004), 'Effect of an amino acid, protein, and carbohydrate mixture on net muscle protein balance after resistance training'. *Int. J. Sport. Nutr. Exerc. Metab.*, vol 14, pp. 255–71.

Bosselaers, I. *et al.* (1994), 'Twenty-four-hour energy expenditure and substrate utiliation in bodybuilders'. *Am. J. Clin. Nutr.*, vol. 59, pp. 10–12.

Bounous, G. and Gold, P. (1991), 'The biological activity of un-denatured whey proteins: role of glutathione'. *Clin. Invest. Med.*, vol. 4, pp. 296–309.

Brand-Miller, J. *et al.* (2003), 'Low GI diet in the management of diabetes'. *Diabetes Care,* vol. 26, pp. 2261–7.

Brand-Miller, J., Foster-Powell, K. and McMillan-Price J., (2005), 'The low GI diet'. (Hodder Mobius).

Brilla, L. R. and Conte, V. (2000), 'Effects of a novel zinc-magnesium formulation on hormones and strength'. *J. Exerc. Physiol. Online*, vol. 3(4), pp. 1–15.

Brinkworth, G. D. *et al.* (2004), 'Effect of bovine colostrum supplementation on the composition of resistance trained and untrained limbs in healthy young men'. *Eur. J. Appl. Physiol.*, vol. 91, pp. 53–60.

Brinkworth, G. D. and Buckley, J. D. (2003), 'Concentrated bovine colostrum protein supplementation reduces the incidence of self-reported symptoms of upper respiratory tract infection in adult males'. *Eur. J. Nutr.*, vol. 42, pp. 228–32.

British Nutrition Foundation (1999), Briefing paper: *n-3 Fatty acids and health.*

Broeder, C. E. *et al.* (2000), 'The Andro Project'. *Arch. Intern. Med.*, vol. 160 (20), pp. 3093–104.

Brouns, F. *et al.* (1998), 'The effect of different rehydration drinks on post-exercise electrolyte excretion in trained athletes'. *Int. J. Sports Med.*, vol. 19, pp. 56–60.

Brown, G. A. *et al.* (1999), 'Effect of oral DHEA on serum testosterone and adaptations to resistance training in young men'. J. A. P. Online, vol. 87(6), pp. 2007–15.

Brown, G. A. *et al.* (2000), 'Effects of anabolic precursors on serum testosterone concentrations and adaptations to resistance training in young men'. *Int. J. Sport Nutr.*, vol. 10, pp. 340–59.

Brown, E. C. *et al.* (2004), 'Soy versus whey protein bars: Effects of exercise training impact on lean body mass and antioxidant status'. *J. Nutr.* vol 3, pp. 22–27.

Bryce-Smith, D. and Simpson, R. (1984), 'Anorexia, depression and zinc deficiency'. *Lancet*, vol. 2, p. 1162.

Bryer S. C. and Goldfarb, A. H. (2006), 'Effect of high dose vitamin C supplementation on muscle soreness, damage, function and oxidative stress to eccentric exercise'. *Int. J. Sport Nutr. Exerc. Metab.*, vol 16, pp. 270–280.

Buckley, J. D. *et al.* (2003), 'Effect of bovine colostrum on anaerobic exercise performance and plasma insulin-like growth factor'. *J. Sports Sci.*, vol. 21, pp. 577–88.

Burd, N. A. *et al.* (2009), 'Exercise training and protein metabolism: influences of contraction, protein intake, and sex-based differences'. *J. Appl. Physiol.*, vol. 106(5), pp. 1692–701.

Burke, L. M. (2001), 'Nutritional practices of male and female endurance cyclists'. *Sports Med.*, vol. 31(7), pp. 521–32.

Burke, L. M. (2010) 'Fueling strategies to optimize performance: training high or training low?'. Scand *J. Med. Sci. Sports*, vol. 20, Suppl 2, pp. 48–58.

Burke, L. M. *et al.* (2011) 'Carbohydrates for training

and competition'. *J. Sports Sci.*, vol. 29, Suppl 1, pp. S17–27.

Burke, D. G. *et al.* (1993), 'Muscle glycogen storage after prolonged exercise: effect of glycaemic index of carbohydrate feedings'. *J. Appl. Physiol.*, vol. 75, pp. 1019–23.

Burke, D. G. *et al.* (1998), 'Glycaemic index – a new tool in sports nutrition'. *Int. J. Sport Nutr.*, vol. 8, pp. 401–15.

Burke, D. G. *et al.* (2000), 'The effect of continuous low dose creatine supplementation on force, power and total work'. *Int. J. Sport Nutr.*, vol. 10, pp. 235–44.

Burke, D. G. *et al.* (2001a), 'The effect of alpha lipoic supplementation on resting creatine during acute creatine loading' (conference abstract). FASEB Journal, vol. 15(5), p. A814.

Burke, D. G. *et al.* (2001b), 'The effect of whey protein supplementation with and without creatine monohydrate combined with resistance training on lean tissue mass and muscle strength'. *Int. J. Sport Nutr.*, vol. 11, pp. 349–64.

Burke, L. (2001) 'Nutritional practices of male and female endurance cyclists'. *Sports Med.*, vol. 31(7), pp. 521–32.

Burke, L. *et al.* (2004), 'Carbohydrates and fat for training and recovery'. *J. Sports Sci.*, vol. 22(1), pp. 15–30.

Burke, L. (2007), *Practical Sports Nutrition*, Human Kinetics.

Burke L. *et al.* (2011), 'Carbohydrates for training and competition'. *J. Sports Sci.*, vol. 29, Suppl 1, pp. S17–27.

Bussau, V. A. *et al.*, (2002), 'Carbohydrate loading in human muscle: an improved 1-day protocol'. *Eur. J. Appl. Physiol.*, vol. 87, pp. 290–5.

Butterfield G. E. (1996), 'Ergogenic Aids: Evaluating sport nutrition products'. *Int. Sport Nutr.*, vol. 6, pp. 191-7.

Cahill, C. F. (1976), 'Starvation in Man'. *J. Clin. Endocrinol. Metab.*, vol. 5, pp. 397–415.

Campbell, W. W. *et al.* (1995), 'Effects of resistance training and dietary protein intake in protein metabolism in older adults'. *Am. J. Physiol.*, Vol 268, pp. 1143–53.

Candow, D. G. *et al.* (2001), 'Effect of glutamine supplementation combined with resistance training in young adults'. *Eur. J. Appl. Physiol.*, vol. 86 (2), pp. 142–9.

Candow, D. G. *et al.* (2006), 'Effect of whey and soy protein supplementation combined with resistance training in young adults'. *Int. J. Sports Nutr. Exerc. Metab.*, vol. 16, pp. 233–44.

Cann, C. E. *et al.* (1984), 'Decreased spinal mineral content in amenhorreic women'. JAMA, vol. 251, pp. 626–9.

Cannell, J. *et al.* (2009), 'Athletic performance and vitamin D'. *Med. Sci. Sports Exerc.*, vol. 41, pp. 1102–10.

Carbon, R. (2002), 'The female athlete triad does not exist'. *Sports Care News*, 26, pp. 3–5.

Carr, A. J. (2011), 'Effects of acute alkalosis and acidosis on performance: a meta-analysis'. *Sports Med.*, vol. 41(10), pp. 801–14.

Carter, J. M. *et al.* (2004), 'The effect of carbohydrate mouth rinse on 1-h cycle time-trial performance'. *Med. Sci. Sports Exerc.*, vol. 36, pp. 2107–11.

Castell, L. M. and Newsholme, E. A. (1997), 'The effects of oral glutamine supplementation on athletes after prolonged exhaustive exercise'. *Nutrition*, vol. 13, pp. 738–42.

Catlin, D. H. *et al.* (2000), 'Trace contamination of over-the-counter androstenedione and positive urine tests for nandrolone metabolite'. *J. Am. Med. Assoc.*, vol. 284, pp. 2618–21.

Cermak N. M. *et al.* (2012) 'Nitrate supplementation's improvement of 10 km time trial performance in trained cyclists'. *Int. J. Sport Nutr. Exerc. Metab.*, vol. 1, pp. 64– 71.

Cheuvront, S. N. (1999), 'The diet zone and athletic performance'. *Sports Medicine*, vol. 27(4), pp. 213–28.

Christensen, E. H. and Hansen, O, (1939), 'Arbeitsfahigheit und Ernahrung'. *Skand Arch Physiol*, vol. 81, pp. 160–71.

Chryssanthopoulos, C. *et al.* (2002), 'The effect of a high carbohydrate meal on endurance running capacity'. *Int. J. Sport Nutr.*, vol. 12, pp. 157–71.

Clark, J. F. (1997), 'Creatine and phosphocreatine: a review'. *J. Athletic Training*, vol. 32 (1), pp. 45–50.

Clark, N. (1995), 'Nutrition quackery: when claims are too good to be true'. *Phys. Sports Med.*, vol. 23, pp. 7–8.

Cobb K. L. *et al.* (2003), 'Disordered eating, menstrual irregularity and bone mineral density in female runners'. *Med. Sci. Sports Exerc.*, vol. 35, pp. 711–19.

Cockburn, E. *et al.* (2008), 'Acute milk-based protein-CHO supplementation attenuates exercise-induced muscle damage'. *Appl. Physiol. Nutr. Metab.*, Aug; 33(4): 775-83.

Cockburn E., Robson-Ansley P, Hayes P. R., Stevenson E. (2012), 'Effect of volume of milk consumed. on the attenuation of exercise-induced muscle damage'. *Eur. J. Appl. Physiol.*, Jan 7. [Epub ahead of print]

Coggan, A. R. and Coyle, E. F. (1987), 'Reversal of fatigue during prolonged exercise by carbohydrate infusion or ingestion'. *J. Appl. Physiol.*, vol. 63, pp. 2388–95.

Coggan, A. R. and Coyle, E. F. (1991), 'Carbohydrate ingestion during prolonged exercise: effects on metabolism and performance'. in J. Holloszy (ed.), *Exercise and Sports Science Reviews*, vol. 19, (Williams and Wilkins), pp. 1–40.

Cole, T. J., Bellizzi, M., Flegal, K. and Dietz W. H. (2000), 'Establishing a standard definition for child overweight and obesity worldwide: international survey'. *British Medical Journal*, vol. 320, pp. 1240–3.

Colgan, M. *et al.* (1991), 'Micronutrient status of endurance athletes affects haematology and performance'. *J. Appl. Nutr.*, vol. 43(1), pp. 17–36.

CompEat 5 (Grantham: Nutrition Systems).

Cook, J. D. (1994), 'The effect of endurance training on iron metabolism'. Sem. Hemat., vol. 31, pp. 146–54.

Costill, D. L. (1986), *Inside Running: Basics of Sports Physiology*, (Benchmark Press), p. 189.

Costill, D. L. (1988), 'Carbohydrates for exercise: dietary demands for optimal performance'. *Int. J. Sports Med.*, vol. 9, pp. 1–18.

Costill, D. L. and Hargreaves, M. (1992), 'Carbohydrate nutrition and fatigue'. *Sports Med.*, vol. 13, pp. 86–92.

Costill, D. L. and Miller, J. (1980), 'Nutrition for endurance sport: carbohydrate and fluid balance'. *Int. J. Sports Med.*, vol. 1, pp. 2–14.

Costill, D. L. (1985), 'Carbohydrate nutrition before, during and after exercise'. *Fed. Proc.*, vol. 44, pp. 364–368.

Costill, D. L. *et al.* (1971), 'Muscle glycogen utilisation during prolonged exercise on successive days'. *J. Appl. Physiol.*, vol. 31, pp. 834–8.

Cox, G. *et al.* (2002), 'Acute creatine supplementation and performance during a field test simulating match play in elite female soccer players'. *Int. J. Sport Nutr.*, vol. 12, pp. 33–46.

Coyle, E. F. (1988), 'Carbohydrates and athletic performance'. *Sports Sci. Exch. Sports Nutr.*, Gatorade Sports Science Institute, vol. 1.

Coyle, E. F. (1991), 'Timing and method of increased carbohydrate intake to cope with heavy training, competition and recovery'. *J. Sports Sci.*, vol. 9 (suppl.), pp. 29–52.

Coyle, E. F. (1995), 'Substrate utilization during exercise in active people'. *Am. J. Clin. Nutr.*, vol. 61 (suppl), pp. 968–79.

Coyle, E. (2004), 'Fluid and fuel intake during exercise'. *J. Sports Sci.*, vol. 22, pp. 39–55.

Crawley, H. (2005), *Eating Well at School: Nutritional and Practical Guidelines*, National Heart Forum and The Caroline Walker Trust. Available from www.heartforum.org.uk or from www.cwt.org.uk.

Cribb P. J. *et al.* (2006), 'The effect of whey isolate and resistance training on strength, body composition and plasma glutamine'. *Int. J. Sports Nutr. Exerc. Metab.*, vol. 16, pp. 494–509.

Crooks, C. V. *et al.* (2006), 'The effect of bovine colostrum supplementation on salivary IgA in distance runners'. *Int. J. Sport Nutr. Exerc. Metab.*, vol. 16, pp. 47–64.

Cupisti, A. *et al.* (2002), 'Nutrition knowledge and dietary composition in Italian female athletes and non-athletes'. *Int. J. Sport Nutr.*, vol. 12, pp. 207–19.

Dangin, M. *et al.* (2000), 'The digestion rate of protein is an independent regulating factor of postprandial protein retention'. *Am. Physiol. Soc. abstracts*, vol. 7: 022E.

Dansinger, M. *et al.* (2005), 'Comparison of the Atkins, Ornish, Weight Watchers, and Zone diets for weight loss and heart disease risk reduction: a randomized trial'. *JAMA.* vol. 293(1) pp. 43–53.

Davey, G. K. *et al.* (2003), 'EPIC-Oxford: Lifestyle characteristics and nutrient intakes in a cohort of 33,883 meat-eaters and 31,546 non meat-eaters in the UK'. *Public Health Nutrition*, vol. 6(3), pp. 259–68.

Davis, C. (1993), 'Body image, dieting behaviours and personality factors: a study of high-performance female athletes'. *Int. J. Sport Psych.*, vol. 23, pp. 179–92.

Davis, J. M. *et al.* (1988), 'Carbohydrate-electrolyte drinks: effects on endurance cycling in the heat'. *Am. J. Clin. Nutr.*, vol. 48, pp. 1023–30.

Davis, K. J. *et al.* (1982), 'Free radicals and tissue damage produced by exercise'. *Biochem. Biophysiol. Res. Commun.*, vol. 107, pp. 1198–205.

DeMarco, H. M. *et al.* (1999), *Med. Sci. Sports Ex.*, vol. 31(1), pp. 164–70.

Department of Health (1994), Nutritional Food Guide (HMSO).

Department of Health (2004), *At least five a week: Evidence on the impact of physical activity and its relationship to health. A report from the chief medical officer.*

Desbrow, B. *et al.* (2004), 'Carbohydrate-electrolyte feedings and 1 h time trial cycling performance'. *Int. J. Sport Nutr. Exerc. Metab.*, vol. 14, pp. 541–9.

Derave, W. *et al.* (2007), 'Beta-alanine supplementation augments muscle carnosine content and attenuates fatigue during repeated isokinetic contraction bouts in trained sprinters'. *J. Appl. Physiol.*, vol. 103, pp 1736–43.

Dodd, S. L. *et al.* (1993), 'Caffeine and exercise performance'. *Sports Med.*, vol. 15, pp. 14–23.

Dodd, H. *et al.* (2011), 'Calculating meal glycaemic index by using measured and published food values compared with directly measured meal glycaemic index'. *Am. J. Clin. Nutr.*, vol. 95, pp. 992–6.

Doherty, M. and Smith, P. M. (2004), 'Effects of caffeine ingestion on exercise testing: a meta-analysis'. *Int. J. Sport Nutr. Exerc. Metab.*, vol. 14, pp. 626–46.

Dreon, D. M. *et al.* (1999), 'A very low-fat diet is not associated with improved lipoprotein profiles in men with a predominance of large low-density lipoproteins'. *Am. J. Clin. Nutr.*, vol. 69, pp. 411–18.

Drinkwater, B. L. (1986), 'Bone mineral content after resumption of menses in amenorrheic athletes'. *JAMA*, vol. 256, pp. 380–2.

Drinkwater, B. L. *et al.* (1984), 'Bone mineral content of amenorrheic and eumenorrheic athletes'. *New England. J. Med.*, vol. 311, pp. 277–81.

Dueck, C. A. *et al.* (1996), 'Role of energy balance in athletic menstrual dysfunction'. *Int. J. Sport Nutr.*, vol. 6, pp. 165–90.

Dulloo, A. G. *et al.* (1999), 'Efficacy of a green tea extract rich in catechins polyphenols and caffeine in increasing 24 hour energy expenditure and fat oxidation in humans'. *Am. J. Clin. Nutr.*, vol. 70, pp. 1040–5.

Durnin, J. V. G. A. and Womersley, J. (1974), *Brit. J. Nutr.*, vol. 32, p. 77.

Easton, C. *et al.* (2007), 'Creatine and glycerol hyperhydration in trained subjects before exercise in the heat'. *Int. J. Sports Nutr. Exerc. Metab.*, vol. 17, pp. 70–91.

Edwards, J. R. *et al.* (1993), 'Energy balance in highly trained female endurance runners'. *Med. Sci. Sports Ex.*, vol. 25(12), pp. 1398–404.

Elliot, T. A. *et al.* (2006), 'Milk ingestion stimulates net muscle protein synthesis following resistance exercise,' *Med. Sci. Sports Exer.*, vol. 38(4) pp. 667–74.

Eisinger, M. (1994), 'Nutrient intake of endurance runners with lacto-ovo vegetarian diet and regular Western diet'. *Z. Ernahrungswiss*, vol. 33, pp. 217–29.

Erasmus, U. (1996), *Fats that Heal: Fats that Kill* (Alive Books).

Erlenbusch, M. *et al.* (2005) 'Effect of high fat or high carbohydrate diets on endurance exercise: a meta-analysis'. *Int. J. Sport Nutr. Exerc. Metab.*, vol. 14, pp. 1–14.

European Federation of Health Product Manufacturers and UK Council for Responsible Nutrition (1997), Report on upper safe levels for supplements.

Faff, J. (2001), 'Effects of antioxidant supplementation in athletes on the exercise-induced oxidative stress'. *Biology of Sport*, vol. 18(1), pp. 3–20.

Fairchild, T. J. *et al.* (2002), 'Rapid carbohydrate loading after a short bout of near maximal-intensity exercise'. *Med. Sci. Sports Exer.*, pp. 980–6.

Farajian, P. *et al.* (2004), 'Dietary intake and nutritional practices of elite Greek aquatic athletes'. *Int. J. Sport Nutr. Exerc. Metab.*, vol 14, pp. 574–85.

Farshchi, H. R., Taylor, M. and McDonald, I. A. (2005) 'Beneficial effects of regular meal frequency on dietary thermogenesis, insulin sensitivity and fasting lipid profiles in healthy obese women'. *Am. J. Clin. Nutr.*, vol. 81, pp. 16–24.

Febbraio, M. A. *et al.* (2000), 'Effects of carbohydrate ingestion before and during exercise on glucose kinetics and performance'. *J. Appl. Physiol.*, vol. 89, pp. 2220–6.

Febbraio, M. A. and Stewart, K. L. (1996), 'CHO feeding before prolonged exercise: effect of glycaemic index on muscle glycogenolysis and exercise performance'. *J. Appl. Phsyiol.*, vol. 81, pp. 1115–20.

Ferguson-Stegall, L. *et al.* (2011), 'Aerobic exercise training adaptations are increased by postexercise carbohydrate-protein supplementation'. *J. Nutr. Metab.*, Epub Jun 9.

Ferreira, M. *et al.* (1998), 'Effects of conjugated linoleic acid supplementation during resistance training on body composition and strength'. *J. Strength Cond. res*, vol. 11, p. 280.

Fiala, K. A. *et al.* (2004), 'Rehydration with a caffeinated beverage during the non-exercise periods of 3 consecutive days of a 2-a-day practices'. *Int. J. Sport Nutr. Exerc. Metab.*, vol 14. pp. 419–429.

Flatt, J. P. (1993), 'Dietary fat, carbohydrate balance and weight maintenance'. Ann NY Acad. Sci., vol. 683, pp. 122–40.

Fleck, S. J. and Reimers, K. J. (1994), 'The practice of making weight: does it affect performance?'. *Strength and Cond.*, vol. 1, pp. 66–7.

Fogelholm, M. (1995), 'Indicators of vitamin and mineral status in athletes' blood: a review'. *Int. J. Sports Nutr.*, vol. 5, pp. 267–84.

Fogelholm, M. (1994), 'Effects of bodyweight reduction on sports performance'. *Sports Med.*, vol. 18 (14), pp. 249–67.

Food Standards Agency (2003), *Safe upper levels for vitamins and minerals*, (HMSO).

Food Standards Agency and Department of Health (2004). *National diet and nutrition survey of adults aged 19–64*, vol. 5, (HMSO).

Forsythe, W. (1995), 'Soy protein, thyroid regulation and cholesterol metabolism'. *J. Nutr.*, vol. 125 (3), pp. 619–23.

Foster-Powell, K. and Brand-Miller, J. C. (1995), 'International tables of glycaemic index'. *Am. J. Clin. Nutr.*, vol. 62 (suppl), pp. 871S–90S.

Foster-Powell, K., Holt, S. and Brand-Miller, J. C. (2002), 'International table of glycaemic index and glycaemic load values: 2002'. *Am. J. Clin. Nutr.*, vol. 76, pp. 5–56.

Fretsos, J. A. and Baer, J. T. (1997), 'Increased energy and nutrient intake during training and competition improves elite triathletes' endurance performance'. *Int. J. Sport Nutr.*, vol. 7, pp. 61–71.

Galloway, S. D. R. and Maughan, R. (2000), 'The effects of substrate and fluid provision on thermoregulatory and metabolic responses to prolonged exercise in a hot environment'. *J. Sports Sci.*, vol. 18(5), pp. 339–51.

Gallup (2001) *The Real Eat Survey* (August 2001).

Garfinkel, P. E. and Garner, D. M. (1982), 'Anorexia nervosa: a multidimensional perspective'. (Brunner/Mazel).

Gatorade Sports Science Institute (GSSI) (1995), 'Roundtable on methods of weight gain in athletes'. *Sports Science Exchange*, vol. 6(3), pp. 1–4.

Gaullier, J. M. *et al.* (2005*)*, 'Conjugated linoleic acid supplementation for 1 y reduces body fat mass in healthy overweight humans'. *J. Nutr.*, vol. 135, pp. 778–84.

Gibala, M. J. (2000), 'Nutritional supplementation and resistance exercise: what is the evidence for enhanced skeletal muscle hypertrophy?'. *Can. J. Appl. Physiol.*, vol. 25(6), pp. 524–35.

Gilson, S.F. *et al.* (2009) 'Effects of chocolate milk consumption on markers of muscle recovery during intensified soccer training'. *Medicine and Science in Sports and Exercise*, 41:S577.

Gisolphi, C. V. *et al.* (1992), 'Intestinal water absorption from select carbohydrate solutions in humans'. *J. Appl. Physiol.*, vol, 73, pp. 2142–50.

Gisolphi, C. V. *et al.* (1995), 'Effect of sodium concentration in a carbohydrate-electrolyte solution on intestinal absorption'. *Med. Sci. Sports Ex.*, vol. 27(10), pp. 1414–20.

Gleeson, M. (2011), 'Nutrition and immunity'. In *Diet, Immunity and Inflammation*, Calder, P. C. and Yaqoob, P (eds) (Woodhead Publishing).

Gleeson, M. *et al* (2008), 'Exercise and immune function: is there any evidence for probiotic benefit for sportspeople?' *Complete Nutrition*, vol. 8, pp. 35–7.

Goldfarb, A. H. (1999), 'Nutritional antioxidants as therapeutic and preventative modalities in exercise-induced muscle damage'. *Can. J. Appl. Physiol.*, vol. 24(3), pp. 249–66.

Gontzea, I. *et al.* (1975), 'The influence of adaptation to physical effort on nitrogen balance in man'. *Nutr. Rep. Int.*, vol. 22, pp. 213–16.

Gonzalez-Alonzo, J. *et al.* (1992), 'Rehydration after exercise with common beverages and water'. *Int. J. Sports Med.*, vol. 13, pp. 399–406.

Goran, M. I. and Astrup, A. (2002), 'Energy metabolism'. *Introduction to Human Nutrition*, Gibney, M., Vorster, II. and Kok, F. (eds) (Blackwell Publishing).

Goulet, E. D. B. (2011), 'Effects of exercise-induced dehydration on time trial exercise performance: a meta-analysis'. *Brit. J. Sports Med.*, vol. 45, pp. 1149–56.

Graham, T. E. and Spriet, L. L. (1991), 'Performance and metabolic responses to a high caffeine dose during prolonged exercise'. *J. Appl. Physiol.*, 71(6): pp. 2292-8.

Graham, T. E. and Spriet, L. L. (1995), 'Metabolic, catecholamine and exercise performance responses to various doses of caffeine'. *J. Appl. Physiol.*, 78: pp. 867–74.

Grandjean, A. (2000), 'The effect of caffeinated, non-caffeinated, caloric and non-caloric beverages on hydration'. *J. Am. Coll. Nutr.*, vol. 19, pp. 591–600.

Green, A. L. *et al.* (1996), 'Carbohydrate augments creatine accumulation during creatine supplementation in humans'. *Am. J. Physiol.*, vol. 271, E821–6.

Greenhaff, P. L. (1997), 'Creatine supplementation and implications for exercise performance and guidelines for creatine supplementation'. In A, Jeukendrup *et al.* (eds), *Advances in Training and Nutrition for Endurance Sports* (Maastrict: Novertis Nutrition Research Unit), pp. 8–11.

Greenwood, M., *et al.* (2003), 'Creatine cramps. Not'. *J. Athletic Training*, vol, 38(3), pp. 216–19.

Greer B. K. *et al.* (2007), 'Branched chain amino acid supplementation and indicators of muscle damage after endurance exercise'. *Int. J. Sports Nutr. Exerc. Metab.*, Vol. 17, pp. 595–607.

Gregory, J. *et al.* (2000), *The National Diet and Nutrition Survey: young people aged 4–18 years,* vol. 1, (HMSO).

Guest, N. S. and Barr, S. (2005), 'Cogitive dietary restraInt. is associated with stress fractures in women runners'. *Int. J. Sports Nutr. Exerc. Metab.*, vol. 15, pp. 147–59.

Halliwell, B. and Gutteridge, J. M. C. (1985), *Free Radicals in Biology and Medicine*, (Clarendon Press), pp. 162–4.

Halliday, T. *et al.* (2011), 'Vitamin D status relative to diet, lifestyle, injury and illness in collge athletes'. *Med. Sci. Sports Exerc.*, vol. 43, pp. 335–43.

Hamilton, B. (2011) Vitamin D and athletic performance: the potential role of muscle'. *Asian J. Sports Med.*, vol. 2(4), pp. 211–219.

Hanne, N., Dlin, R. and Rotstein, A. (1986), 'Physical fitness, anthropometric and metabolic parameters in vegetarian athletes'. *J. Sports Med. Phys. Fitness.*, vol. 26, pp. 180–5.

Hargreaves, M. and Snow, R. (2001), 'Amino acids and endurance exercise'. *Int. J. Sport Nutr.*, vol. 11, pp. 133–145.

Hargreaves, M. *et al.* (2004), 'Pre-exercise carbohydrate and fat ingestion: effects on metabolism and performance'. *J. Sports Sci.*, vol. 22 (1), pp. 31–38.

Harris, R. C. *et al.* (2006), 'The absorption of orally supplied beta-alanine and its effect on muscle carnosine synthesis in human vastus lateralis'. Amino Acids vol. 30(3) pp. 279–89.

Hartman, J. W. *et al.* (2007), 'Consumption of fat-free fluid milk after resistance exercise promotes greater lean mass accretion than does consumption of soy or carbohydrate in young, novice, male weightlifters'. *Am. J. Clin. Nutr.*, vol. 86(2), pp. 373-81.

Harris, R. C. (1998), 'Ergogenics 1'. *Peak Performance*, vol. 112, pp. 2–6.

Harris, R. C. *et al.* (1992), 'Elevation of creatine in resting and exercised muscle of normal subjects by creatine supplementation'. *Clin. Sci.*, vol. 82, pp. 367–74.

Haub, M. D. (1998), 'Acute l-glutamine ingestion does not improve maximal effort exercise'. *J. Sport Med. Phys. Fitness*, vol. 38, pp. 240–4.

Haub, M. D. *et al.* (2002), 'Effect of protein source on resistive-training-induced changes in body composition and muscle size in older men'. *Am. J. Clin. Nutr.*, vol. 76, pp. 511–17.

Haussinger, D. *et al.* (1996), 'The role of cellular hydration in the regulation of cell functioning'. *Biochem. J.*, vol. 31, pp. 697–710.

Hawley, J. *et al.* (1997), 'Carbohydrate loading and exercise performance'. *Sports Med.*, vol. 24(1), pp. 1–10.

Hawley, J. A. and Burke, L. M. (2010) 'Carbohydrate availability and training adaptation: effects on cell metabolism'. *Exerc. Sports Sci. Rev.*, vol. 38, pp. 152–160.

Hawley *et al.* (2011) 'Nutritional modulation of training-induced skeletal muscle adaptations'. *J. Appl. Physiol.*, vol. 100, pp. 834–45.

Helge, J. W. *et al.* (2001), 'Fat utilisation during exercise: adaptation to a fat rich diet increases utilisation of plasma fatty acids and very low density lipoprotein-triacylglycerol in humans'. *J. Physiol.*, vol. 537; 3, pp. 1009–20.

Herman, P. and Polivy, J. (1991), 'Fat is a psychological issue'. *New Scientist*, 16 Nov., pp. 41–5.

Hickey, H. S. *et al.* (1994), 'Drinking behaviour and exercise-thermal stress: role of drink carbonation'. *Int. J. Sport Nutr.*, vol. 4, pp. 8–12.

Hitchins, S. *et al.* (1999), 'Glycerol hyperhydration improves cycle time trial performance in hot humid conditions'. *Eur. J. Appl. Physiol. Occup. Physiol.*, vol. 80(5), pp. 494–501.

Hoffman, J. R. *et al.* (2008), 'Short-duration beta-alanine supplementation increases training volume and reduces subjective feelings of fatigue in college football players'. *Nutr. Res.*, vol. 28, pp. 31–5.

Holt, S. J. (1992), 'Relationship of satiety to post-prandial glycaemic, insulin and cholecystokinin responses'. *Appetite*, vol. 18, pp. 129–41.

Horton, T. J. *et al.* (1995), 'Fat and carbohydrate overfeeding in humans: different effects on energy storage'. *Am. J. Clin. Nutr.*, vol. 62, pp. 19–29.

Houtkooper, L. B. (2000), 'Body composition'. in Manore, M. M. and Thompson, J. L., *Sport Nutrition for Health and Performance*, Human Kinetics, pp. 199–219.

Howard, B. V. *et al.* (2006), 'Low-fat dietary pattern and risk of cardiovascular disease: the Women's Health Initiative Randomized Controlled Dietary Modification Trial'. JAMA., vol. 295(6), pp. 655–66.

Howarth, K. R. *et al.* (2009), 'Coingestion of protein with carbohydrate during recovery from endurance exercise stimulates skeletal muscle protein synthesis in humans'. *J. Appl. Physiol.*, vol. 106, pp. 1394–1402.

Hultman, E. *et al.* (1996), 'Muscle creatine loading in man'. *J. Appl. Physiol.*, vol. 81, pp. 232–9.

Hunter, A. M. *et al.* (2002), 'Caffeine ingestion does not alter performance during a 100-km cycling time trial performance'. *Int. J. Sport Nutr.*, vol. 12, pp. 438–52.

Hytten, F. E. and Leitch, I. (1971), *The Physiology of Human Pregnancy*, 2nd ed. (Blackwell Scientific Publications).

Institute of Medicine (1990), *Nutrition during Pregnancy*. Part 1: Weight Gain (National Academy Press).

International Association of Athletic Federations (IAAF) (2007), Nutrition for athletics: The 2007 IAAF Consensus Statement.

International Olympic Committee (IOC) (2011), Consensus Statement on Sports Nutrition 2010, 4,29 Suppl 1: S3-4. http://www.olympic.org/Documents/Reports/EN/CONSENSUS-FINAL-v8-en.pdf.

International Olympic Committee (IOC) (2004), Consensus on Sports Nutrition, 2003, *J. Sports Sci.*, vol. 22(1): X.

Ivy, J. L. *et al.* (1988b), 'Muscle glycogen storage after different amounts of carbohydrate ingestion'. *J. Appl. Physiol.*, vol. 65, pp. 2018–23.

Ivy, J. L. *et al.* (1988a), 'Muscle glycogen synthesis after exercise: effect of time of carbohydrate ingestion'. *J. Appl. Physiol.*, vol. 64, pp. 1480–5.

Ivy, J. L. *et al.* (2002), 'Early post-exercise muscle glycogen recovery is enhanced with carbohydrate-protein supplement'. *J. Appl. Physiol.*, vol 93, pp. 1337–1344.

Ivy, J. L. *et al.* (2003), 'Effect of a carbohydrate-protein supplement on endurance performance during exercise of varying intensity'. *Int. J. Sport Nutr. Exerc. Metab.*, vol 13, pp. 388–401.

Jacobs, K. A. and Sherman, W. M. (1999), 'The efficacy of carbohydrate supplementation and chronic high-carbohydrate diets for improving endurance performance'. *Int. J. Sport Nutr.*, vol. 9, pp. 92–115.

Jäger, R. *et al*, (2011), 'Analysis of the efficacy, safety, and regulatory status of novel forms of creatine'. Amino Acids vol. 40 (5), pp. 1369–83.

Jamurtas, A. Z. *et al.* (2011), 'The effects of low and high glycemic index foods on exercise performance and beta-endorphin responses'. *J. Int. Soc. Sports Nutr.*, vol. 8, p. 15.

Janelle, K. C. and Barr, S. I. (1995), 'Nutrient intakes and eating behavior scores of vegetarian and nonvegetarian women'. *J. Am. Diet. Assoc.*, vol. 95, pp.180–6, 189.

Jebb, S. *et al.* (2004), 'New body fat reference curves for children'. *Obesity Reviews* (NAASO Suppl) A146.

Jenkins, D. J. *et al.* (1987), 'Metabolic effects of a low GI diet'. *Am. J. Clin. Nutr.*, vol. 46, pp. 968–75.

Jeukendrup, A. *et al.* (1997) 'Carbohydrate-electrolyte feedings improve 1-hour time trial cycling performance'. *Int. J. Sports Med.*, vol. 18, pp. 125–9.

Jeukendrup, A. (2004) 'Carbohydrate intake during exercise and performance'. *Nutrition*, vol. 20, pp. 669–677.

Jeukendrup, A. (2008) 'Carbohydrate feeding during exercise'. *Eur. J. Sports Sci.*, vol. 8 (2), pp. 77–86.

Jeukendrup, A. (2010) 'Carbohydrate and exercise performance: the role of multiple transportable carbohydrates'. *Curr. Opin. Clin. Nutr. Metab. Care*, vol. 13(4), pp. 452–457.

Ji, L. L. (1999), 'Antioxidants and oxidative stress in exercise'. *Proc. Soc. Exp. Biol. Med.,* vol. 222, pp. 283–292.

Jonnalagadda, S. S. *et al.* (2004), 'Food preferences, dieting behaviours, and body image perceptions of elite figure skaters'. *Int. J. Sports Nutr. Exerc. Metab.*, vol. 14, pp. 594–606.

Josse A. R. *et al.* (2010), 'Body composition and strength changes in women with milk and resistance exercise'. *Med. Sci. Sports Exerc.*, vol. 42(6), pp. 1122–30.

Jowko, E. *et al.*, (2001) 'Creatine and HMB additively increase lean body mass and muscle strength during a weight training programme'. *Nutrition*, vol. 17(7), pp. 558–66.

Kamber, M. *et al.* (2001), 'Nutritional supplements as a source for positive doping cases?'. *Int. J. Sports Nutr.*, vol. 11, pp. 258–63.

Kammer L. *et al.* (2009), 'Cereal and non-fat milk support muscle recovery following exercise'. *J. Int. Soc. Sports Nutr.*, vol. 6, pp. 11.

Jouris K. *et al.* (2011), 'The effect of omega-3 fatty acid supplementation on the inflammatory response to eccentric strength exercise'. *J. Sports Sci. Med.*, vol. 10, pp. 432–38.

Kanter, M. M. and Eddy, D. M. (1992), 'Effect of antioxidant supplementation on serum markers of lipid peroxidation and skeletal damage following eccentric exercise'. *Med. Sci. Sports Ex.*, vol. 24 (supp.), S17.

Kanter, M. M. *et al.* (1993), 'Effects of an antioxidant mixture on lipid peroxidation at rest and post-exercise'. *J. Appl. Physiol.*, vol. 74, pp. 965–9.

Karlsson, J. and Saltin, B. (1971), 'Diet, muscle glycogen and endurance performance'. *J. Appl. Physiol.*, vol. 31, pp. 201–6.

Keizer, H. A. *et al.* (1986), 'Influence of liquid or solid meals on muscle glycogen resynthesis, plasma fuel hormone response and maximal physical working capacity'. *Int. J. Sports Med.*, vol. 8, pp. 99–104.

Kennerly, K. *et al.* (2011), Influence of banana versus sports beverage ingestion on 75 km cycling performance and exercise-induced inflammation'. *Med. Sci. Sports Exerc.*, vol. 43(5), pp. 340–341.

Key, T. J. A. *et al.* (1996), 'Dietary habits and mortality in a cohort of 11,000 vegetarians and health conscious people: results of a 17-year follow-up'. *Br. Med. J.,* vol. 313, pp. 775–9.

Kiens, B. *et al.* (1990), 'Benefit of simple carbohydrates on the early post-exercise muscle glycogen repletion in male athletes'. *Med., Sci. Sports Ex.* (suppl.), S88.

King, D. S. *et al.* (1999), 'Effects of oral androstenedione on serum testosterone and adaptations to resistance training in young men'. *J. Am. Med. Assoc.*, vol. 281 (21), pp. 2020–8.

Kreider, R. (2003) 'Effects of whey protein supplementation with casein or BCAA and glutamine on training adaptations: body composition'. *Med. Sci. Sport Exerc.*, vol. 35(5), suppl 1, p. S395.

Kreider, R. B. *et al.* (1996), 'Effects of ingesting supplements designed to promote lean tissue accretion on body composition during resistance training'. *Int. J. Sport Nutr.*, vol. 63, pp. 234–46.

Kreider, R. B. *et al.* (2000), 'Effects of calcium-HMB supplementation during training on markers of catabolism, body composition, strength and sprint. performance'. *J. Exerc. Physiol.*, vol. 3 (4), pp. 48–59.

Kristiansen, M. *et al.* (2005), 'Dietary supplement use by varsity athletes at a Canadian University'. *Int. J. Sport Nutr. Exerc. Metab.*, vol. 15, pp. 195–210.

Krotkiewski, M. *et al.* (1994), 'Prevention of muscle soreness by pre-treatment with antioxidants'. *Scand. J. Med. Sci. Sports*, vol. 4, pp. 191–9.

Krumbach, C. J. *et al.* (1999), 'A report of vitamin and mineral supplement use among University Athletes in a division I Institution'. *Int. J. Sport Nutr.*, vol. 9, p. 416–25.

Lambert, E. V. *et al.* (1994) 'Enhanced endurance in trained cyclists during moderate intensity exercise following 2 weeks adaptation to a high fat diet'. *Eur. J. Appl. Physiol*, vol. 69, pp. 287–293.

Lansley K. I. *et al.* (2011), 'Dietary nitrate supplementation reduces the O2 cost of walking and running: a placebo-controlled study'. *J. Appl. Physiol.*, vol. 110, pp. 591-600.

Lansley K. I., *et al.* (2011), 'Acute dietary nitrate supplementation improves cycling time trial performance'. *Med. Sci. Sports Exerc.*, vol. 43, pp. 1125–1131.

Larson-Meyer, D. E. and Willis, K. S. (2010), 'Vitamin D and athletes'. *Curr. Sports Med. Rep.*, vol. 9(4), pp. 220–6.

Laursen, P. B. *et al.* (2006), 'Core temperature and hydration status during an Ironman triathlon'. *Br. J. Sports Med.* 2006 Apr; 40(4):320–5; discussion 325.

Layman, D. K. *et al.* (2005), 'Dietary protein and exercise have additive effects on body composition during weight loss in adult women'. *J. Nutr.* vol. 35(8), pp. 1903–10.

Lean, M. E. J. *et al.* (1995), 'Waist circumference as a measure for indicating need for weight management'. *BMJ*, vol. 311, pp. 158–61.

Leeds, A., Brand Miller, J., Foster-Powell, K. and Colagiuri, S. (2000), *The Glucose Revolution* (London: Hodder and Stoughton), p. 29.

Lemon, P. W. R. (1992), 'Protein requirements and muscle mass/ strength changes during intensive training in novice bodybuilders, *J. Appl. Physiol.*, vol. 73, pp. 767–75.

Lemon, P. W. R. (1998), 'Effects of exercise on dietary protein requirements'. *Int. J. Sport Nutr.*, vol. 8, pp. 426-47.

Lemon, P. W. R. (1995), 'Do athletes need more dietary protein and amino acids?'. *Int. J. Sport Nutr.*, vol. 5 pp. s39–61.

Lloyd, T. *et al.* (1986), 'Women athletes with menstrual irregularity have increased musculo-skeletal injuries'. *Med. Sci. Sports Ex.*, vol. 18, pp. 3427–9.

Lohman, T. G. (1992), 'Basic concepts in body composition assessment'. In *Advances in Body Composition Assessment*, Human Kinetics, pp. 109–118.

Loucks, A. B. *et al.* (1989), 'Alterations in the hypothalamic-pituitary-ovarian and the hypothalamic-pituitary axes in athletic women'. *J. Clinical Endocrinol. Metab.*, vol. 68, pp. 402–22.

Loucks, A. B. (2003), 'Energy availability, not body fatness, regulates reproductive function in women'. *Exerc. Sport Sci. Rev.*, vol. 31, pp. 144–148.

Lovell, G. (2008), 'Vitamin D status of females in an elite gymnastic programme'. *Clin. J. Sports Med.*, vol. 18, pp. 159–61.

Lowery, L. M. *et al.* (1998), 'Conjugated linoleic acid enhances muscle size and strength gains in novice bodybuilders'. *Med. Sci. Sports Exerc.*, vol. 30(5), p. s182.

Luden, N. D. *et al.* (2007), 'Post-exercise carbohydrate-protein-antioxidant ingestion increase CK and muscle soreness in cross-country runners'. *Int. J. Sports Exerc. Metab.*, vol. 17, pp. 109–122.

Macintosh, B. R. *et al.* (1995), 'Caffeine ingestion and performance of a 1500-metre swim'. *Can. J. Appl. Physiol.*, vol. 20 (2): pp. 168–77.

Madsen, K. *et al.* (1996), 'Effects of glucose and glucose plus branched chain amino acids or placebo on bike performance over 100 km'. *J. Appl. Physiol.*, vol. 81, pp. 2644–50.

MAFF/RSC (1991), McCance and Widdowson's *The Composition of Foods*, 5th ed. (Cambridge: MAFF/RSC).

Maffucci, D. M. and McMurray, R. G. (2000), 'Towards optimising the timing of the pre-exercise meal'. *Int. J. Sport Nutr.*, vol. 10, pp. 103–13.

Martinez, L. R. and Haymes, E. M. (1992), 'Substrate utilisation during treadmill running in prepubescent girls and women'. *Med. Sci. Sports Exerc.*, vol. 24, pp. 975–83.

Mason, W. L. *et al.* (1993), 'Carbohydrate ingestion during exercise: liquid vs solid feedings'. *Med. Sci. Sports Ex.*, vol. 25, pp. 966–9.

Maughan, R. J. (1995), 'Creatine supplementation and exercise performance'. *Int. J. Sport Nutr.*, vol. 5, pp. 94–101.

Maughan, R. J. *et al.* (1996), 'Rehydration and recovery after exercise'. *Sports Sci. Ex.*, vol. 9(62), pp. 1–5.

Maughan, R. J. and Shireffs, S. M. (2012) 'Nutrition for sports performance: issues and opportunities'. *Proc. Nutr. Soc.*; vol. 71 (1), pp. 112–19.

Maughan, R. J. *et al.* (2011), 'Dietary supplements for athletes: emerging trends and recurring themes'. *J. Sports Sci.*, vol. 29 suppl 1, S57–66.

Mayhew, D. L. *et al.* (2002), 'Effects of long term creatine supplementation on liver and kidney function in American Football players'. *Int. J. Sport Nutr.*, vol. 12, pp. 453–60.

McConnell, G. K. *et al.* (1997), 'Influence of ingested fluid volume on physiological responses during prolonged exercise'. *Acta. Phys. Scand.*, vol. 160, pp. 149–56.

McLean, D. A. *et al.* (1994), 'Branch-chain amino acids augment ammonia metabolism while attenuating protein breakdown during exercise'. *Am. J. Physiol.*, vol. 267, E1010–22.

McNaughton, L. R. *et al.* (1998), 'The effects of creatine supplementation on high intensity exercise performance in elite performers'. *Eur. J. Appl. Physiol.*, vol. 78, pp. 236–40.

Meier, C. *et al.* (2004), 'Supplementation with oral vitamin D and calcium during winter prevents seasonal bone loss: a randomnised controlled open-label prospective trial'. *J. Bone Mineral Res.*, vol. 19, pp. 1221–30.

Melby, C. *et al.* (1993), 'Effect of acute resistance exercise on resting metabolic rate'. *J. Appl. Physiol.*, vol. 75, pp. 1847–53.

Mihic, S. *et al.* (2000), 'Acute creatine loading increases fat free mass but does not affect blood pressure, plasma creatinine or CK activity in men and women'. *Med. Sci. Sport. Exerc.*, vol. 32, pp. 291–6.

Millard-Stafford, M. L. *et al.* (2005), 'Should carbohydrate concentration of a sports drink be less than 8% during exercise in the heat?'. *Int. J. Sport Nutr. Exerc. Metab.*, vol. 15, pp. 117–130.

Miller, S. L. *et al.* (2002), 'Metabolic responses to provision of mixed protein-carbohydrate supplementation during endurance exercise attenuate the increases in cortisol'. *Int. J. Sport Nutr.*, vol. 12, pp. 384–97.

Minehan, M. R. *et al.* (2002), 'Effect of flavour and awareness of kilojoule content of drinks on preference and fluid balance in teAm. sports'. *Int. J. Sport Nutr.*, vol. 12, pp. 81–92.

Moore, D. R. *et al.* (2009), 'Ingested protein dose response of muscle and albumin protein synthesis after esistence exercise in young men'. *Am. J. Clin. Nutr.*, vol. 89, pp. 161–8.

Morrison, L. J. *et al.* (2004), 'Prevalent use of dietary supplements among people who exercise at a commercial gym'. *Int. J. Sport Nutr. Exerc. Metab.*, vol. 14, pp. 481–92.

Morton, J. P. *et al.* (2009), 'Reduced carbohydrate availability does not modulate training-induced heat shock protein adaptations but does upregulate oxidative enzyme activity in human skeletal muscle'. *J. Appl. Physiol.*, vol. 106 (5), pp. 1513–21. Epub 2009 Mar 5.

Mountain, S. J. and Coyle, E. F. (1992), 'The influence of graded dehydration on hyperthermia and cardiovascular drift during exercise'. *J. Appl. Physiol.*, vol. 73, pp. 1340–50.

Mujika, I. *et al.* (1996), 'Creatine supplementation does not improve sprInt. performance in competitive swimmers'. *Med. Sci. Sports. Exerc.*, vol. 28, pp. 1435–41.

Mullins, V. A. *et al.* (2001), 'Nutritional status of US elite female heptathletes during training'. *Int. J. Sport Nutr.*, vol. 11, pp. 299–314.

Muoio, D. M. *et al.* (1994), 'Effect of dietary fat on metabolic adjustments to maximal VO$_2$ and endurance in runners'. *Med. Sci. Sports Exerc.*, vol. 26(1), pp. 81–8.

Murphy, M. *et al.* (2012), 'Whole beetroot consumption acutely improves running performance'. *J. Acad. Nutr. Diet.*, vol. 112, pp. 548–52.

Murray, R. *et al.* (1999), 'A comparison of the gastric emptying characteristics of selected sports drinks'. *Int. J. Sports Nutr.*, vol. 9, pp. 263–74.

National Institute of Health (1994), 'Weight cycling'. *J. Am. Med. Assoc.*, vol. 272 (15), pp. 1196–202.

Nelson, A. *et al.* (1997), 'Creatine supplementation raises anaerobic threshold'. FASEB J., vol. 11, A586 (abstract).

Nelson, M. E. *et al.* (1986), 'Diet and bone status in amenorrheic runners'. *Am. J. Clin. Nutr.*, vol. 43, pp. 910–16.

Neufer, P. D. *et al.* (1987), 'Improvements in exercise performance: effects of carbohydrate feedings and diet'. *J. Appl. Physiol.*, vol. 62, pp. 983–8.

Nichols, J. F. *et al.* (2007), 'Disordered eating and menstrual irregularity in high school athletes in lean-build and non lean-build sports'. *Int. J. Sport Nutr. Exerc. Metab.*, vol. 17, pp. 364–77.

Nieman, D. C. (1999), 'Physical fitness and vegetarian diets: is there a relation?' *Am. J. Clin. Nutr.*, (Sep) vol. 70 (3 suppl), pp. 570S–5S.

Nieman, D. C. *et al.* (1989), 'Hematological, anthropometric, and metabolic comparisons between vegetarian and nonvegetarian elderly women'. *Int. J. Sports Med.*, vol. 10, pp. 243–50.

Nieman, D. C. *et al.* (2007), 'Quercetin reduces illness but not immune perturbations after intense exercise'. *Med. Sci. Sports Exerc.*, vol. 39, pp. 1561–69.

Nissan, S. *et al.* (1996), 'Effect of leucine metabolite HMB on muscle metabolism during resistance exercise training'. *J. Appl. Physiol.*, vol. 81, pp. 2095–104.

Nissan, S. *et al.* (1997), 'Effect of feeding HMB on body composition and strength in women'. FASEB J., vol. 11, A150 (abstract).

Noakes, T. D. (1993), 'Fluid replacement during exercise'. *Exerc. Sport Sci. Rev.*, vol. 21, pp. 297–330.

Noakes, T. D. (2000), 'Hyponatremia in distance athletes: pulling the IV on the dehydration myth'. *Phys. Sportsmed.*, vol. 26 (Sept), pp. 71–6.

Noakes, T. (2002), 'IMMDA advisory statement on guidelines for fluid replacement during marathon running'. *New Studies in Athletics: The IAAF Technical Quarterly.*, vol. 17 (1), pp. 15–24.

Noakes, T. D. (2007), 'Drinking guidelines for exercise: what evidence is there that athletes should drink as much as possible to replace the weight lost during exercise or ad libitum?'. *J. Sports Sci.*, vol. 25 (7), pp. 781–96.

Noakes, T. D. (2010), 'Is drinking to thirst optimum?' *Ann. Nutr. Metab.*, vol, 57, Suppl 2, pp. S9–17.

Noakes, T. D. (2012), *Waterlogged: The Serious Problem of Overhydration in Endurance Sports*, (Champaign, IL:/Human Kinetics).

Nosaka, K. *et al.* (2006), 'Effects of amino acid supplementation on muscle soreness and damage'. *Int. J. Sports Nutr. Exerc. Metab.*, vol. 16, pp. 620–35.

Oh, K. *et al.* (2005), 'Dietary fat intake and risk of coronary heart disease in women: 20 years of follow-up of the nurses' health study'. *Am. J. Epidemiol.*, vol. 161(7), pp. 672–9.

Ostoic, S. (2004), 'Creatine supplementation in young soccer players'. *Int. J. Sport Nutr. Exerc. Metab.*, vol. 14, pp. 95–103.

Otis, C. L. *et al.* (1997), 'American College of *Sports Medicine* position stand. The Female Athlete Triad'. *Med. Sci. Sport Exerc.*, vol. 29, pp. i–ix.

Owens, B. M. (2007), 'The potential effects of pH and buffering capacity on dental erosion'. *Gen. Dent.*, vol. 55(6), pp. 527–31.

Paddon-Jones, D. *et al.* (2001), 'Short term HMB supplementation does not reduce symptoms of eccentric muscle damage'. *Int. J. Sport Nutr.*, vol. 11, pp. 442–50.

Pannomans, D. L. *et al.* (1997), 'Calcium excretion, apparent calcium absorption and calcium balance in young and elderly subjects: influence of protein intake'. *Brit. J. Nutr.*, vol. 77(5), pp. 721–9.

Parry-Billings, M. *et al.* (1992), 'Plasma amino acid concentrations in over-training syndrome: possible effects on the immune system'. *Med. Sci. Sport Ex.*, vol. 24, pp. 1353–8.

Passe, D. H. *et al.* (2004), 'Palatability and voluntary intake of sports beverages, diluted orange juice and water during exercise'. *Int. J. Sport Nutr. Exerc. Metab.*, vol. 14, pp. 272–84.

Patterson S. D. and Gray, S. C. (2007), 'Carbohydrate-gel supplementation and endurance performance during intermittent high-intensity shuttle running'. *Int. J. Sports Nutr. Exerc. Metab.*, vol. 17 pp. 445–55.

Pereira, M. *et al.* (2004), 'Effects of a low glycaemic load diet on resting energy expenditure and heart disease risk factors during weight loss'. JAMA, vol. 292, pp. 2482–90.

Peters, E. M. *et al.* (1993), 'Vitamin C supplementation reduces the incidence of post-race symptoms of upper-respiratory-tract infection in ultra-marathon runners'. *Am. J. Clin. Nutr.*, vol. 57, pp. 170–4.

Peters, E. M. *et al.* (2001), 'Vitamin C supplementation attenuates the increases in circulating cortisol, adrenaline and anti-inflammatory polypeptides following ultra-marathon running'. *Int. J. Sports Med.*, vol. 22(7), pp. 537–43.

Petrie, T. A. (1993), 'Disordered eating in female collegiate gymnasts'. *J. Sport Ex. Psych.*, vol. 15, pp. 434–6.

Phillips, S. M. *et al.* (1997), 'Mixed muscle protein synthesis and breakdown after resistance training in humans'. *Am. J. Physiol.*, vol. 273(1), pp. E99–E107.

Phillips, S. M. *et al.* (1999), 'Resistance training reduces acute exercise-induced increase in muscle protein turnover'. *Am. J. Physiol.*, vol. 276(1), pp. E118–24.

Phillips, S. M. *et al.* (2005), 'Dietary protein to support anabolism with resistance exercise in young men,' *J. Am. Coll. Nutr.*, vol. 24 (2), pp. 134S–9S.

Phillips, S. M *et al.* (2007), 'A critical examination of dietary protein requirements, benefits and excesses in athletes'. *Int. J. Sports Nutr. Exerc. Metab.*, vol. 17, pp. 58–78.

Phillips, S. M. and Van Loon, L. J. (2011), 'Dietary protein for athletes: from requirements to optimum adaptation'. *J. Sports Sci.*, vol. 29, Suppl 1:S29–38.

Phillips, S. M., *et al.* (2011), 'Nutrition for weight and resistance training'. In: Lanham – new, S. A. *et al.* (eds), *Sport and Exercise Nutrition*. (Oxford:/ Wiley-Blackwell).

Pollock, M. L. and Jackson, A. S. (1984), 'Research progress invalidation of clinical methods of assessing body composition'. *Med. Sci. Sport Ex.*, vol. 16, pp. 606–13.

Poortmans, J. R. and Francaux, M. (1999), 'Long-term oral creatine supplementation does not impair renal function in healthy athletes'. *Med. Sci. Sports Ex.*, vol. 31(8), pp. 1103–10.

Powers, M. E. (2002), 'The safety and efficacy of anabolic steroid precursors: what is the scientific evidence?'. *J. Athol. Training*, vol. 37(3), pp. 300–5.

Powers S. K. *et al.* (2004), 'Dietary antioxidants and exercise'. *J. Sports Sci.*, vol. 22, pp. 81–94.

Powers, S. *et al.* (2011), 'Antioxidant and vitamin D supplements for athletes: sense or nonsense?'. *J. Sports Sci.*, vol. 29, Suppl. 1, S47–55.

Prentice, A. M. *et al.* (1989), 'Metabolism or appetite: questions of energy balance with particular reference to obesity'. *J. Hum. Nutr. Diet.*, vol. 2, pp. 95–104.

Ready, S. L. *et al.* (1999), 'The effect of two sports drink formulations on muscle stress and performance'. *Med. Sci. Sports Exerc.*, vol. 31(5), p. S119.

Res, P. T. *et al.* (2012), 'Protein ingestion prior to sleep improves post-exercise overnight recovery'. *Med. Sci. Sports Exerc.*, Feb 9. [Epub ahead of print]

Richter, E. A. *et al.* (1991), 'Immune parameters in male athletes after a lacto-ovo-vegetarian diet and a mixed Western diet'. *Med. Sci. Sports Exerc.*, vol. 23, pp. 517–21.

Rivera-Brown, A. M. *et al.* (1999), 'Drink composition, voluntary drinking and fluid balance in exercising trained heat-acclinatized boys'. *J. Appl. Physiol.*, vol. 86, pp. 78–84.

Rizkalla, S. *et al.* (2004), 'Improved plasma glucose control, whole body glucose utilisation and lipid profile on a low glycaemic index diet in type 2 diabetic men: a randomised controlled trial'. *Diab. Care*, vol. 27, pp. 1866–72.

Robertson, J. *et al.* (1991), 'Increased blood antioxidant systems of runners in response to training load'. *Clin. Sci.*, vol. 80, pp. 611–18.

Robinson. T. M. *et al.* (2000), 'Dietary creatine supplementation does not affect some haematological indices, or indices of muscle damage and hepatic and renal function'. *Brit. J. Sports Med.*, vol. 34, pp. 284–8.

Rogers, J. *et al.* (2005), 'Gastric emptying and intestinal absorption of a low carbohydrate sport drink during exercise'. *Int. J. Sport Nutr. Exerc. Metab.*, vol. 15, pp. 220–35.

Rokitzki, L. *et al.* (1994), 'a-tocopherol supplementation in racing cyclists during extreme endurance training'. *Int. J. Sports Nutr.*, vol. 4, pp. 235–64.

Rolls, B. J. *et al.* (2004), 'Salad and satiety: energy density and portion size of a first-course salad affect energy intake at lunch'. *J. Am. Diet. Assoc.*, vol. 104(10), pp. 1570–6.

Rolls, B. J. and Shide, D. J. (1992), 'The influence of fat on food intake and body weight'. *Nutr. Revs.*, vol. 50(10), pp. 283–90.

Romarno-Ely, B. C. *et al.* (2006), 'Effects of an isocaloric carbohydrate-protein-antioxidant drink on cycling performance'. *Med. Sci. Sports Exerc.*, vol. 38, pp. 1608–16.

Rosen, L. W. *et al.* (1986), 'Pathogenic weight-control behavior in female athletes'. *Phys. Sports Med.*, vol. 14, pp. 79–86.

Rowbottom, D. G. *et al.* (1996), 'The energizing role of glutamine as an indicator of exercise stress and overtraining'. *Sports Med.*, vol. 21(2), pp. 80–97.

Samaha, F. F. *et al.* (2003), 'A low-carbohydrate as compared with a low-fat diet in severe obesity'. *New England J. Med*, vol. 348, pp. 2074–81.

Saunders, M. J. *et al.* (2004), 'Effects of a carbohydrate-protein-beverage on cycling endurance and muscle damage'. *Med. Sci. Sports Exerc.*, vol. 36, pp. 1233–8.

Saunders, M. J. (2007), 'Coingestion of carbohydrate-protein during endurance exercise: influence on performance and recovery'. *Int. J. Sports Nutr. Exerc. Metab.*, vol. 17, S87–S103.

Sawka, M. N. *et al.* (2007), 'American College of *Sports Medicine* Position stand. Exercise and fluid replacement'. *Med. Sci. Sports Exerc.*, vol. 39, pp. 377–90.

Schokman, C. P. *et al.* (1999), 'Pre- and post game macronutrient intake of a group of elite Australian Football Players'. *Int. J. Sport Nutr.*, vol. 9, pp. 60–9.

Seifert J. *et al.* (2007), 'Protein added to a sports drink improves fluid retention'. *Int. J. Sport Nutr. Exerc. Metab.*, vol. 16, pp. 420–9.

Seiler, D. *et al.* (1989), 'Effects of long-distance running on iron metabolism and hematological parameters'. *Int. J. Sports Med.*, vol. 10, pp. 357–62.

Sen, C. K. (2001), 'Antioxidants in exercise nutrition'. *Sports Med.*, vol. 31(13), pp. 891–908.

Sherman, W. M. *et al.* (1981), 'Effect of exercise-diet manipulation on muscle glycogen and its subsequent utilisation during performance'. *Int. J. Sports Med.*, vol. 2, pp. 114–18.

Sherman, W. M. *et al.* (1991), 'Carbohydrate feedings 1 hour before exercise improve cycling performance'. *Am. J. Clin. Nutr.*, vol 54, pp. 866–70.

Shimomura, Y. *et al.* (2006), 'Nutraceutical effects of branched chain amino acids on skeletal muscle'. *J. Nutr.*, vol. 136, pp. 529–32.

Shing C.M. *et al.* (2007), 'Effects of bovine colostrum supplementation on immune variables in highly trained cyclists'. *J. Appl. Physiol.*, vol. 102, pp. 1113–22.

Shirreffs, S. M., *et al.* (1996), 'Post-exercise rehydration in man: effects of volume consuMed. and drink sodium content'. *Med. Sci. Sports Ex.*, vol. 28, pp. 1260–71.

Shirreffs S. M. *et al.* (2004), 'Fluid and electrolyte needs for preparation and recovery from training and competition.' *J. Sports Sci.*, vol. 22(1), pp. 57–63.

Shirreffs, S. M. *et al.* (2007), 'Milk as an effective post-exercise rehydration drink'. *Br. J. Nutr.*, vol. 98, pp. 173–180.

Shirreffs, S. M. and Sawka, M. N (2011), 'Fluid and electrolyte needs for training, competition, and recovery'. *J. Sports Sci.*, vol. 29 suppl1, S39–46.

Short, S. H. and Short, W. R. (1983), 'Four-year study of university athletes' dietary intake'. *J. Am. Diet. Assoc.*, vol. 82, p. 632.

Simopoulos, A. P. and Robinson, J. (1998). *The Omega Plan* (New York, HarperCollins).

Sinning, W. E. (1998), 'Body composition in athletes'. In Roche, A. F. *et al.* (eds.) *Human Body Composition*, (Champaign, IL: Human Kinetics), pp. 257–73.

Slater, G. *et al.* (2001), 'HMB supplementation does not affect changes in strength or body composition during resistance training in trained men'. *Int. J. Sport Nutr.*, vol. 11, pp. 383–96.

Sloth, B. *et al.* (2004), 'No difference in body weight decrease between a low GI and high GI diet but reduced LDL cholesterol after 10 wk ad libitum intake of the low GI diet'. *Am. J. Clin Nutr.*, vol. 80, pp. 337–47.

Snyder, A. C. *et al.* (1989), 'Influence of dietary iron source on measures of iron status among female runners'. *Med. Sci. Sports Exerc.*; vol. 21, pp. 7–10.

Sohlstrom, A. *et al.* (1992), 'Evaluation of simple methods to estimate total body fat in healthy women'. *Scand. J. Sci. Med. Sport*, vol. 2(4), pp. 207–11.

Speedy, D. B. *et al.* (1999), 'Hyponatremia in ultra-distance triathletes'. *Med. Sci. Sports Exerc.*, vol. 31, pp. 809–15.

Spriet, L. (1995), 'Caffeine and performance'. *Int. J. Sport Nutr.*, vol. 5, pp. S84–S99.

Steen, S. N. and McKinney, S. (1986), 'Nutrition assessment of college wrestlers'. *Phys. Sports Med.*, vol. 14, pp. 100–6.

Steenge, G. R. *et al.* (1998), 'The stimulatory effect of insulin on creatine accummulation in human skeletal muscle'. *Am. J. Physiol.*, vol. 275, pp. E974–9.

Stevenson, E. *et al.* (2005), 'Improved recovery from prolonged exercise following the consumption of low glycaemic index carbohydrate meals'. *Int. J. Sport Nutr. Exerc. Metab.*, vol. 15, pp. 333–49.

Stunkard, A. J. *et al.* (1986), 'An adoption study of human obesity'. *New England J. Med.*, vol. 314, pp. 193–8.

Stunkard, A. J. *et al.* (1990), 'The body mass index of twins who have been reared apart'. *New England J. Med.*, vol. 322, pp. 1483–7.

Subudhi, A. W. *et al.* (2001), 'Antioxidant status and oxidative stress in elite Alpine ski racers'. *Int. J. Sport Nutr.*, vol. 11, pp. 32–41.

Sun G. *et al.* (2005), 'Comparison of multifrequency bioelectrical impedance analysis with dual-energy X-ray absorptiometry for assessment of percentage body fat in a large, healthy population'. *Am. J. Clin Nutr.*, vol. 81, pp. 74–8.

Sundgort-Borgen, J. (1994a), 'Eating disorders in female athletes'. *Sports Med.*, vol. 17(3), pp. 176–88.

Sundgort-Borgen, J. (1994b), 'Risk and trigger factors for the development of eating disorders in female elite athletes'. *Med. Sci. Sports Ex.*, vol. 26, pp. 414–19.

Sundgort-Borgen, J. and Larsen, S. (1993), 'Nutrient intake and eating behaviour in elite female athletes suffering from anorexia nervosa, anorexia athletica and bulimia nervosa'. *Int. J. Sport Nutr.*, vol. 3, pp. 431–42.

Sundgot-Borgen J. and Torstveit M. K. (2004), 'Prevalence of eating disorders in elite athletes is higher than the general population'. *Clin. J. Sport Nutr.*, vol. 14, pp. 25–32.

Swaminathan, R. *et al.* (1985), 'Thermic effect of feeding carbohydrate, fat, protein and mixed meal in lean and obese subjects'. *Am. J. Clin. Nutr.*, vol. 42, pp. 177–81.

Tang, J. E. *et al.* (2009), 'Ingestion of whey hydrolysate, casein, or soy protein isolate: effects on mixed muscle protein synthesis at rest and following resistance exercise in young men'. *J. Appl. Physiol.*, vol. 107(3), pp. 987–92.

Tarnopolsky, M. and MacLennan, D. P. (1988), 'Influence of protein intake and training status in nitrogen balance and lean body mass'. *J. Appl. Physiol*, vol. 64, pp. 187–93.

Tarnopolsky, M. and MacLennan, D. P. (1992), 'Evaluation of protein requirements for trained strength athletes'. *J. Appl. Physiol*, vol. 73, pp. 1986–95.

Tarnopolsky, M. and MacLennan, D. P. (1997), 'Post exercise protein-carbohydrate and carbohydrate supplements increase muscle glycogen in males and females'. *J. Appl. Physiol.*, Abstracts, vol. 4, p. 332A.

Tarnopolsky, M. and MacLennan, D. P. (2000), 'Creatine monohydrate supplementation enhances high-intensity exercise performance in males and females'. *Int. J. Sport Nutr.*, vol. 10, pp. 452–63.

Thom E. *et al.* (2001), 'Congugated linoleic acid reduces body fat in healthy exercising humans.' *J. Int. Med. Res.*, vol. 29, pp. 392–6.

Thomas, D. E. *et al.* (1991), 'Carbohydrate feeding before exercise: effect of glycaemic index'. *Int. J. Sports Med.*, vol. 12, pp. 180–6.

Thomas, D. E. *et al.* (1994), 'Plasma glucose levels after prolonged strenuous exercise correlate inversely with glycaemic response to food consuMed. before exercise'. *Int. J. Sports Nutr.*, vol. 4, pp. 261–73.

Thompson, D. *et al.* (2001), 'Prolonged vitamin C supplementation and recovery from demanding exercise'. *Int. J. of Sport Nutr.*, vol. 11(4), pp. 466–81.

Thomson, J. L. *et al.* (1996), 'Effects of diet and diet-plus-exercise programs on resting metabolic rate: a meta analysis'. *Int. J. Sport Nutr.*, vol. 6, pp. 41–61.

Tipton, C. M. (1987), 'Commentary: physicians should advise wrestlers about weight loss'. *Phys. Sports Med.*, vol. 15, pp. 160–5.

Tipton K. and Wolfe R. (2007), 'Protein needs and amino acids for athletes'. *J. Sports Sci.*, vol 22(1), pp. 65–79.

Tipton, K. D. *et al.* (2004), 'Ingestion of casein and whey proteins result in muscle analbolism after resistance exercise'. *Med. Sci. Sports Exerc.*, vol. 36 (12), pp. 2073–81.

Tipton, K. D *et al.* (2007), 'Stimulation of net protein sythesis by whey protein ingestion before and after exercise'. *Am. J. Physiol. Endocrinol. Metab.*, vol. 292(1), pp. E71–6.

Tipton, K. D. and Witard, O. C. (2007), 'Protein requirements and recommendations for athletes: relevance of ivory tower arguments for practical recommendations'. *Clin. Sports Med.*, vol. 26(1), pp. 17–36.

Torstveit, M. K. and J. Sundgot-Borgen (2005), 'Participation in leanness sports but not training volume is associated with menstrual dysfunction: a national survey of 1276 athletes and controls'. *Br. J. Sports Med.*, vol. 39, pp. 141–7.

Truby, H. *et al.* (2008), 'Commercial weight loss diets meet nutrient requirements in free living adults over 8 weeks: a randomised controlled weight loss trial'. *Nutrition Journal* 2008, vol. 7, p. 25.

Tsintzas, O. K. *et al.* (1995), 'Influence of carbohydrate electrolyte drinks on marathon running performance'. *Eur. J. Appl. Physiol.*, vol. 70, pp. 154–60.

Unnithan, V. B. *et al.* (2001), 'Is there a physiologic basis for creatine use in children and adolescents?'. *J. Strength Cond. Res.*, vol. 15(4) pp. 524–8.

Vahedi, K. (2000), 'Ischaemic stroke in a sportsman who consuMed. mahuang extract and creatine monohydrate for bodybuilding'. *J. Neur., Neurosurgery and Psych.*, vol. 68, pp. 112–13.

Van Essen M. and Gibala, M. J. (2006), 'Failure of protein to improve time trial performance when added to a sports drink'. *Med. Sci. Sports Exerc.*, vol. 38(8), pp. 1476–83.

Van Loon, L. J. C. (2007), 'Application of protein or protein hydrolysates to improve postexercise recovery'. *Int. J. Sports Nutr. Exerc. Metab.*, vol. 17, S104–17.

Van Someren, K. A. *et al.* (2005), 'Supplementation with HMB and KIC reduces signs and symptoms of exercise-induced muscle damage in man'. *Int. J. Sport Nutr. Exerc. Metab.*, vol. 15, pp. 413–24.

Venables, M. *et al.* (2005), 'Erosive effect of a new sports drink on dental enamel during exercise'. *Med. Sci. Sports Exerc.*, vol. 37(1), pp. 39–44.

Volek, J. S. (1997), 'Response of testosterone and cortisol concentrations to high-intensity resistance training following creatine supplementation'. *J. Strength Cond. Res.*, vol. 11, pp. 182–7.

Volek, J. S. and Kraemer, W. J. (1996), 'Creatine supplementation: its effects on human muscular performance and body composition'. *J. Strength Cond. Res.*, vol. 10(3), pp. 200–10.

Volek, J. S. *et al.* (1996), 'Creatine supplementation enhances muscular performance during high intensity resistance exercise'. *J. Am. Diet Assoc.*, vol. 97, pp. 765–70.

Volek, J. S. *et al.* (1999), 'Performance and muscle fibre adaptations to creatine supplementation and heavy resistance training'. *Med. Sci. Sports Ex.*, vol. 31(8), pp. 1147–56.

Wagenmakers, A. J. M. *et al.* (1996), 'Carbohydrate feedings improve one-hour time-trial cycling performance'. *Med. Sci. Sports Ex.*, vol. 28, supp. 37.

Walberg-Rankin, J. (2000), 'Forfeit the fat, leave the lean: optimising weight loss for athletes'. *Gatorade Sports Science Exchange*, vol. 13(1).

Wang, Y. *et al.* (2005), 'Comparison of abdominal adiposity and overall obesity in predicting risk of type 2 diabetes among men'. *Am. J. Clin. Nutr.*, vol. 8, pp. 555–63.

Wansink, B. (2005), 'Bad popcorn in big buckets: portion size can influence intake as much as taste'. *J. Nutr. Educ. Behav.*, vol. 37(5), pp. 42–5.

Wansink, B. *et al.* (2005), 'Bottomless bowls: why visual cues of portion size may influence intake'. *Obes. Res.*, vol. 13(1), pp. 93–100.

Warren, J. *et al.* (2003), 'Low glycaemic index breakfasts and reduced food intake in preadolescent children'. *Paediatrics*, vol. 112, pp. 414–19.

Watt, K. K. O. *et al.* (2004), 'Skeletal muscle total creatine content and creatine transporter gene expression in vegetarians prior to and following creatine supplementation'. *Int. J. Sport Nutr. Exerc. Metab.*, vol. 14, pp. 517–31.

Welbourne, T. (1995), 'Increased plasma bicarbonate and growth hormone after an oral glutamine load'. *Am. J. Clin. Nutr.*, vol. 61, pp. 1058–61.

Wemple, R. D. *et al.* (1997), 'Caffeine vs. Caffeine-free sports drinks: effects on urine production at rest and during prolonged exercise'. *Int. J. Sports Med.*, vol. 18(1), pp. 40–6.

Wilk, B. and Bar-Or, O. (1996), 'Effect of drink flavour and NaCl on voluntary drinking and rehydration in boys exercising in the heat'. *J. Appl. Physiol.*, vol. 80, pp. 1112–17.

Wilkinson, S. B. *et al.* (2007), 'Consumption of fluid skim milk promotes greater protein accretion after resuistece exercise than does consumption of an isonitrogenous and isoenergetic soy-protein beverage'. *Am. J. Clin. Nutr.*, vol. 85(4), pp.1031–40.

Williams, M. H. (1985), *Nutritional Aspects of Human Physical and Athletic Performance*, (Springfield, IL: Charles C Thomas Publisher).

Williams, C. and Devlin, J. T. (eds) (1992), *Foods, Nutrition and Performance: An International Scientific Consensus* (London: Chapman and Hall).

Williams, M. H. (1992), *Nutrition for Fitness and Sport* (Dubuque, IO: WilliAm. C. Brown).

Williams, M. H. (1999), *Nutrition for Health, Fitness and Sport*, 5th ed. (New York: McGraw-Hill).

Williams, M. H. *et al.* (1999), *Creatine: The Power Supplement* (Champaign, IL: Human Kinetics).

Williams, M. H. (1998), *The Ergogenics Edge* (Champaign, IL: Human Kinetics).

Wilmore, J. H. (1983), 'Body composition in sport and exercise'. *Med. Sci. Sports Ex.*, vol. 15, pp. 21–31.

Wright, D. W. *et al.* (1991), 'Carbohydrate feedings before, during or in combination improve cycling endurance performance'. *J. Appl. Physiol.*, vol. 71, pp. 1082–88.

Wu, C. L. *et al.* (2003), 'The influence of high carbohydrate meals with different glycaemic indices on substrate utilisation during subsequent exercise'. *Br. J. Nutr.*, vol. 90(6), pp. 1049–56.

Wu, C. L and Williams, C. (2006), 'A low glycaemic index meal before exercise improves endurance running capacity in men'. *Int. J. Sports Nutr. Exerc. Metab.*, vol 16, pp. 510–27.

Yeo, W. K. *et al.* (2008), 'Skeletal muscle adaptation and performance responses to once a day versus twice-every-second-day endurance training regimens'. *J. Appl. Physiol.*, vol. 105, pp. 1462–70.

Zawadzki, K. M. *et al.* (1992), 'Carbohydrate-protein complex increases the rate of muscle glycogen storage after exercise'. *J. Appl. Physiol.*, vol. 72, pp. 1854–9.

Ziegenfuss, T. *et al.* (1997), 'Acute creatine ingestion: effects on muscle volume, anaerobic power, fluid volumes and protein turnover'. *Med. Sci. Sports Ex.*, vol. 29, supp. 127.

Ziegler, P. J. *et al.* (1999), 'Nutritional and physiological status of US National Figure Skaters'. *Int. J. Sport Nutr.*, vol. 9, pp. 345–60.

Ziegler, P. J. *et al.* (1998), 'Nutritional status of nationally ranked junior US figure skaters'. *J. Am. Diet. Assoc.*, vol. 98, pp. 809–11.

Zucker, N. L. *et al.* (1999), 'Protective factors for eating disorders in female college athletes'. *Eating Disord.*, vol. 7, pp. 207–18.

FURTHER READING

Applegate, L. (2001), *Eat Smart Play Hard*, Rodale.

Beals, K. (2004), *Disordered Eating among Athletes – A Comprehensive Guide for Health Professionals*, Human Kinetics.

Bean, A. (2007), *Food for Fitness*, 3rd ed., London: A and C Black.

Burke, L. (2007), *Practical Sports Nutrition*, Human Kinetics.

Costain, L. *et al.* (2008), *The Calorie, Carb and Fat Bible 2011*, Weight Loss Resources.

Dunford, M. (2010), *Fundamentals of Sport and Exercise Nutrition*, Human Kinetics.

Food Standards Agency (2002), *McCance and Widdowson's The Composition of Foods*, 6th summary ed., Royal Society of Chemistry.

Gastelu, D. and Hatfield, F. (1997), *Dynamic Nutrition for Maximum Performance*, Avery Publishing Group.

Jeukendrup, A. and Glesson, M. (2010), *Sport Nutrition*, 2nd ed., Human Kinetics.

Lanham-New, S. *et al.* (eds) (2011), *Sport and Exercise Nutrition*, Wiley-Blackwell

McArdle, W. *et al.* (2006), *Exercise Physiology: Energy, Nutrition, and Human Performance*, 6th ed. Lippincott, Williams and Wilkins.

Wilmore, J. and Costill, D. (2005), *Physiology of Sport and Exercise*, 3rd ed., Human Kinetics.

USEFUL ADDRESSES

British Dietetic Association
5th floor, Charles House
148–9 Great Charles Street
Queensway
Birmingham   B3 3HT
www.bda.uk.com

British Nutrition Foundation
High Holborn House
52–54 High Holborn
London   WC1V 6RQ
www.nutrition.org.uk

Beat (Beating Eating Disorders)
1st floor, Wensum House
103 Prince of Wales Road
Norwich   NR1 1DW
www.beat.co.uk

Association for Nutrition
28 Portland Place
London   W1B 1LY
www.associationfornutrition.org

National Sports Medicine Institute of the UK
32 Devonshire Street
London   W1G 6PX
www.nsmi.org.uk

The Nutrition Society
10 Cambridge Court
210 Shepherds Bush Road
London   W6 7NJ
www.nutritionsociety.org

Vegetarian Society
Parkdale
DunhAm. Road
Altrincham
Cheshire   WA14 4QG
www.vegsoc.org

ONLINE RESOURCES

British Nutrition Foundation
www.nutrition.org.uk
The website of the British Nutrition Foundation, contains information, fact sheets and educational resources on nutrition and health.

Food Standards Agency
www.eatwell.gov.uk
The website of the government's Food Standards Agency has news of nutrition surveys, nutrition and health information.

American Dietetic Association
www.eatright.org
The website of the American Dietetic Association, gives nutrition news, tips and resources.

British Dietetic Association
www.bda.uk.com
The website of the British Dietetic Association includes fact sheets and information on healthy eating for children. It also provides details of Registered Dieticians working in private practice.

Gatorade Sports Science Institute
www.gssiweb.com
This website provides a good database of articles and consensus papers on nutritional topics written by experts.

Runners World
www.runnersworld.co.uk
The website of the UK edition of *Runner's World* magazine provides an extensive library of excellent articles on nutrition, training and sports injuries, and sports nutrition product reviews.

The Fit Map
www.thefitmap.com
UK health, fitness and exercise portal with articles about healthy living, interactive tools, and details of health clubs and gyms throughout the UK.

BBC Healthy living
www.bbc.co.uk/health/healthy_living/
This website provides good clear information on lots of health, fitness, and nutrition topics.

Vegetarian Society
www.vegsoc.org
This website provides information on vegetarian nutrition for children as well as general nutrition, health and recipes.

Weight Concern
www.weightconcern.com
Excellent information on obesity issues, including a section on children's health and a BMI calculator.

Health Supplements Information Service
www.hsis.org

This website provides balanced information on vitamins, minerals and supplements.

Weight Loss Resources
www.weightlossresources.co.uk

This UK website provides excellent information on weight loss, fitness and healthy eating as well as a comprehensive calorie database and a personalised weight loss programme.

Diabetes UK
www.diabetes.org.uk

Diabetes UK is the leading charity for people with diabetes and this website provides authoritative information on living with diabetes, as well as sections for children, teenagers and young adults.

The Mayo Clinic
www.mayoclinic.com

Written by medical experts, this US site offers good nutrition and health information, as well as advice on medical conditions in a user-friendly format.

WebMD
www.webmd.com

This comprehensive US website has an A–Z dictionary of health topics and advice on many aspects of nutrition and fitness.

Health Status
www.healthstatus.com

This US website provides useful health calculators and assessments that help you work out your body mass index, body fat percentage, number of calories burned during exercise and daily calorie intake.

Nutrition Data
http://nutritiondata.self.com

This US website provides a detailed nutrition database together with nutritional information from food manufacturers and restaurants.

Net Doctor
www.netdoctor.co.uk/dietandnutrition

This UK website provides excellent advice on healthy eating. weight loss, health conditions, weight problems and lifestyle management.

Beat (Beat Eating Disorders)
www.b-eat.co.uk

The website of Beat (the working name of the Eating Disorders Association) provides helplines, online support and a network of UK-wide self-help groups as well as information sheets and booklets, which can be downloaded free.

Australian Institute of Sport
www.ausport.gov.au/ais/nutrition

The website of AIS provides excellent and up-to-date factsheets on sports nutrition written by sports dietitians.

Sports Dietitians UK
www.sportsdietitians.org.uk/

Find a Sports Dietitian near you, also accessed from www.senr.org.uk/

Sports Dietitians Australia
www.sportsdietitians.com.au

The SDA website provides excellent fact sheets on a wide range of sports nutrition topics.

INDEX

sweating 104
sweatsuits 107–8

T
taurine supplements 101–2
teeth 115
testosterone boosters 101
thermogenesis 153
thermogenic supplements 94–5
thirst 109–10

V
vegetables 10, 11
vegetarianism 209–17, 249–63, 271–80
vitamins 8–9, 292–303
    requirements 65–76
    supplements 67–8, 71–3, 199–200
    types of 68–71

W
weather, effect on performance of 117, 118
weight gain 164–70
    calories and 166–7
    carbohydrates and 167
    dietary fat and 167
    exercise for 164, 165
    pregnancy and 182–5
    protein and 167
    snacks for 170, 207
    speed of 165–6
    supplements 168–9
    young athletes and 206–7
weight loss 59, 141–63, 220–22
    alcohol and 145
    calories and 145–8
    carbohydrates and 143–4, 145, 147, 161
    commercial diets 161–2
    by dehydration 143

    dietary fat and 144–5, 147
    effect on performance 142–3
    exercise for 157–60
    protein and 59, 144, 145, 147
    psychology of 148
    repeated 143
    speed of 142, 148
    strategy 148–54
    training during 143
    weight training for 158–60
    young athletes and 200–5, 206

Y
young athletes
    carbohydrates for 190–5
    creatine for 200
    dehydration 195–9
    energy requirements of 187–9
    protein for 190
    snacks for 191–5, 205, 207
    strength training for 207–8
    weight gain for 206–7
    weight loss for 200–5, 206
yo-yo dieting 141–2, 143

Z
zinc 214–15
ZMA (zinc monomethionine aspartate and magnesium aspartate) 102